Health Promotion in Long-Term Care Facilities

Kallol Kumar Bhattacharyya
Editor

Health Promotion in Long-Term Care Facilities

The Present Scenario and Future Demands

Springer

Editor
Kallol Kumar Bhattacharyya
School of Public Health
University of Memphis
Memphis, TN, USA

ISBN 978-3-031-91037-1 ISBN 978-3-031-91038-8 (eBook)
https://doi.org/10.1007/978-3-031-91038-8

This Springer imprint is published by the registered company Springer Nature Switzerland AG
The registered company address is: Gewerbestrasse 11, 6330 Cham, Switzerland

Dedication
This work and accomplishment are dedicated to my adored Gurudev, late Sri Sri Manimohan Goswami.

Foreword

I am honored to write the foreword for this book. Dr. Kallol Kumar Bhattacharyya has brought together a distinguished group of experts to provide a comprehensive exploration of the barriers and opportunities associated with health promotion in long-term care facilities. As global life expectancy rises, often outpacing gains in healthy life expectancy, focusing on the health and well-being of the most vulnerable older adults—like those in long-term care—is both timely and essential. Long-term care facilities face unique challenges to implementing health promotion strategies that stem from both the cognitive and physical frailty of residents as well as staffing, resources, and geographical and other unique circumstances.

Readers will gain practical insights into the factors influencing health promotion in long-term care through discussions of key themes, such as the relationship between quality of care and quality of life, the challenges posed by cognitive deficits and polypharmacy, the complexities of direct care staffing, and the effects of adverse events, including natural disasters and the COVID-19 pandemic.

Whether you are a caregiver, a family member, a resident, or simply someone seeking to better understand this vital topic, this book is an invaluable resource. I am confident it will leave a lasting impact and deepen your appreciation for the importance of promoting health among vulnerable older adults in long-term care settings.

Edson College of Nursing and Health Innovation
Arizona State University,
Phoenix, AZ, USA

Ross Andel

Foreword

Preface

I started my professional journey as a family physician in India nearly two and a half decades ago. As a clinician, a substantial amount of my time was spent educating my patients about taking care of their health in a holistic way. However, after many years of clinical practice, I realized that the world of health is more than just being a physician or a nurse…I had been seeking a new challenge. I reentered academia with an interest in studying health from a biopsychosocial perspective to improve the quality of life of older adults, particularly those with cognitive impairment living in the community and long-term care.

In the United States, the aging population is increasingly diverse; many of them suffer from multiple chronic morbidities and need post-acute care. Further, for older adults, a person-centered approach to care, particularly post-acute care, shifts the mindset of care partners from a traditional medical model to a promising social model in managing various chronic conditions, including dementia, aiming to maintain personal autonomy, comfort, dignity, preferences, and purposeful living. Given the growing demand for care expectations, the concept of long-term care is constantly changing to provide most care needs. Currently, we are serving many people at a time, including residents, families, staff, and others; this needs urgent collaboration.

Health promotion enables people to enhance control over their own health. As an umbrella term, it includes a wide range of socio-behavioral interventions designed to improve an individual's quality of life by managing the primary causes of ill health instead of focusing only on curative treatment. This book discusses various biopsychosocial barriers and facilitators of long-term care services, focusing on health promotional activities targeting to maximize the quality of life in long-term care. In this book, with the support of well-known scholars of diverse backgrounds and career stages, I have tried to illustrate the paradigm shift in interdisciplinary long-term care. The introductory chapter will discuss the factors that have the most powerful impact on long-term care residents, particularly the most vulnerable ones' quality of life and the potential of health promotional practices. The following chapters will attempt to tie various disparate themes together, focusing on the current quality of services, emphasizing the possible role of cross-cultural health promotional practices in maintaining the quality of life and promoting a person-centered holistic biopsychosocial approach to aging that maximizes their quality of life while living with different chronic conditions. I hope this book will benefit a wide group of readers, including formal and informal caregivers and policymakers. Further, I believe this book, with a strong academic value from a multidisciplinary perspective, will be highly relevant reading for gerontology graduate and undergraduate students; however, it will also be beneficial for specialized courses in psychology, public health, health management and policy, and health services research.

Memphis, TN, USA Kallol Kumar Bhattacharyya

Acknowledgments

I want to thank my former professors, Drs. Kathryn Hyer and Victor Molinari (both deceased), who nurtured my interest in long-term care and encouraged me to broaden my dissemination and implementation-related ideas for interdisciplinary aging research. I am thankful to Drs. Ross Andel, Lindsay Peterson, Jennifer Craft Morgan, Elizabeth Fauth, and Gizem Hueluer for their input and guidance. I am grateful to all my friends, colleagues, and professors with whom I was able to work during my professional and academic journeys to achieve my goals. I also want to express my sincere gratitude to all co-authors who contributed to this book.

I am thankful to the entire Springer team. My special thanks to Ms. Janet Kim, executive editor of Springer, for her patient cooperation throughout the publication process. I am grateful to my parents, late Mr. Kalyan Kumar Bhattacharyya and late Mrs. Gita Bhattacharyya, and my grandparents for their continuous blessings. I would not have been able to complete this book without their love and support.

I must acknowledge, my wife, Paramita Bhattacharya, and my son, Shailpik Bhattacharyya, as my main strengths and constant source of support. I was amazed at how Paramita helped me edit multiple documents in this book and was consistently patient with me. This book may be my official achievement, but all credit goes to them unofficially.

Finally, I want to express my heartiest gratitude to all those individuals with or without disorders who came to me for clinical suggestions on different occasions. Without their blessings, it would not have been possible for me to come to the point where I am today.

Contents

1 **Introduction: Health Promotion in the Context of Long-Term Care** 1
Kallol Kumar Bhattacharyya

2 **Are Quality of Care and Quality of Life Synonymous in Long-Term Care?** 9
Kallol Kumar Bhattacharyya

3 **Cognitive Decline and Polypharmacy in Long-Term Care** 25
Mia E. Lussier and Gail B. Rattinger

4 **Dementia Citizenship in Mitigating Global Challenges of Polypharmacy in Long-Term Care** 41
Panagiota Tragantzopoulou and Vaitsa Giannouli

5 **Health Promotion in Long-Term Care Services and Supports: Increasing the Numbers and Extending the Capacity of Direct Care Workers** 49
Alfred Boakye and Jennifer Craft Morgan

6 **Impact of Disasters and Pandemics on Residents' Behavioral Health in Long-Term Care: Implications for Health Promotion** 61
Lisa M. Lind and Lisa M. Brown

7 **Critical Staffing Issues and the Impact of COVID-19 on Long-Term Care Workforce Management** 77
Jessica Vanderwerf and Lindsay J. Peterson

8 **Palliative Care in Long-Term Care** 97
Frances M. Hawes and Lisa Quinn-Lee

9 **Cognitive and Mental Health Issues in Long-Term Care from a Health Disparities Perspective** 111
Solange M. Marcel

10 Cultural Perspectives for Promoting Residents' Quality of Life in Long-Term Care 121
David Hage

11 How Social Determinants of Health Influence Health Promotion in Long-Term Care 137
Romil Rakesh Parikh

12 Aging in Place *or* Long-term Care? Changing the Narrative to Promote Aging in Place *in* Long-Term Care 155
Elizabeth Braungart Fauth, Gavin Green, and Josey Batura

13 Person-Centered Care and the Culture Change Movement in Long-Term Care 165
Michelle Goonasekera, Kristina M. Kokorelias, Erica Dove, and Maurita T. Harris

14 Extending the Age-Friendly Movement to Long-Term Care 181
Patricia Oh, Mary Lou Ciolfi, and Kimberly Snow

15 Potentials of Health Promotional Practices in Long-Term Care 203
Sean N. Halpin and Joshua Saul

Index 221

Editor and Contributors

About the Editor

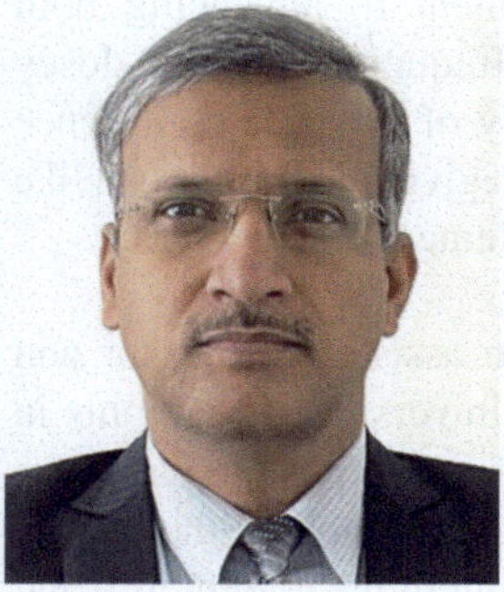

Kallol Kumar Bhattacharyya MBBS, MA, PhD, is an assistant professor and health economist at the University of Memphis School of Public Health in Tennessee. Dr. Bhattacharyya considers himself a physician gerontologist interested in studying health from a biopsychosocial perspective to improve the quality of life of older adults, especially those with dementia, living in the community and long-term care. Dr. Bhattacharyya received his master's degree in gerontology from Georgia State University and completed his PhD in aging sciences at the School of Aging Studies, University of South Florida. He also worked as a postdoctoral fellow in the Alzheimer's Disease and Dementia Research Center at Utah State University. Kallol is particularly focused on the individualized care provided in long-term care, especially nursing homes, and the economics of long-term care, especially how regulatory oversight and resident choices in the nursing home market affect health outcomes. He is also interested in the risk factors and alternative therapeutic interventions for Alzheimer's disease and related dementia.

Kallol has been an active member of the Gerontological Society of America. He has several publications in well-known peer-reviewed journals, book chapters, and many conference presentations. His first book with Springer was *Rethinking the Aging Transition: Psychological, Health, and Social Principles to Guide*

Aging Well. His innovative research has won many awards in scholarly platforms, including the Gerontological Society of America, Southern Gerontological Society, etc. He is serving in the editorial teams of *Gerontology and Geriatric Medicine*, *BMC Geriatrics*, and *PLOS ONE*. Finally, Kallol has extensive clinical, leadership, and administrative experience working as a family physician in India before rejoining academia.

Contributors

Josey Batura is a PhD student in Human Development and Family Services at Utah State University, specializing in Alzheimer's and dementia research. Josey is actively involved in innovative research utilizing fNIRS hyperscanning to examine neural activity in family caregivers and care recipients, with a focus on how caregiving dynamics impact neural plasticity. With several articles in preparation for peer-reviewed publication, Josey's work reflects a commitment to advancing both scientific understanding and real-world applications. A frequent presenter, Josey has shared research insights at the Gerontological Society of America conference and other academic platforms, emphasizing innovative caregiving interventions like online Acceptance and Commitment Therapy (ACT) for dementia caregivers.

Kallol Kumar Bhattacharyya MBBS, MA, PhD, is an assistant professor and health economist in the School of Public Health at the University of Memphis in Tennessee. Dr. Bhattacharyya considers himself a physician gerontologist interested in studying health from a biopsychosocial perspective to improve the quality of life of older adults, especially those with dementia, living in the community and long-term care. Dr. Bhattacharyya received his master's degree in Gerontology from Georgia State University and completed his PhD in Aging sciences from the School of Aging Studies, University of South Florida. He also worked as a postdoctoral research fellow in the Alzheimer's Disease and Dementia Research Center at Utah State University. Kallol is particularly focused on the individualized care provided in long-term care, especially nursing homes, and the economics of long-term care, especially how regulatory oversight and resident choices in nursing home market affect health outcomes. He is also interested in the risk factors and alternative therapeutic interventions for Alzheimer's disease and related dementia. Dr. Bhattacharyya also has extensive clinical, leadership, and administrative experience working as a family physician in India before rejoining academia.

Alfred Boakye is a doctoral student in Gerontology at the University of Maryland, Baltimore (UMB). His research explores the interplay between trauma and resilience among minority Direct Care Workers (DCWs) who are Black, Indigenous, and Persons of Color (BIPOC) and examines how their experiences shape the care and support provided to People Living with Dementia (PLWD). Mr. Boakye's work seeks to develop innovative strategies that empower DCWs to improve their health outcomes and enhance care delivery, enabling them to provide person-centered care to nursing home residents with dementia. Through his leadership roles and achievements, Mr. Boakye continues to bridge the gap between research, policy, and practice to advance equitable health and dementia care. He holds an MA in Gerontology from Georgia State University and an MPhil in Human Resource Management from the University of Ghana-Accra.

Lisa M. Brown PhD, ABPP, is a Professor Emeritus of Clinical Psychology at Palo Alto University and an Adjunct Clinical Professor at Stanford University School of Medicine in California. Her clinical and research focus is on trauma, human rights, and vulnerable populations. She has authored more than 200 journal articles, book chapters, and program evaluations. Dr. Brown has served on numerous states, national, and international boards, committees, and commissions, including the Disaster Mental Health Subcommittee of the National Biodefense Science Board Federal Advisory Committee. She is currently serving as a voting member on the National Advisory Committee on Seniors and Disasters, Health and Human Services.

Mary Lou Ciolfi JD, MS, is Assistant Director of Policy and Education at the University of Maine Center on Aging where she conducts research and analysis on various aspects of aging-related policy and long-term care service delivery. She is also Co-Director of the Consortium for Aging Policy Research and Analysis (CAPRA), a partnership between the University of Maine and the University of Southern Maine. Mary Lou is a licensed Maine attorney with a master's degree in health policy. She practiced law in Maine for many years and then operated a long-term care community as a residential care administrator. She has worked in aging policy research with colleagues at the University of Southern Maine's Muskie School of Public Service, and she is an adjunct faculty member at the University of New England and teaches Public Health Law and Public Health Policy. Mary Lou is a national facilitator for the National Center to Reframe Aging, housed at The Gerontological Society of America. She frequently presents on ageism and related issues. Mary Lou received her undergraduate degree from the University of Chicago, her law degree from the University of New Hampshire Franklin Pierce School of Law, and her master's degree from the University of Southern Maine's Muskie School of Public Service.

Erica Dove is a final-year PhD candidate in the Rehabilitation Sciences Institute (RSI) at the University of Toronto in Canada. Erica earned her MSc from the RSI at the University of Toronto in 2021. Erica's research focuses on the creative application of technology to support the health, function, and well-being of people living with dementia.

Elizabeth (Beth) Braungart Fauth PhD, is a Utah State University professor in the Department of Human Development and Family Studies. She is also Director of

Utah's state-funded Alzheimer's Disease and Dementia Research Center. Her research primarily focuses on reducing stress for dementia caregivers, the interface between physical function and cognitive function in late life, and rural mental health. She has over 60 publications in scientific journals and a history of securing external funding for her research, including an active grant from the National Institute of Health. She has received awards for excellence in teaching, research, and service and is a Fellow of the Gerontological Society of America.

Vaitsa Giannouli holds a BSc in Psychology, an MSc in Cognitive Psychology and Neuropsychology from the Aristotle University of Thessaloniki, and an MSc in Health Care Management from the Hellenic Open University in Greece. She has received a PhD in Neuroscience from the Aristotle University of Thessaloniki. Her clinical and research interests focus on the application of neuropsychological methods and advanced neuroimaging techniques for both structural and functional evaluation of the brain–behavior relationship in neurological and psychiatric diseases in old age. Her research examines topics from different fields such as cognitive psychology, neuropsychology, biopsychology, geropsychology, health psychology, and quantitative/qualitative methods of research.

Michelle Goonasekera is a Master of Public Health candidate at the Dalla Lana School of Public Health, University of Toronto, Canada, specializing in aging and health policy. She holds a Bachelor of Science from the University of Alberta. With a deep commitment to advancing the health and well-being of older adults, Michelle's research interests are at the intersections of aging, caregiving, and social support systems, aiming to address the unique challenges faced by older adults through evidence-based policy solutions.

Gavin Green is a master's student at Utah State University in the Human Development and Family Studies department, specializing in gerontology research. A dedicated presenter, he recently shared his work at the Gerontological Society of America conference, highlighting the strong acceptance of an innovative Acceptance and Commitment Therapy caregiving intervention. Early in his academic career, Gavin is already making meaningful contributions to the field, with several publications in preparation for peer-reviewed journals. His research focuses on enhancing emotional closeness between caregivers and care recipients, using fNIRS hyperscanning to explore its utility as a protective factor. At the Alzheimer's Disease and Dementia Research Center, under Dr. Beth Fauth, he examines how improving caregiver mental health through acceptance enhances caregiving relationships and cognitive health outcomes.

David Hage PhD, MSW, serves as Assistant Professor of Social Work and is an Affiliate Faculty member of the Shady Rest Institute on Positive Aging at Florida Gulf Coast University and is experienced in long-term care and clinical social work, gerontological education, research, and consulting. He is a Licensed Clinical Social Worker (LCSW), a Fellow of the American College of Healthcare Executives

(FACHE), a Jewish Healthcare Foundation Feinstein Death & Dying Fellow, a member of the Academy of Certified Social Workers (ACSW), a Certified Advanced Social Work Case Manager (C-ASWCM), Certified Advanced Aging Life Care Professional™, and a Certified Dementia Practitioner (CDP).

Sean N. Halpin PhD, is a Gerontologist and Qualitative Analyst with RTI International on the Genomics, Ethics, and Translational Research team. Dr. Halpin has over a decade of experience leading socio-behavioral studies across chronic and infectious disease areas, with a focus on older adults in various long-term care settings. He has published widely on mind–body practices, alternative therapies, and physical activity for older adults, including acupuncture and movement-based therapies. At RTI, Dr. Halpin's responsibilities include preparing research proposals, developing and executing protocols, overseeing data collection and analysis, interpreting research results to support sponsors' strategic goals, and managing both operational and financial aspects of studies. He holds a Ph.D. in qualitative research and evaluation methodologies from the University of Georgia and an MA in developmental psychology from Teachers College, Columbia University.

Maurita T. Harris PhD, is an Assistant Professor in the Faculty of Liberal Arts at the Wilfrid Laurier University in Canada, holding appointments in User Experience Design and Social Justice & Community Engagement. She earned her B.A. from North Carolina State University in Psychology, and her M.S. and Ph.D. in Community Health from the University of Illinois Urbana-Champaign. Dr. Harris' research explores the way technology can support the well-being of people as they age from a Human Factors perspective focusing on design for aging; digital health; health and racial equity; and the technology lifecycle. As the director of the Well-Tech Research & Design Laboratory, she leads a team who collaborates with researchers across the world to ensure the integration of interdisciplinary approaches and thinking from diverse fields (e.g., community health, design, engineering, gerontology, leisure, psychology, and social justice).

Frances M. Hawes PhD, is an Assistant Professor in the Health Administration Program at the University of Wisconsin—Eau Claire, a program dedicated to educating future senior care leaders. She holds an MS and PhD in gerontology from the University of Massachusetts Boston and is a certified grief support specialist, with over 15 years of experience in the long-term care field.

Kristina M. Kokorelias PhD, works as the Geriatrics Program Manager and Associate Scientist for the Department of Medicine's Healthy Ageing and Geriatrics Program at Sinai Health and the University Health Network. Kristina also has status appointments as Assistant Professor, Occupational Science and Occupational Therapy and in the Rehabilitation Sciences Institute at the University of Toronto in Canada. Kristina is also an Associate Fellow of the National Institute on Ageing. Her program of research aims to understand the evolving experiences and needs of family caregivers and older adults with complex care needs with the aim of using this information to develop, evaluate, and implement timely family-centered care programs and services. Kristina received her PhD from the Rehabilitation Sciences Institute at the University of Toronto and completed postdoctoral fellowships in Implementation Science and Alzheimer's Diseases with St. John's Rehab within the Sunnybrook Health Sciences Center.

Lisa M. Lind PhD, ABPP, is a board-certified Geropsychologist who serves as Chief Clinical Officer for Deer Oaks Behavioral Health in Texas. She serves on several committees focused on long-term care and aging, including immediate past president of Psychologists in Long-Term Care (PLTC), Chair of the Post-Acute and Long-Term Care Medical Association's (PALTmed) Behavioral Health Subcommittee, and member of the American Psychological Association's (APA) Committee on Aging (CONA). Dr. Lind was selected as the 2024 Clinician of the Year by The Foundation for Post-Acute and Long-Term Care Medicine and received PLTC's George Georgoulakis Award for Outstanding Contributions to Psychology in Long-Term Care in 2022. Her current research interests include examining the behavioral health impact of the COVID-19 pandemic on LTC residents.

Mia E. Lussier obtained her PharmD from Wilkes University in 2020 and her Master's in Business Analytics from the University of Maryland in 2023. Following her PharmD, Dr. Lussier completed a two-year postdoctoral fellowship focused on pharmacy outcomes research from Geisinger. At this time, Dr. Lussier is a clinical assistant professor at Binghamton University in the School of Pharmacy and Pharmaceutical Sciences where she teaches in the integrated pharmacotherapy and social and administrative sciences curriculums. Dr. Lussier also maintains a clinical site at United Health Services where she practices as an ambulatory care pharmacist with a focus on optimizing medication therapy for chronic diseases and an interest in deprescribing medications in older adults.

Solange M. Marcel DNP, PMHNP-BC, ANP-BC, is an adult nurse practitioner with a gerontological specialty from Vanderbilt University School of Nursing and a post-master psychiatric mental health nursing certification along with a Doctorate of Nursing Practice from Georgia Southern University School of Nursing. Additionally, Dr. Marcel is a PhD candidate at Hunter-Bellevue's School of Nursing in New York, NY. Dr. Marcel is an advanced nursing professional with over 20 years dedicated to the care of the geriatric patient population with a current geropsychiatric and severe mental illness focus. Her expertise includes inpatient and long-term care settings for behavioral crisis stabilization via consult-liaison services in both rural and urban communities. Improving access to psychiatric care in the inpatient, long-term care, and post-acute care hospitalization settings while encouraging a strong interdisciplinary team of healthcare professionals to ensure continuity of care is a personal priority. Focused research in the areas of dementia, delirium, and decisional capacity with a solid commitment to bioethical principles is at the forefront of her advanced clinical practice. Dr. Marcel's personal mission is to ease the stresses our severely mentally ill population encounter across the age continuum by diligently addressing today's healthcare issues—from bedside to policy.

Jennifer Craft Morgan PhD, is a Professor and the Director of the Gerontology Institute at Georgia State University. Her research focuses on jobs and careers, attempting to understand how policy, population, workplace, and individual level factors shape how work is experienced and how work is organized across care settings. Dr. Morgan is a national expert on recruitment, training, and retention of direct care workers. She serves, since 2016, as the co-chair for Workforce Development working group of the Georgia Alzheimer's and Related Dementia Collaborative. Dr. Morgan has led several major evaluation efforts focused on sharing lessons learned, in real time, to inform and improve model development for practice and education-based intervention work. Dr. Morgan holds an MA and PhD in Sociology from the University of North Carolina at Chapel Hill.

Patricia Oh PhD, MSW, is Assistant Director for Community Innovation & Research at the Center on Aging at the University of Maine. She coordinates its Lifelong Maine initiative, which includes providing technical support and programming for the AARP Network of Age-Friendly States and Communities (NAFSC) in Maine, advising AARP Livable about its rural outreach efforts, and supporting the AARP NAFSC nationally. In her role as Co-Director of the Consortium on Aging Policy, Research, and Analysis, Dr. Oh studies the impact of policy on the lives of older Mainers. She is a frequent speaker at community events and has been invited to present age-friendly community development and healthy aging at state, regional, national, and international venues. Dr. Oh obtained a Ph.D. in Gerontology from the University of Massachusetts, Boston and MSW from the University of Southern Maine. As a practitioner and researcher, her expertise is in translational research, program development, evaluation, research, and professional and community education. Since 2012, she has focused on age-friendly community development at the national and state levels, with a particular interest in rural communities. Currently, her research focuses on climate and aging, municipal motivation to join the AARP NAFSC, the impact of joining on the social and service environments, and multisector collaborations to advance age-friendly community development, and specifically, higher education's role. Based on her research with communities, Dr. Oh has authored more than a dozen book chapters and articles about aging in community and is lead author to the award-winning AARP Roadmap to Livability Series and Rural Livability Report.

Romil Rakesh Parikh MBBS, MPH, PhD, is a clinical epidemiologist and a physician-scientist with a passion for advancing evidence-based, equitable, and person-centered care for older adults. He is senior research scientist and manager at the AHRQ Minnesota Evidence-Based Practice Center, where he leads evidence synthesis projects commissioned by professional medical societies for clinical guideline development and by federal and non-federal agencies for the development of public health recommendations. He holds a joint appointment as a research fellow in the Equity and Quality in Long-term care Supports and Services (EQuaLS) lab in the Division of Health Policy and Management at the University of Minnesota School of Public Health. In this capacity he leads several research studies on health inequities and quality measurement in various long-term care settings. He has coauthored research manuscripts published in leading journals such as the JAMA, the Lancet, the Journal of American Geriatrics Society, and the Journal of American Medical Directors Association. He also serves as an invited reviewer for several academic journals as well as a conference abstract reviewer for the American Geriatrics Society annual meetings.

Lindsay J. Peterson PhD, is a research associate professor in the School of Aging Studies at the University of South Florida. She began studying gerontology at USF in 2012 after working as a daily newspaper reporter for more than two decades, covering a wide range of topics, including aging in Florida. Department. She received her PhD from USF in 2016. Lindsay directs the USF School of Aging Studies internship/AIT program. She also conducts research, with primary interests in long-term care policy, quality of care in nursing homes and assisted living communities, and disaster preparedness for older adults and caregivers in long-term care and community-based settings.

Lisa Quinn-Lee PhD, is a Professor and Chair in the Social Work Department at the University of Wisconsin—Eau Claire. She has a BSW from University of Wisconsin-Eau Claire, an MSSW from University of Wisconsin-Madisons, and a PhD in social work from University of Minnesota. She has over 20 years of experience in hospice and palliative care and continues to teach and research in these areas.

Gail B. Rattinger obtained her PhD in the chemical sciences from University of Illinois Urbana-Champaign and her PharmD from University of California, San Francisco. Moreover, she completed a postdoctoral fellowship in health outcomes research, pharmacoepidemiology, and pharmacoeconomics at University of Maryland School of Pharmacy. Currently, Dr. Rattinger is a professor at Binghamton University in the School of Pharmacy and Pharmaceutical Sciences where she teaches across multiple Economic, Social, and Administrative Sciences as well as epidemiology and public health courses. Her research interests include medication use and disease management in older adults with a focus on dementia and factors associated with dementia progression and costs of informal dementia care.

Joshua Saul DACM, LAc., is a doctor of Acupuncture and Chinese medicine and 2nd generation acupuncturist with a focus on functional nutrition, digestive disorders and pain management. He is NCCAOM board-certified Acupuncture and Oriental Medicine practitioner and also holds certification in Applied Clinical Nutrition from the Texas Chiropractic College. He received a first professional doctorate from the Pacific College of Oriental Medicine, a Master's degree from AOMA's Graduate School of Integrative medicine.

Kimberly Snow MHSA, is a Senior Research Associate at the Catherine Cutler Institute, Muskie School of Public Service, University of Southern Maine, where she conducts program evaluation and research and analysis on Medicare and

Medicaid policy, elder abuse, caregiving, and workforce issues impacting older adults. She is also Co-Director of the Consortium for Aging Policy Research and Analysis (CAPRA), a partnership between the University of Maine and the University of Southern Maine. Her work has assisted state and federal partners understand how public resources are used to their best effect in helping older adults live healthy, active, secure, and engaged lives. With a particular interest in elder abuse detection, prevention, and impact, she is a member of the Maine Council for Elder Abuse Prevention. She has investigated the impact of elder abuse on service use and cost among older adults who are dually eligible for Medicare and Medicaid. Kimberly received her undergraduate degree from Oberlin College and her master's degree in health services administration from the University of Michigan School of Public Health.

Panagiota Tragantzopoulou serves as a visiting lecturer at the University of Westminster and as an associate lecturer at the University of Wolverhampton in the United Kingdom. Her research interests are focused on eating disorders, psychotherapy, and chronic illnesses. She received a BA from Aristotle University of Thessaloniki, an MA in Educational Psychology from UCL Institute of Education, an MSc in Integrative counselling and psychotherapy from the University of Derby, and a PhD in Psychology from the University of Westminster.

Jessica "Jess" VanderWerf is a PhD student in the School of Aging Studies at the University of South Florida. Before and while attending college, Jess worked as a certified nursing assistant, activities assistant, food aide, and hospital aide, working in and out of long-term care. Her current research focus is on disaster and emergency preparedness involving first responders. She has also researched environmental gerontology, gerontological education, and the individualized experience of aging as it relates to diversity topics. Jess is an active member of the Gerontological Society of America, and as a Master's student, she served as president of Sigma Phi Omega, the gerontological honors society.

List of Figures

Fig. 3.1 Timeline of Centers for Medicare and Medicaid Services Regulations Related to Antipsychotics (2013–2023) (Sources: Lucas & Bowblis, 2017; CMS, 2017; CMS, 2024) 33
Fig. 5.1 Percentages of combined data sources on the demographic profiles of direct care workers by industry. Note: All data (2022) except unpaid family caregiving status was pooled by Ruggles et al. (2024). Unpaid family caregiving status (2021) was pooled by Flood et al. (2023). All the data presented here were analyzed by PHI (June 2023; 2024) 52
Fig. 11.1 Examples of social determinants of health in long-term care 138

List of Table

Table 14.1 Summary of activities in the Community Supports and Health Services Domain 192

Chapter 1
Introduction: Health Promotion in the Context of Long-Term Care

Kallol Kumar Bhattacharyya

I remember that evening when I first saw her …an older adult woman who visited my clinic with multiple chronic morbidities. After a brief conversation, I came to know that she belonged to a low socioeconomic status and lived in solitary …an ideal example of multiple jeopardy. She came with a pale face …two high-powered glasses in a broken black frame were trying to cover her hesitation. After a couple of weeks, after at least three rounds of treatment, she became much …much better compared to the day I first saw her. In another couple of weeks, I saw a signing glow in her eyes that even made her broken black spectacle frame go unnoticed. I should mention here that by that time, I already started comparing her with my grandmother, and probably for that, during the entire treatment, I did not take any fees from her and tried to provide her medications as much as possible from my desk. I do not know whether for that reason or maybe I am wrong …on her last visit to my clinic, she presented me a handkerchief with the letter "K" stitched in one corner. I still remember the smile I saw on her face while presenting me the handkerchief …a smile of appreciation that still encourages me to continue providing my services to older adults as a clinician.

The current global *aging in place* movement supports older adults with the idea of staying in their home and community as they age instead of moving into a long-term care facility, i.e. an assisted living facility or nursing home. According to Forbes Health (Hip, 2024), 92% of older adults want to stay in their homes later in life. However, about 1.3 million residents reside in one of the 1.7 million beds in nearly 15,500 nursing homes in the United States (CDC, 2020; Harris-Kojetin et al., 2019). Considering the massively increasing cost of long-term care, "age in place" is probably the ideal option for any older adult regarding the cost efficacy. However, is it only because of cost-effectiveness? Probably, the answer is a big NO. In later

K. K. Bhattacharyya (✉)
School of Public Health, University of Memphis, Memphis, TN, USA
e-mail: kkbhttch@memphis.edu

K. K. Bhattacharyya (ed.), *Health Promotion in Long-Term Care Facilities*,
https://doi.org/10.1007/978-3-031-91038-8_1

life, an individual's healthcare needs often become more complex and chronic (World Health Organization [WHO], 2007). Possibly, the most important reason for opting for "age in place" is that people want to maintain their independence and quality of life as they get older.

In the United States, the aging population is increasingly diverse; many of them suffer from multiple chronic morbidities and need post-acute care (Ward & Schiller, 2013). Given the growing demand for care expectations, the concept of long-term care is constantly changing to provide most care needs. Further, the growing demand also argues for more equitable, innovative, inclusive, and accessible healthcare (Jones & Dolsten, 2024). We are serving many people at a time, including residents, families, staff, and others; this needs urgent collaboration (Rosen et al., 2018). However, the healthcare system does not effectively address many relevant factors, such as the social determinants of health, including individuals' education, financial status, living status, and social supports, strongly affecting the health outcomes of older adults (Chetty et al., 2016; Jones & Dolsten, 2024).

Nonetheless, the care needs of older adults in long-term care are different from community living individuals and are primarily influenced by restrictions on autonomy (De Biasi et al., 2020). Loneliness, helplessness, and boredom are the classic triad responsible for the deteriorating mental health conditions in long-term care residents, further giving rise to insufficient satisfaction with care (Bergman-Evans, 2004; Desai & Grossberg, 2001). Resident satisfaction is integral to the quality of care in long-term care settings. Indeed, although technical competence is the prime aspect of any healthcare service, it is evident that autonomy, environment, meaningful activities, and interpersonal quality of professionals are the most important predictors for older adults' self-reported satisfaction in a long-term care institution (Bhattacharyya et al., 2022). Further, such satisfaction is only possible if the needs of all the stakeholders, such as caregivers and care recipients, are addressed. The current care system requires more to correspond to many older adult residents' care preferences and needs (Bartels, 2003). In reality, person-centered care in long-term care facilities should exceed merely meeting stipulated quality measures (Edelman et al., 2021). As documented in care plans, what matters to residents needs to be aligned with standard person-centered care practices (Johnson et al., 2021; Koren, 2010). Therefore, education and training of gerontologists from diverse backgrounds in the principles of person-centered care to improve the quality of care and quality of life in long-term care is an urgent need to extend the culture change movement to long-term care by identifying and detailing its components in a holistic way. From this perspective, the growing demand for health promotional practices is an essential issue that also supports implementing an age-friendly initiative in long-term care facilities.

The current 4Ms model of an age-friendly health system attempts to incorporate the care values of older adults and family caregivers, focusing on what matters to them (Fulmer & Li, 2018; Fulmer et al., 2018). *What matters* to residents is broad and complex, and the 4Ms model needs to embrace the concept of person-centered care holistically, focusing on the barriers and facilitators of caregiving. In fact, the 4Ms model primarily reflects the residents' context, focusing on identifying and managing care preferences relative to residents' physical health outcomes. However, residents' care preferences do not always emphasize a specific clinical health outcome. Therefore, only person-centered and more comprehensive care can meet the proper implementation of "what matters" in long-term care that includes all levels of caregivers (Edelman et al., 2021). Tailoring healthcare conversations according to residents' and their families' requirements is a crucial component of person-centered care (Edelman et al., 2021; Jazieh et al., 2018). Person-centered care does not only require a "culture change" in how residents and caregivers work as a unit to achieve the same goal, but it also requires that long-term care facilities ensure staff deliver care with the best possible level of empathy and adopt meaningful care practices. A recently proposed "8Ms" framework addresses resident and family concerns and also satisfies the needs and roles of paid caregivers and administration personnel in making long-term care facilities friendly for older residents and staff (Bhattacharyya et al., 2023b).

Several scholars found the *quality of life* indicators superior in predicting resident outcomes than the *quality of care* indicators; they believe the former taps into the residents' perceptions and is more closely associated with their health (Kane, 2003). The 8Ms framework best describes both. The 8Ms framework may result in multiple benefits in long-term care by assuring good quality of care to residents, caregivers' job satisfaction, and assisting nursing home administration in providing residents with the best possible quality of life (Bhattacharyya et al., 2023b). Constructing an architecturally favorable environment in long-term care settings to ensure the easy movability of residents is a vital issue; however, it is not the ultimate one. Residents' quality of life could only be enhanced with their active involvement, and it needs enthusiastic human support, i.e. zestful support from the surrounding persons. Both caregivers, including direct care workers and nursing home administrators, and care recipients, i.e., residents and family members, must understand their roles and expectations. The idea of age-friendly long-term care could be best illustrated by a triangular model, involving care receivers' (resident), direct caregivers' (staff), and care supervisors' (administrative personnel) perspectives, respectively.

One scoping review, focusing on standards and quality of care for older adults in long-term care facilities globally, found the effectiveness of prompted voiding interventions for urinary incontinence, professional support to facility staff, and pressure ulcer prevention programs, with a dearth of research on psychosocial care standards (Kalideen et al., 2021). The study concluded that although much research focuses on intervention effectiveness, they provide limited attention to people-centeredness and safety. The authors suggested the need for global implementation of effective interventions, more research on psychosocial care, and more studies in low-to-middle-income countries are essential to improve long-term care standards (Kalideen et al., 2021).

Another recent study that focuses on long-term care facilities in Canada examined the shift from biomedically-oriented care to a person-centered model of care and found that safety, security, and order are often prioritized over other quality of life measures, such as individuality and autonomy, with significant variation in policy language and implementation across jurisdictions (Irwin et al., 2023). The study concluded that while person-centered policies exist, they are often underutilized or overshadowed by more dominant safety-focused policies. The authors suggested that enhancing the visibility and implementation of person-centered policies could significantly improve the quality of life for long-term care residents (Irwin et al., 2023).

The other study, focusing on the impact of volunteer activities on the quality of life of older adult residents, employees, and volunteers in a long-term care institution in Brazil, found significant improvements in personal relationships for volunteers, overall health for residents, and overall quality of life for employees after the return of volunteer activities (de Sandes-Guimarães et al., 2023). The study concludes that the return of volunteer activities positively impacted various quality of life aspects for all three groups, with specific benefits linked to increased social interaction and reduced workload. The authors suggested that incorporating volunteer activities in long-term care facilities can enhance the overall quality of care and well-being for residents, employees, and volunteers (de Sandes-Guimarães et al., 2023). Relatedly, another study found that more extensive social networks are associated with better cognitive function, while the frequency and type of service activities did not predict cognitive performance (Dodds et al., 2024). Therefore, it is evident that quality of life in long-term care facilities does not only focus on certain medical care to be provided but instead demands care that satisfies residents' autonomy, social connection, and meaningfulness in life.

Tying Diverse Threads Together

I remember, in one of the initial days after I got my medical degree, I prescribed an antibiotic to a newly admitted patient with enteric fever based on his blood report. When my mentor came to visit the patient, he first asked me to reexamine the patient and scolded me for prescribing the medicine based on his blood report. He criticized me for whether I would treat blood reports or a human being in my future career as a clinician. Indeed, the person was diagnosed with some other problem later, not enteric fever. Often, we never think the way we see an issue may not be exactly the same as it belongs in reality. For example, we learned that "white" is the opposite of "black," "father" is the opposite of "mother," and "student" is the opposite of "teacher." Now, the question is whether they are opposite or complement each other (Sisodia, 2019). Is this a flaw in our education system that gave a wrong impression to our brain when we were in elementary school? Or is this knowledge that we learned from our environment? Nonetheless, we need to update our methods of educating children; opposite words are not always opposing each other; instead, they complement each other in most cases (Sisodia, 2019). We should not prejudice anything based on what we see in the naked eye. Long-term care quality is also relevant from this perspective.

In recent years, we have emphasized long-term care quality based on what services are provided to care recipients but often forget the other side of the coin, the way residents accept the care. Health services research mostly captures how a solitary issue dissatisfies a resident regarding care quality. For example, a bitter tablet in the morning spoils the mood of an older adult resident, thereby dissatisfying her regarding the quality of care. However, we often ignore the urge to dive deeper into this matter. Suppose the older adult resident's son did not visit her for the last 4 days, which increased her anger. When the son came during lunch on the fifth day and explained to her why he could not visit due to a serious health issue of her grandson, it automatically changed her mind; when the same nurse gave her the same medicine in the evening, she took that gladly because now she wants to return home quickly to see her grandson. She realized that this bitter medicine is the best for her recovery, and now she is satisfied with care. Furthermore, a clinical factor may come into play: the diurnal variation of adrenalin, a hormone that impacts our emotions. Maybe for a higher serum adrenalin level, the resident's level of satisfaction changed from morning to evening. Likewise, the level of optimistic outlook, personality traits, and many other internal psychosocial factors can also influence a resident's decision on quality of care. Relatedly, it is true that teaching students starts from outside the classroom and ends outside the classroom; classroom teaching is only a portion in between. Likewise, an individual's quality of life standard starts long before they enter a long-term care facility and, for most, continues long after they are discharged from the facility; the quality of life in long-term care is only a portion in between. Therefore, the time has come to pay serious attention to other relevant but less apparent issues from a holistic perspective; in this context, the importance of health promotional practices should be integral to health services research.

The relocation of older adults from their homes to an entirely new long-term care facility environment can be challenging. This transition impacts the health and well-being of the concerned individual remarkably from economic, physical, and psychological perspectives. All these issues considerably influence the morbidity and lifespan of the individual in later life. Although the importance of long-term care and its socioeconomic significance is increasing as a fast-growing portion of US healthcare, a substantial number of facilities continue to have significant quality problems (Bhattacharyya et al., 2024; Harrington et al., 2016). A good quality of life does not depend only on providing good medical care. Residents' demands are increasing. Relatedly, a recent study found older adults feel themselves successful agers when they are physically and socially active, have basic aspects of well-being, have satisfaction with life, can participate in meaningful activities, and are financially secure (Bhattacharyya et al., 2023a). This psychological outlook exists even in long-term care environments. Here comes the importance of health promotional practices.

The concept of health promotion varies by the differences in the definition of health. The World Health Organization (WHO) defined *health* as "a state of complete physical, mental, and social well-being and not merely the absence of disease or infirmity" (Sartorius, 2006, p. 1). From a broad perspective, health promotion supports individuals and communities in preventing, coping with, and addressing health challenges, and enables people to enhance control over their health. The selection-optimization-compensation (SOC) framework (Baltes & Baltes, 1990) could provide important guidance related to adaptation in long-term care in later ages. The process of selection in our daily life is needed to focus our efforts, while compensatory processes are required to counteract age-related deficits and losses; the process of optimization balances between these two (Baltes, 1993; Wahl, 2020). Long-term care requires adopting a culture change, which enhances resident choice, empowers staff, and should be promoted to improve resident care and health outcomes (Miller et al., 2014). Residents do not just want to add years in their later life but life to later years (Wahl, 2020). Health promotional activities are essential in providing good supportive care to add life in later years.

Health promotion enables people to enhance control over their own health. As an umbrella term, it includes a wide range of socio-behavioral interventions designed to improve individuals' quality of life by managing the underlying causes of ill health instead of focusing only on curative treatment. The current book discusses various biopsychosocial barriers and facilitators of long-term care services, focusing on health promotional activities targeting to maximize the quality of life in long-term care. This awareness of the landscape of activities may help us rectify and develop strategies for better supporting long-term care residents living with various chronic disorders, including dementia, at a more dignified and meaningful level. Further, although no consensus has yet been developed to build an all-encompassing theory of caregiving, multiple theories currently represent several domains of long-term care practices. In this book, various theoretical formulations, such as structure-process-outcome (by Donabedian), selective optimization with compensation (SOC) model (Baltes & Baltes, 1990), person-centered, activity-disengagement, biopsychosocial, and positive psychology, would be the central aspect to address the subject matter in different chapters and the book in its entirety.

The aim of the current book is consonant with the WHO's concept of health that emphasizes basic strategies for health promotion, i.e., advocate (boost the factors that encourage health), enable (support people in achieving health equity), and mediate (collaborate across sectors) (Carlisle, 2000; WHO, 1986). The following chapters will attempt to tie various diverse threads together, focusing on the current quality of services (discussed in the chapters on Quality of Care and Quality of Life, Cognitive Decline and Polypharmacy, Direct Care Workforce, and The Impact of Disasters and COVID-19), emphasizing the possible role of cross-cultural health promotional practices in maintaining the quality of life (the central aspects in Cultural perspectives, Social Determinants of Health, and Health Promotional Practices chapters), and promoting a person-centered holistic biopsychosocial approach to aging that maximizes their quality of life while living with different chronic conditions (the key element in Aging In Place or Long-Term Care, Person-Centered Care and Culture Change Movement, and Palliative Care). Although the book focuses on nursing homes and assisted living facilities, we will also consider other spaces (environments) according to their relevancy.

References

Baltes, P. B., & Baltes, M. M. (1990). Psychological perspectives on successful aging: The model of selective optimization with compensation. In P. B. Baltes & M. M. Baltes (Eds.), Successful aging: Perspectives from the behavioral sciences (pp. 1–34). Cambridge University Press. https://doi.org/10.1017/CBO9780511665684.003

Baltes P. B. (1993). The aging mind: Potential and limits. *The Gerontologist, 33*(5), 580–594. https://doi.org/10.1093/geront/33.5.580

Bartels, S. J. (2003). Improving the system of care for older adults with mental illness in the United States. *The American Journal of Geriatric Psychiatry, 11*(5), 486–497. https://doi.org/10.1176/appi.ajgp.11.5.486

Bergman-Evans, B. (2004). Beyond the basics. Effects of the Eden alternative model on quality of life issues. *Journal of Gerontological Nursing, 30*(6), 27–34. https://doi.org/10.3928/0098-9134-20040601-07

Bhattacharyya, K. K., Molinari, V., & Andel, R. (2023a). Longevity is not an ingredient of successful aging as self-reported by community-dwelling older adults: A scoping review. *Aging & Mental Health, 27*(2), 217–229. https://doi.org/10.1080/13607863.2022.2033696

Bhattacharyya, K. K., Molinari, V., Black, K., & Whitbourne, S. K. (2023b). Creating age-friendly nursing homes: The time is now. *Gerontology & Geriatrics Education, 44*(4), 613–630. https://doi.org/10.1080/02701960.2022.2106981

Bhattacharyya, K. K., Molinari, V., & Hyer, K. (2022). Self-reported satisfaction of older adult residents in nursing homes: Development of a conceptual framework. *The Gerontologist, 62*(8), e442–e456. https://doi.org/10.1093/geront/gnab061

Bhattacharyya, K. K., Peterson, L., Molinari, V., Fauth, E. B., & Andel, R. (2024). The importance of zero-deficiency complaints in nursing homes: A mere consequence or serious concern?. *Journal of Applied Gerontology, 43*(7), 945–955. https://doi.org/10.1177/07334648241229548

Carlisle, S. (2000). Health promotion, advocacy and health inequalities: A conceptual framework. *Health Promotion International, 15*(4), 369–376. https://doi.org/10.1093/heapro/15.4.369

Centers for Disease Control and Prevention (CDC). (2020). *National Center for Health Statistics—Nursing home care*. Assessed on October 16, 2020 from https://www.cdc.gov/nchs/fastats/nursing-home-care.htm

Chetty, R., Stepner, M., Abraham, S., Lin, S., Scuderi, B., Turner, N., Bergeron, A., & Cutler, D. (2016). The association between income and life expectancy in the United States, 2001-2014. *JAMA, 315*(16), 1750–1766. https://doi.org/10.1001/jama.2016.4226

De Biasi, A., Wolfe, M., Carmody, J., Fulmer, T., & Auerbach, J. (2020). Creating an age-friendly public health system. *Innovation in Aging, 4*(1), igz044. https://doi.org/10.1093/geroni/igz044

de Sandes-Guimarães, L. V., Dos Santos, P. C., Alves, C. P. G. P., Cervato, C. J., Silva, A. P. A., & Leão, E. R. (2023). The effect of volunteer-led activities on the quality of life of volunteers, residents, and employees of a long-term care institution: A cohort study. *BMC Geriatrics, 23*(1), 151. https://doi.org/10.1186/s12877-023-03898-y

Desai, A. K., & Grossberg, G. T. (2001). Recognition and management of behavioral disturbances in dementia. *Primary Care Companion to the Journal of Clinical Psychiatry, 3*(3), 93–109. https://doi.org/10.4088/pcc.v03n0301

Dodds, L., Brayne, C., & Siette, J. (2024). Associations between social networks, cognitive function, and quality of life among older adults in long-term care. *BMC Geriatrics, 24*(1), 221. https://doi.org/10.1186/s12877-024-04794-9

Edelman, L. S., Drost, J., Moone, R. P., Owens, K., Towsley, G. L., Tucker-Roghi, G., & Morley, J. E. (2021). Applying the age-friendly health system framework to long term care settings. *The Journal of Nutrition, Health & Aging, 25*(2), 141–145. https://doi.org/10.1007/s12603-020-1558-2

Fulmer, T., & Li, N. (2018). Age-friendly health systems for older adults with dementia. *The Journal for Nurse Practitioners, 14*(3), 160–165. https://doi.org/10.1016/j.nurpra.2017.09.001

Fulmer, T., Mate, K. S., & Berman, A. (2018). The age-friendly health system imperative. *Journal of the American Geriatrics Society, 66*(1), 22–24. https://doi.org/10.1111/jgs.15076

Harrington, C., Schnelle, J. F., McGregor, M., & Simmons, S. F. (2016). The need for higher minimum staffing standards in U.S. nursing homes. *Health Services Insights, 9*, 13–19. https://doi.org/10.4137/HSI.S38994

Harris-Kojetin, L., Sengupta, M., Lendon, J. P., Rome, V., Valverde, R., & Caffrey, C. (2019). *Long-term care providers and services users in the United States, 2015–2016*. (Vol. 3). National Center for Health Statistics. Vital and Health Statistics.

Hip, D. (2024). Aging in place statistics and facts in 2024. Forbes Health. Retrieved September 27, 2024, from https://www.forbes.com/health/healthy-aging/aging-in-place-statistics/.

Irwin, P., Taylor, D., & Keefe, J. M. (2023). Provincial policies affecting resident quality of life in Canadian residential long-term care. *BMC Geriatrics, 23*(1), 362. https://doi.org/10.1186/s12877-023-04074-y

Jazieh, A. H., Volker, S., & Taher, S. (2018). Involving the family in patient care: A culturally tailored communication model. *Global Journal on Quality and Safety in Healthcare, 1*(2), 33–37. https://doi.org/10.4103/JQSH.JQSH_3_18

Johnson, B. P., Dyck, M. J., Hovey, S., & Shropshire, M. D. (2021). Gerontological nursing competencies: A crosswalk with the 4Ms framework of the age-friendly initiative. *Gerontology & Geriatrics Education*, 1–8. Advance online publication. https://doi.org/10.1080/02701960.2021.1974430

Jones, C. H., & Dolsten, M. (2024). Author correction: Healthcare on the brink: Navigating the challenges of an aging society in the United States. *NPJ Aging, 10*(1), 25. https://doi.org/10.1038/s41514-024-00153-5

Kalideen, L., Govender, P., van Wyk, J. M., & Kuupiel, D. (2021). Mapping evidence on standards and quality of care for older persons in long-term care facilities: A scoping review protocol. *Systematic Reviews, 10*(1), 153. https://doi.org/10.1186/s13643-021-01709-2

Kane, R. A. (2003). Definition, measurement, and correlates of quality of life in nursing homes: Toward a reasonable practice, research, and policy agenda. *The Gerontologist, 43*, 28–36. https://doi.org/10.1093/geront/43.suppl_2.28

Koren, M. J. (2010). Person-centered care for nursing home residents: The culture-change movement. *Health Affairs (Project Hope), 29*(2), 312–317. https://doi.org/10.1377/hlthaff.2009.0966

Miller, S. C., Lepore, M., Lima, J. C., Shield, R., & Tyler, D. A. (2014). Does the introduction of nursing home culture change practices improve quality? *Journal of the American Geriatrics Society, 62*(9), 1675–1682. https://doi.org/10.1111/jgs.12987

Rosen, M. A., DiazGranados, D., Dietz, A. S., Benishek, L. E., Thompson, D., Pronovost, P. J., & Weaver, S. J. (2018). Teamwork in healthcare: Key discoveries enabling safer, high-quality care. *The American Psychologist, 73*(4), 433–450. https://doi.org/10.1037/amp0000298

Sartorius, N. (2006). The meanings of health and its promotion. *Croatian Medical Journal, 47*(4), 662–664.

Sisodia, M. (2019, September 29). *Manish Sisodia's powerful speech on education at Goa* [video]. YouTube. https://youtu.be/3mav0o5uJoA?si=TuUlYgceEd4jj8yP.

Wahl, H. W. (2020). Aging successfully: Possible in principle? Possible for all? Desirable for all? *Integrative Psychological & Behavioral Science, 54*, 251–268. https://doi.org/10.1007/s12124-020-09513-8

Ward, B. W., & Schiller, J. S. (2013). Prevalence of multiple chronic conditions among US adults: Estimates from the National Health Interview Survey, 2010. *Preventing Chronic Disease, 10*, E65. https://doi.org/10.5888/pcd10.120203

World Health Organization. (1986). *The Ottawa Charter for Health Promotion*. Retrieved on September 27, 2024, from: https://www.who.int/teams/health-promotion/enhanced-wellbeing/first-global-conference.

World Health Organization. (2007). *Age-friendly environments*. Retrieved on March 7, 2021, from: https://www.who.int/ageing/projects/age-friendly-environments/en/.

Chapter 2
Are Quality of Care and Quality of Life Synonymous in Long-Term Care?

Kallol Kumar Bhattacharyya

Consistent with the surge in the aging population, in recent years, the healthcare industry, particularly long-term care, has shown tremendous growth with multiple amenities aiming toward meeting the growing demands of residents' care needs. Long-term care constitutes a variety of services, including preventive, rehabilitative, restorative, and post-acute nursing care, to facilitate individualized health, focusing on the social and personal care of older adults (Kalideen et al., 2021; National Institute on Aging, 2023). Long-term care is offered in formal or informal settings through a variety of trained or untrained caregivers. Skilled nursing facilities, commonly called nursing homes, and assisted living facilities are vital components of the growing long-term care industry. Nursing homes are state-regulated and licensed healthcare institutions providing long-term housing and round-the-clock care to debilitated individuals, including functionally independent older adults (Heiks & Sabine, 2022; National Institute on Aging, 2023). In contrast, assisted living facilities are distinct long-term care settings designed to promote maximum autonomy to residents, with round-the-clock assistance with personal care, social and recreational engagements, and limited healthcare services (National Center for Health Statistics, 2013). Compared to nursing homes, fewer services and staffing resources are available in assisted living facilities, with registered nurses usually available on call (Hoben et al., 2024). Recent data suggests that, in the United States, 50% of assisted living facility residents are 85 years or older, 30% have dementia, and 67% have multiple comorbidities (Hua et al., 2022). Nursing home residents, who are more vulnerable, have more physical and cognitive impairments than assisted living facility residents; however, many demographics (e.g., age, sex, etc.) and morbidity (e.g., dementia, diabetes, COPD, and heart problems) profiles do not have much difference between the two (Hoben et al., 2024). Remarkably, the

K. K. Bhattacharyya (✉)
School of Public Health, University of Memphis, Memphis, TN, USA
e-mail: kkbhttch@memphis.edu

K. K. Bhattacharyya (ed.), *Health Promotion in Long-Term Care Facilities*,
https://doi.org/10.1007/978-3-031-91038-8_2

purpose and measures to maintain the residents' quality of life match between the two.

Although long-term care quality measures have shown improvement in recent years, residents' care needs have continued to become more complex (Castle & Ferguson, 2010; Tinetti et al., 2012; Zimmerman et al., 2024). Long-term care, particularly nursing home, services are often scanned due to growing concerns regarding the quality of care and quality of life from professionals, including policymakers, consumers, or researchers (Grabowski et al., 2008; Harrington et al., 2001, 2016). "Quality" is a multifaceted term that is impacted by a compound effect of several factors (Hansen et al., 2019). Measuring long-term care quality is a multidimensional arena in which investigating residents' complaints plays a crucial role (McGregor et al., 2011). Thus, the quality of service in long-term care, specifically in nursing homes, mainly relies on the quality of care the facilities provide, which aims to maintain the quality of life of care recipients. In this context, compared to the way states monitor and enforce nursing home regulations, less was researched about state efforts in monitoring and enforcing assisted living facilities regulations (Kaskie et al., 2022). In many states, oversight of assisted living facilities was distributed across three or more agencies, and administrative support varied depending on staffing and budget allocations; despite the significant growth of the industry, agency staff in many states are not sufficiently dedicated to assisted living oversight (Kaskie et al., 2022). Most importantly, unlike nursing homes, information regarding the quality of assisted living facilities is not easily accessible to the public. Many scholars ardently argued for redesigning assisted living models regarding their financing, regulation, workforce, and resident care patterns (Zimmerman et al., 2022). In the current chapter, we will focus mainly on the quality of nursing homes and discuss the quality of assisted living facilities where appropriate.

Quality of Care in Long-Term Care Facilities

Quality of care is one of the main determinants of the standard of service nursing homes provide. Thus, it has been a primary concern in public policy initiatives for an extended period. The effort to standardize the quality of care was initiated in 1965 with the implementation of Medicare and Medicaid programs to maintain a good quality of care for debilitated individuals in nursing homes (Marjoua & Bozic, 2012; Walshe, 2001). However, research revealed that a considerable number of nursing facilities still need to meet those care standards (Walshe, 2001). The Omnibus Budget Reconciliation Act (OBRA), 1987, was introduced to improve the quality of care and, thereby, the quality of life for nursing home residents by providing adequate services toward achieving and maintaining their highest possible physical, psychological, and social well-being (Walshe, 2001; Walshe & Harrington, 2002). However, the entire implementation and accomplishment of the OBRA still remain elusive. At the same time, there is very scant evidence to discern whether the benefits mentioned in the act justified the costs. Although several reforms and redesigning efforts have been conducted through the Senate Special Committee on Aging, the United States Government Accountability Office (US GAO), and other federal regulatory bodies, the best possible nursing home care remains unaccomplished and a complex domain in healthcare (Grabowski et al., 2008; Marjoua & Bozic, 2012; Walshe, 2001). Academicians are still trying to rectify the best quality indicators to support policymakers in creating policies ensuring nursing home residents receive optimal quality care.

Quality of care is often interpreted as "care that consistently contributes to the improvement or maintenance of quality and/or duration of life" (American Medical Association, 1986). The Centers for Medicare & Medicaid Services (CMS) informs the public about nursing home quality through its Five-Star Quality Rating System, comparing a nursing facility based on state and national averages for scores on the quality of care. The ratings are based on scores generated from health inspections, quality measures, and staffing (CMS, 2015; 2016). The critical component of the Five-Star system, the health inspection scores, is calculated by evaluating the results of annual recertification surveys and consumer complaint investigations (CMS, 2015; 2016; Peterson & Bowblis, 2023). State survey agencies carry out recertification surveys of all CMS-certified skilled nursing facilities every 9 to 15 months to assess their compliance with federal standards (Hansen et al., 2019; US GAO, 2011); however, sometimes they are predictable (Bhattacharyya et al., 2024a, 2024b; Williams et al., 2016). Nevertheless, the violation of a standard often leads to a deficiency citation. Furthermore, state survey agencies investigate consumer complaints, i.e. complaints lodged by residents, family members, staff, and others such as long-term care ombudsmen. When a complaint is received, after a subsequent investigation, state surveyors decide whether the complaint is substantiated, i.e., viable, and if a regulatory violation is found to warrant a deficiency citation (Bhattacharyya et al., 2024a, 2024c). When a deficiency citation is issued, irrespective of the result of an annual recertification survey or complaint investigation, the concerned nursing home is required to develop a rectification plan to remedy the noted deficiency. It may also need payment of a fine, termination from the Medicare or Medicaid programs, or a combination of all these possibilities (Castle, 2011). Researchers have found in the last few decades that using the proxy measure of deficiency citations a facility receives is a good option for evaluating the quality of care in nursing homes.

According to the structure-process-outcome (SPO) model, quality is associated with a system being analyzed (Donabedian, 2005). Measuring nursing home quality is a multidimensional field; many researchers used Donabedian's structure-process-outcome (SPO) model to identify the "quality of care" indicators obtained from annual recertification surveys. In the SPO model, "structure" is considered as the characteristics of an organization or nursing home, such as profit status, chain membership, the number of residents/beds, and residents' reimbursement status. The "process" component is defined as the factors essential in delivering services, such as the clinical and non-clinical care provided by different categories of staff (e.g., medical director, nurse, and nursing assistant) to the residents. However, "outcomes" largely depend on the purpose of the study and the research question, such as the number of deficiency citations, the scope and severity of deficiency citations, and other factors relevant to resident health outcomes. In addition, Donabedian (1988) argued for analyzing the relationship between care provider (staff) and care recipient (residents) to assess how the process (staff-to-resident interactions) influences the outcome, assessing both residents' health (objective) and satisfaction with care (subjective) (Bhattacharyya et al., 2022). Residents' health outcomes, such as the presence of pressure ulcers and the usage of catheters, feeding tubes, and restraints, are standard measures to assess the quality of care; however, deficiency citations are also vital as a proxy indicator to evaluate the quality of care in nursing homes.

From the perspective of Donabedian's SPO model, structural factors in nursing homes are critical to affecting the quality of care. Although deficiency citations often elucidate nursing home's organizational infrastructure, such as profit status, chain membership, or many other structural factors (Castle et al., 2011), they may not be altered easily. Research revealed that nursing homes that are for-profit, members of chain facilities (i.e., facilities allied with the same corporate parent body), and have higher resident occupancy receive a higher number of complaints (Stevenson, 2006). Studies also found that for many clinical quality measures, for example, pressure sores, indwelling catheters, feeding tubes, and physical restraints, the nursing homes identified as poor-quality facilities remained in the same status over 10 years, and this is evident even in high-quality facilities (Grabowski & Castle, 2004). Further, nursing homes with higher Medicaid funding provided better care, suggesting that reimbursements should be considered quality of care factors (Grabowski & Castle, 2004). Regarding the "process" factors, nursing homes with a higher proportion of registered nurses (RNs) and certified nursing assistants (CNAs) among staff members provide better quality of care (Bowblis & Roberts, 2018). Further, a higher number of CNAs significantly predicted lower aggregated deficiency scores within nursing homes and lowered quality of care deficiency scores (Hyer et al., 2011). In contrast, Castle (2008) found that about 40% of the quality indicators in nursing facilities were significantly positively related to staffing levels when measuring the quality of care based on staffing patterns. Additionally, staff skill mix and delivery of care have a more direct impact on the quality of care over the number of staff members on duty; thus, every quality indicator has the potential to show the policymakers and practitioners its association with the quality of care in nursing homes (Castle, 2008).

Quality of Life in Long-Term Care Facilities

Quality of life is considered a state that supports an individual in maintaining good health and well-being and enjoying life events weighted by a personal set of values (Felce & Perry, 1995). Assessing quality of life is also complex; many tools and scales have been used to measure quality of life from different perspectives, such as the World Health Organization Quality of Life (WHOQOL) instrument, EuroQol 5-Dimension (EQ-5D), Quality of Life Enjoyment and Satisfaction Questionnaire (Q-LES-Q), Long-Term Care Quality Of Life assessment scale (LTC-QOL), and the Satisfaction with Life Scale (SWLS) (Alomari & Steinke, 2024; Arensberg et al., 2023). Although in long-term care, quality of life significantly depends on the quality of care the residents are offered, it is more than only the clinical care they receive. More research is needed on the associations between residents and staff to determine how provider–resident interactions affect resident outcomes regarding their health and well-being (Donabedian, 1988). It is also argued that nursing home "quality of life" indicators are parallel to residents' functional abilities, aggressive behaviors, and physical restraints used in the facility (Castle, 2002). Researchers found "quality of life" indicators better in predicting resident outcomes than "quality of care" indicators because they are directly associated with residents' statuses (Kane, 2003). In this context, some federally available datasets, such as the complaint dataset and the Certification and Survey Provider Enhanced Reports (CASPER) survey dataset, are not considered to measure resident quality of life directly; however, several researchers have studied to assess the "quality of life" factors by examining proxy variables from those datasets. Castle et al. (2011) tried to reveal the relation between organizational (facility characteristics), internal (operating characteristics of nursing homes), and external (outside factors that influence facilities) factors associated with deficiency citations that impact residents' quality of life. They also estimated the scope and severity of deficiency citations to evaluate the extent of potential harm for each citation possibly associated with the quality of life of residents. However, the information enlisted in those administrative datasets is mainly derived from outside sources, such as surveyor assessments, rather than directly from residents.

Measuring quality of life should be a comprehensive assessment that includes psychological, social, environmental, and functional perspectives of a resident's life (Shippee et al., 2015). Not only the facility characteristics, such as paying status, ownership status, location, and staffing pattern, but resident characteristics, such as physical and cognitive abilities, duration of stay, payment source, disability status, age, and race, also impact the quality of life of residents directly (Shippee et al., 2015). Also, functional statuses and meaningful involvement with nursing facilities' social environment influence their quality of life (Shippee et al., 2015). Additionally, the information on resident abuse and neglect is also important in assessing the quality of life in nursing homes. The reimbursement for care through Medicaid impacts the quality of nursing home care because research has found that nursing homes reimbursed mainly through Medicaid were prone to have a higher number of deficiency citations related to resident abuse (Castle, 2011). Further, resident abuse in nursing facilities that affects the quality of life draws significant concerns for residents' health and safety (Castle, 2011). Using four abuse-related deficiency citations available in the OSCAR dataset, Castle (2011) also found that around 30% of nursing homes in the United States received citations for resident abuse in 1999–2000; those abuses and neglect directly affected resident quality of life, as well as life expectancy.

Psychiatric polypharmacy, i.e., taking multiple drugs concurrently that leads to substantial drug interactions, is another example that further dwindles already debilitated residents' quality of life. Research revealed that 85% of newly admitted residents persistently received psychoactive medication even 3 months after admission, proving psychopharmacological therapy is the treatment of choice in most long-term care facilities (Molinari et al., 2011). CMS's steps to reduce unnecessary antipsychotic usage in long-term care (Bhattacharyya et al., 2023a; Lucas & Bowblis, 2017), particularly in managing behavioral symptoms of dementia, proved to benefit residents; however, it still needs to go a long way.

Many researchers found resident satisfaction to be more accurate in accessing quality of life (Kane, 2003). Hirschman was probably the first individual to show the two options from the consumer's point of view, i.e., "exit," for instance, stop buying from a firm, or "voice" against the concerned management (Hirschman, 1970; Stevenson, 2006). If dissatisfied, residents may either relocate to another nursing facility, or lodge a complaint against the concerned facility (Kane, 2003). One related study found that in four US states, the first option was limited to only 3.3% because of the resident's poor health condition (Hirth et al., 2003). The other option is also not very rewarding for the residents because most of them hesitate to report a valid complaint because of their debilitated health and, more importantly, their anxious nature regarding retaliation from nursing home staff. Many scholars consider consumers' complaints as the best assessment tool for the residents' quality of life and nursing home quality as a whole because, to them, regular surveys (i.e., annual recertification surveys) are carried out to maintain a uniform and persistent standard of care (Grabowski, 2005; Stevenson, 2006). Further, several factors diminish the potential effectiveness of consumer complaints (Grabowski, 2005); for instance, a more straightforward complaint-lodging system may generate more complaints in the database than in earlier years. However, complaints are considered an essential tool for improving resident care in nursing facilities. Complaint investigation renders a unique opportunity for long-term care consumers to notify regulators regarding the potential loopholes in the quality of care (Grabowski, 2005). Moreover, complaints may yield timely alerts regarding potential care-related issues because they can be lodged and investigated at any time, not only during the annual survey.

Consumer Complaints as a Measure of Quality

Nursing Home Quality data has revealed mixed results in the last few years. On the one hand, some Federal reports indicate that one of the four data sets that measure residents' quality of care in nursing homes, consumer complaints, demonstrates that residents' concerns over quality have increased. On the other hand, the other three datasets, i.e., annual recertification survey deficiencies, staffing levels, and clinical quality measures, show potential improvement in nursing homes' quality of services. Therefore, analyses of the current complaint data will assess how the complaint investigation process assists in providing essential information to the public on nursing homes'quality of services and rectifying the gaps to improve nursing home care.

Complaints, as a measure of quality in long-term care, were not very popular in earlier studies because many thought that complaints were nothing but emotional outbursts, not the most accurate reflection of the underlying issue. Stevenson was among the first to use nursing home complaints to assess the quality of nursing home care; he reported that 35% of nursing homes had no complaints, and 18% had five/more complaints during 1998–2002 (Stevenson, 2006). In another study, Hansen et al. (2019) found that 23% of nursing homes had no complaints, and 47.5% had five/more complaint allegations during 2007–2011; notably, one complaint may contain multiple allegations. A more recent study analyzing data from 2013–2017 found that about 20% of nursing homes, on average, had zero complaints annually, 38% of facilities had five/more complaints, and 55% of facilities had five/more complaint allegations in a given year (Bhattacharyya et al., 2023b); this study also revealed that 42% of nursing homes with at least one complaint received no deficiencies. In this context, research has found evidence that many substantiated complaints prioritized as immediate jeopardy (IJ) lead to no deficiencies (Bhattacharyya et al., 2024b); this study provides a possible explanation for these inconsistencies, which further points toward the possibility that the failure to investigate complaints in a timely way may lead to severe quality deficits going undetected and unremedied (Bhattacharyya et al., 2024c). The Inspector General for the U.S. Department of Health and Human Services has frequently highlighted the tendency of late investigations in some states, raising questions about states' abilities to address serious complaints (Office of Inspector General, 2020). Vital shreds of evidence can be lost when a serious complaint is not quickly investigated.

The prevalence of consumer complaints registered between 2005 and 2014 reveals an escalating trend; however, it still needs to be determined how far this affects an actual change in the quality of care due to the state variation in recording complaints (US GAO, 2015). For instance, consumers may be complaining more due to the current user-friendly complaint lodging options, which reflects higher complaints in the database compared to the earlier years. This trend, on the one hand, may explain why nursing home complaints have been increasing over time. On the other hand, the average number of deficiency citations listed per nursing facility shows a decreasing pattern; however, multiple survey types and challenges faced by the state survey agencies constitute a big concern about the validity of extracting nursing home quality measures from this data. For example, allegations without any citation indicate flaws in the current complaint process that require further investigation and improvement, including staff training. It is evident that a substantial number of complaint allegations are related to quality of care, resident abuse, and neglect (Bhattacharyya et al., 2024b). Moreover, many of them led to no deficiencies, even though they were prioritized as immediate jeopardy at intake. This inconsistency indicates the possibility of failure to investigate complaints in a timely manner may assist facilities in hiding the issue, which could lead to a deficiency. These facts further indicate why facilities with a higher proportion of residents with dementia were associated with fewer substantiated complaints and deficiency citations, although after receiving complaints from consumers. Additionally, because the facilities self-report data on staffing levels and clinical quality measures, it may further describe the possible inconsistencies in the dataset in measuring actual quality (US GAO, 2015).

Complaints can be viewed from a different perspective. The state Medicaid programs are the primary form of insurance for nursing home utilization and cover nearly half of nursing home expenditures and around two-thirds of all bed days, reimbursing nursing home costs for certain low-income individuals. That means roughly one-third of those who do not meet a certain income threshold pay out-of-pocket nursing home costs (Grabowski & Gruber, 2007). In fact, Medicare-paying residents usually stay for a shorter duration than Medicaid-paying individuals in nursing homes (Stevenson, 2006). Further, research has found that nursing homes with a higher proportion of residents with dementia had a higher proportion of Medicaid-paying residents but had a lower proportion of Medicare-paying residents. In contrast, nursing homes with a lower proportion of residents with dementia had more Medicare-paying residents (Bhattacharyya et al., 2024a), indicating that nursing homes with more short-term residents (e.g., post-surgical care) may complain more perhaps their more cognitive capability and have more family members' support and visitation with more responsiveness to quality. This discrepancy explains why nursing homes with a lower prevalence of residents with dementia are associated with higher numbers of complaints (Bhattacharyya et al., 2024a). Indeed, research revealed that the average demand for nursing home quality is still low; residents who were younger, more educated, without dementia, and who opted for long-term care after the introduction of the five-star rating system have shown higher care expectations (Cheng, 2023).

Relatedly, the ombudsmen and the state survey agency have different responsibilities, and they respond to consumer complaints in a different manner; for example, survey agencies investigate complaints, issue deficiency citations, and instruct for correction plans; in contrast, the ombudsmen investigate resident rights. Troyer and Sause (2011) analyzed the association between those two sources of complaints for North Carolina nursing homes and the roles of the ombudsman and state certification agency in receiving and assessing the complaints. They found that the substantiation rates of complaints investigated by the two agencies differed; however, both revealed that most complaints were lodged on quality of care. The researchers concluded that even though the two agencies' investigation processes differed, involving no duplication in the investigatory process, the ultimate goals emphasized the quality measure indicators (Troyer & Sause, 2011). In another study, the authors found inspection violations to be positively associated with state certification agency complaints but not with ombudsman complaints (Troyer & Sause, 2013). The results also revealed a weak or no association between ombudsman complaints and deficiencies, suggesting that the ombudsman complaint information was not duplicating the information of the state survey agency. It is suggested that CMS should consider adding information on all ombudsman complaints against nursing homes in Nursing Home Compare data in order to complement presently available nursing home quality measures (Troyer & Sause, 2013).

Although CMS has made several amendments to the nursing home oversight activities in recent years, it still needs to monitor the long-term consequences of those on nursing home quality oversight. Several new oversight activities have been added, and some existing activities have been modified or removed. CMS elucidated that most exclusion measures of oversight activities are opted in response to a recent escalation in oversight responsibilities and inadequate availability of human and financial resources; however, they have not explained how these steps might impact its ability to assess nursing home quality. In the last few years, CMS and state survey agencies have taken various measures to oversee nursing home quality. As a result, some potential improvements in nursing home quality have been evidenced in recent years, such as reduced deficiency citations. Further, improvements in specific clinical measures in nursing facilities, such as reductions in pressure ulcers, have been noticed as a measure of improved quality of care. However, it is still unclear whether this indicates a genuine improvement (US GAO, 2003). The CMS has also recently introduced federal monitoring surveys and special focus surveys (SFS) for nursing homes with a history of persistent poor performance (one survey at least every 6 months) (US GAO, 2015). Policymakers, consumers, and even academicians often criticize nursing facilities due to concerns regarding the quality of service (Harrington et al., 2001). However, as mentioned, complaints are not always the systematic evaluation of faults; often, they are emotional expressions of residents' dissatisfaction. If meticulously scrutinized, the complaints are potential predictors of nursing homes'quality of care and are often considered important resources for consumers in recognizing their health choices.

Evaluating consumer complaints is vital as the voices of individuals point out certain neglected areas of assuring the quality of care in nursing homes. Thus, assessing the current trends of nursing home complaints, their significance, and which allegations lead to deficiency citations are critical public concerns. Many complaints that are substantiated head to further investigations and potentially receive deficiency citations. Although research has found an increasing trend in consumer complaints in recent years (Bhattacharyya et al., 2023b; Liu et al., 2019), little has been performed on the rigorous examination of resident complaints. Further, one complaint may give rise to multiple allegations, which may further yield multiple deficiencies; however, none of the earlier research emphasized examining which allegation, at the intake point, leads to a specific deficiency citation. In other words, multiple allegations within a complaint create more confusion in precisely tracking the gaps in nursing home care. Thus, it is clear that the way residents' perspectives align with surveyors' findings enables researchers to understand nursing home care better.

In a complaint, tracking a specific allegation to a deficiency citation is only possible when the complaint contains only one substantiated allegation (Bhattacharyya et al., 2024b). This information is crucial for confirming that the particular nursing home is accountable for its service quality to make sure the quality of care is existing, standard, and best. Although complaint investigation divulges many happenings behind the screen, it should be uniform throughout the investigation process to maintain federal standards nationwide. In this context, people seek long-term care when their chronic conditions impair their physical and/or cognitive function. According to the CMS, in 2014, 36.6% of nursing home residents had severe cognitive impairment, 24.8% had moderate, and 38.7% had mild or no cognitive impairment (CMS, 2015). Because many nursing homes provide accommodation for a large number of residents with dementia, it is also vital to assess the relationship between the number of complaints and the proportion of residents with dementia in that facility. This knowledge is essential to evaluate what matters for residents when choosing a living option in order to maintain a good quality of life.

Many studies emphasizing residents' quality of life showed that facility-level factors, such as profit status, chain affiliation, and location, e.g., urban/rural, differentiate high- and low-quality facilities based on residents' self-reports (Kane et al., 2004). Research already demonstrated that an increase in nursing staff in facilities might directly affect residents' health outcomes and thereby be more likely to meet regulatory standards (Bowblis, 2011). CMS has already made some modifications in the Minimum Data Set (MDS) in order to obtain information on nursing home care and evaluate residents' preferences regarding quality of life in nursing facilities. Although only two states, Minnesota and Ohio, conducted care and services surveys in nursing facilities to assess quality of life, these activities were not uniform. It is already evidenced that many nursing homes with a Five-Star rating in Nursing Home Compare had very low consumer scores; in contrast, some nursing homes with a 1-star rating had very high consumer satisfaction (Williams et al., 2016). Thus, a higher score on health inspections, quality measures, and staffing patterns may speculate consumer satisfaction; however, those measures do not proxy consumer input. Discerning consumers' satisfaction is a complex issue, and therefore, consumers' self-reported satisfaction measures should be integrated into the complaint investigation process. Future research should address that direction.

However, this is only one side of the coin. Quality of life can be viewed from an individual's perspective, too. For example, unless caregivers (or the concerned institutional management) feel the urge of their responsibility, caregiving will remain, for some, a mere duty and, for others, a business. Therefore, a few more criteria need to be fulfilled. For example, considering everyone with equal respect and dignity and providing services by favorably modifying the surrounding environment safe, secure, and livable for older adults with the highest health and willingness is essential. In long-term care facilities, using various complementary and alternative approaches to provide an alternative to traditional models of care by supplementing conventional medical management (i.e., complementary) and using these techniques instead of traditional ones (i.e., alternative) are also vital. These techniques "are not promoted to cure disease. Rather, they alleviate symptoms and improve well-being and quality of life"(Takeda et al., 2012, p. 2). These include (but are not limited to) mindfulness practices like yoga, laughter therapy, animal-assisted therapy, music therapy, gardening, and so on (National Center for Complementary and

Integrative Health, 2016). Also, meaningful engagement in everyday life through social interaction and close companionship is vital for individual well-being. Relatedly, policies and payment reform are urgently needed at the state and nationwide federal levels. The goal should be to identify and improve strategies and create a sustainable model for improving the quality of life for nursing home residents living with or without dementia.

Conclusion

Because the evaluation of every resident is distinct, the care approach should be unique. According to the growing trends of person-centered care plans, which need the active participation of both care partners and the residents themselves, resident's satisfaction regarding the quality of care should be guided by the determinants of person-centered care (Liu et al., 2019; Rozenblum & Bates, 2013). Moreover, changing patterns in allegation categories is also vital. Therefore, future research should emphasize the trends of allegation types and the prevalence of complaints highlighting those allegation types to recognize changes in residents' care demands over time. In this context, resident characteristics are probably the equally important, perhaps more important, factors regarding resident satisfaction with the quality of care. Long-term care deserves growing attention in the sector of health economics, especially how regulatory oversight and resident choices in the nursing home market affect health outcomes. Although sociodemographic characteristics are routine inclusion in most research studies, unless we include residents' psychosocial factors (variables) in our analysis, we will miss a big chunk of information and continue to see discrepancies in datasets, even those coming from the same source. The quality of care and the quality of life are not synonymous in long-term care; instead, they often depend on and impact each other, and the regulatory process needs to recognize that association to provide older adult residents adding life to their later years. Therefore, our future research needs to go beyond simply analyzing administrative datasets, instead exploring their real-world applications and emphasizing the quality of individualized care provided in long-term care, especially in nursing homes. Toward that direction, we should consider several confounding factors, including internal, such as psychosocial factors, and external, such as meaningful engagement, impacting residents' quality of life in long-term care.

Acknowledgments This chapter is based on an independent study conducted during dissertation coursework at the University of South Florida. I am thankful to my dissertation committee members, including Drs. Kathryn Hyer (now deceased), Victor Molinari (now deceased), Lindsay Peterson, and Ross Andel, for their guidance.

References

Alomari, E., & Steinke, C. (2024). Quality of life in assisted living facilities for seniors: A descriptive exploratory study. *Nursing Open, 11*(3), e2084. https://doi.org/10.1002/nop2.2084

American Medical Association. (1986). Quality of care council on medical service. *JAMA, 256*, 1032–1034.

Arensberg, M. B., Gahche, J., Clapes, R., Kerr, K. W., Merkel, J., & Dwyer, J. T. (2023). Research is still limited on nutrition and quality of life among older adults. *Frontiers in Medicine, 10*, 1225689. https://doi.org/10.3389/fmed.2023.1225689

Bhattacharyya, K. K., Molinari, V., Black, K., & Whitbourne, S. K. (2023a). Creating age-friendly nursing homes: The time is now. *Gerontology & Geriatrics Education, 44*(4), 613–630. https://doi.org/10.1080/02701960.2022.2106981

Bhattacharyya, K. K., Molinari, V., & Fauth, E. B. (2023b). Trends in nursing home complaints: Prevalence and variation across Center for Medicare and Medicaid Services regions. *Journal of Applied Gerontology, 42*(7), 1600–1610. https://doi.org/10.1177/07334648231159648

Bhattacharyya, K. K., Molinari, V., & Hyer, K. (2022). Self-reported satisfaction of older adult residents in nursing homes: Development of a conceptual framework. *The Gerontologist, 62*(8), e442–e456. https://doi.org/10.1093/geront/gnab061

Bhattacharyya, K. K., Molinari, V., Peterson, L., Fauth, E. B., & Andel, R. (2024a). Do nursing homes with a higher proportion of residents with dementia have greater or fewer complaints? *Aging & Mental Health, 28*(3), 448–456. https://doi.org/10.1080/13607863.2023.2277265

Bhattacharyya, K. K., Peterson, L., Molinari, V., & Bowblis, J. R. (2024b). Consumer complaints in nursing homes: Analyzing substantiated single-allegation complaints to deficiency citations. *Journal of Aging & Social Policy, 36*(1), 174–188. https://doi.org/10.1080/08959420.2023.2297599

Bhattacharyya, K. K., Peterson, L., Molinari, V., Fauth, E. B., & Andel, R. (2024c). The importance of zero-deficiency complaints in nursing homes: A mere consequence or serious concern?. *Journal of Applied Gerontology, 43*(7), 945–955. https://doi.org/10.1177/07334648241229548

Bowblis, J. R. (2011). Staffing ratios and quality: An analysis of minimum direct care staffing requirements for nursing homes. *Health Services Research, 46*(5), 1495–1516. https://doi.org/10.1111/j.1475-6773.2011.01274.x

Bowblis, J. R., & Roberts, A. R. (2018). Cost-effective adjustments to nursing home staffing to improve quality. *Medical Care Research and Review, 77*(3), 274–284. https://doi.org/10.1177/1077558718778081

Castle, N. G. (2002). Nursing homes with persistent deficiency citations for physical restraint use. *Medical Care, 40*(10), 868–878. https://doi.org/10.1097/00005650-200210000-00005

Castle, N. G. (2008). Nursing home caregiver staffing levels and quality of care: A literature review. *Journal of Applied Gerontology, 27*(4), 375–405. https://doi.org/10.1177/0733464808321596

Castle, N. G. (2011). Nursing home deficiency citations for abuse. *Journal of Applied Gerontology, 30*, 719–743. https://doi.org/10.1177/0733464810378262

Castle, N. G., & Ferguson, J. C. (2010). What is nursing home quality and how is it measured? *The Gerontologist, 50*(4), 426–442. https://doi.org/10.1093/geront/gnq052

Castle, N. G., Wagner, L. M., Ferguson, J. C., & Handler, S. M. (2011). Nursing home deficiency citations for safety. *Journal of Aging and Social Policy, 23*(1), 34–57. https://doi.org/10.1080/08959420.2011.532011

Centers for Medicare & Medicaid Services (CMS). (2015). Nursing home data compendium 2015 edition. https://www.cms.gov/Medicare/Provider-Enrollment-andCertification/CertificationandComplianc/Downloads/nursinghomedatacompendium_508-2015.pdf.

Centers for Medicare and Medicaid Services (CMS). (2016). *Design for nursing home compare Five-Star Quality Rating System: Technical users' guide.* Retrieved from https://www.cms.gov/Medicare/Provider-Enrollment-and-Certification/CertificationandComplianc/downloads/usersguide.pdf.

Cheng, A. (2023). Demand for quality in the presence of information frictions: Evidence from the nursing home market. Available at SSRN: https://ssrn.com/abstract=4470002 or https://doi.org/10.2139/ssrn.4470002.

Donabedian, A. (1988). The quality of care: How can it be assessed? *JAMA, 260*(12), 1743–1748. https://doi.org/10.1001/jama.260.12.1743

Donabedian, A. (2005). Evaluating the quality of medical care. 1966. *The Milbank Quarterly, 83*(4), 691–729. https://doi.org/10.1111/j.1468-0009.2005.00397.x

Felce, D., & Perry, J. (1995). Quality of life: Its definition and measurement. *Research in Developmental Disabilities, 16*(1), 51–74. https://doi.org/10.1016/0891-4222(94)00028-8

Grabowski, D. C. (2005). Consumer complaints and nursing home quality. *Medical Care, 43*(2), 99–101. https://doi.org/10.1097/00005650-200502000-00002

Grabowski, D. C., & Castle, N. G. (2004). Nursing homes with persistent high and low quality. *Medical Care Research and Review, 61*(1), 89–115. https://doi.org/10.1177/1077558703260122

Grabowski, D. C., & Gruber, J. (2007). Moral hazard in nursing home use. *Journal of Health Economics, 26*(3), 560–577. https://doi.org/10.1016/j.jhealeco.2006.10.003

Grabowski, D. C., Gruber, J., & Angelelli, J. J. (2008). Nursing home quality as a common good. *The Review of Economics and Statistics, 90*(4), 754–764. https://doi.org/10.1162/rest.90.4.754

Hansen, K. E., Hyer, K., Holup, A. A., Smith, K. M., & Small, B. J. (2019). Analyses of complaints, investigations of allegations, and deficiency citations in United States. *Medical Care Research and Review, 76*(6), 736–757. https://doi.org/10.1177/1077558717744863

Harrington, C., Schnelle, J. F., McGregor, M., & Simmons, S. F. (2016). The need for higher minimum staffing standards in U.S. nursing homes. *Health Services Insights, 9*, 13–19. https://doi.org/10.4137/HSI.S38994

Harrington, C., Woolhandler, S., Mullan, J., Carrillo, H., & Himmelstein, D. U. (2001). Does investor ownership of nursing homes compromise the quality of care? *American Journal of Public Health, 91*(9), 1452–1455. https://doi.org/10.2105/ajph.91.9.1452

Heiks, C., & Sabine, N. (2022). Long term care and skilled nursing facilities. *Delaware Journal of Public Health, 8*(5), 144–149. https://doi.org/10.32481/djph.2022.12.032

Hirschman, A. O. (1970). *Exit, voice, and loyalty: Responses to decline in firms, organizations, and states*. Harvard University Press.

Hirth, R. A., Banaszak-Holl, J. C., Fries, B. E., & Turenne, M. N. (2003). Does quality influence consumer choice of nursing homes? Evidence from nursing home to nursing home transfers. *Inquiry, 40*(4), 343–361. https://doi.org/10.5034/inquiryjrnl_40.4.343

Hoben, M., Dymchuk, E., Doupe, M. B., Keefe, J., Aubrecht, K., Kelly, C., Stajduhar, K., Banerjee, S., O'Rourke, H. M., Chamberlain, S., Beeber, A., Salma, J., Jarrett, P., Arya, A., Corbett, K., Devkota, R., Ristau, M., Shrestha, S., & Estabrooks, C. A. (2024). Counting what counts: Assessing quality of life and its social determinants among nursing home residents with dementia. *BMC Geriatrics, 24*(1), 177. https://doi.org/10.1186/s12877-024-04710-1

Hua, C. L., Cornell, P. Y., Zimmerman, S., Carder, P., & Thomas, K. S. (2022). Excess mortality among assisted living residents with dementia during the COVID-19 pandemic. *Journal of the American Medical Directors Association, 23*(10), 1743–1749.e6. https://doi.org/10.1016/j.jamda.2022.07.023

Hyer, K., Thomas, K. S., Branch, L. G., Harman, J. S., Johnson, C. E., & Weech-Maldonado, R. (2011). The influence of nurse staffing levels on quality of care in nursing homes. *The Gerontologist, 51*(5), 610–616. https://doi.org/10.1093/geront/gnr050

Kalideen, L., Govender, P., van Wyk, J. M., & Kuupiel, D. (2021). Mapping evidence on standards and quality of care for older persons in long-term care facilities: A scoping review protocol. *Systematic Reviews, 10*(1), 153. https://doi.org/10.1186/s13643-021-01709-2

Kane, R. A. (2003). Definition, measurement, and correlates of quality of life in nursing homes: Toward a reasonable practice, research, and policy agenda. *The Gerontologist, 43*, 28–36. https://doi.org/10.1093/geront/43.suppl_2.28

Kane, R. L., Bershadsky, B., Kane, R. A., Degenholtz, H. H., Liu, J. J., Giles, K., & Kling, K. C. (2004). Using resident reports of quality of life to distinguish among nursing homes. *The Gerontologist, 44*(5), 624–632. https://doi.org/10.1093/geront/44.5.624

Kaskie, B., Xu, L., Taylor, S., Smith, L., Cornell, P., Zhang, W., Carder, P., & Thomas, K. (2022). Promoting quality of life and safety in assisted living: A survey of state monitoring and enforcement agents. *Medical Care Research and Review: MCRR, 79*(5), 731–737. https://doi.org/10.1177/10775587211053410

Liu, J., Hou, S., Evans, R., Xia, C., Xia, W., & Ma, J. (2019). What do patients complain about online: A systematic review and taxonomy framework based on patient centeredness. *Journal of Medical Internet Research, 21*(8), e14634. https://doi.org/10.2196/14634

Lucas, J. A., & Bowblis, J. R. (2017). CMS strategies to reduce antipsychotic drug use in nursing home patients with dementia show some progress. *Health Affairs (Project Hope), 36*(7), 1299–1308. https://doi.org/10.1377/hlthaff.2016.1439

Marjoua, Y., & Bozic, K. J. (2012). Brief history of quality movement in US healthcare. *Current Reviews in Musculoskeletal Medicine, 5*(4), 265–273. https://doi.org/10.1007/s12178-012-9137-8

McGregor, M. J., Cohen, M., Stocks-Rankin, C. R., Cox, M. B., Salomons, K., McGrail, K. M., Spencer, C., Ronald, L. A., & Schulzer, M. (2011). Complaints in for-profit, non-profit and public nursing homes in two Canadian provinces. *Open Medicine, 5*(4), e183–e192.

Molinari, V. A., Chiriboga, D. A., Branch, L. G., Schinka, J., Schonfeld, L., Kos, L., Hyer, K. (2011). Reasons for psychiatric medication prescription for new nursing home residents. *Aging & Mental Health, 15*(7), 904–912. https://doi.org/10.1080/13607863.2011.569490

National Center for Complementary and Integrative Health. (2016). *Complimentary, alternative or integrative health: What's in a name?* U.S. Department of Health and Human Services. Retrieved on December 7, 2020, from: https://nccih.nih.gov/health/integrative-health#cvsa.

National Center for Health Statistics. (2013). Long-term care services in the United States: 2013 overview. Washington, D.C.: Government Printing Office. Accessed October 2, 2023. Available from: https://www.cdc.gov/nchs/data/nsltcp/long_term_care_services_2013.pdf

National Institute on Aging. (2023). Long-term care facilities: Assisted living, nursing homes, and other residential care. Bethesda, MD. Accessed October 2, 2024. Available from: https://www.nia.nih.gov/health/assisted-living-and-nursing-homes/long-term-care-facilities-assisted-living-nursing-homes.

Office of Inspector General. (2020). States continued to fall short in meeting required timeframes for investigating nursing home complaints: 2016–2018 (OIG publication No. OEI-01-19-00421). Washington, DC: Office of the Inspector General. Retrieved from https://oig.hhs.gov/oei/reports/OEI-01-19-00421.asp.

Peterson, L. J., & Bowblis, J. R. (2023). Assessment of consumer complaint investigation scores, recertification survey scores, and overall nursing home health inspection star quality rating. *JAMA Network Open, 6*(2), e2253952. https://doi.org/10.1001/jamanetworkopen.2022.53952

Rozenblum, R., & Bates, D. W. (2013). Patient-centred healthcare, social media and the internet: The perfect storm? *BMJ Quality & Safety, 22*(3), 183–186. https://doi.org/10.1136/bmjqs-2012-001744

Shippee, T. P., Henning-Smith, C., Kane, R. L., & Lewis, T. (2015). Resident- and facility-level predictors of quality of life in long-term care. *The Gerontologist, 55*(4), 643–655. https://doi.org/10.1093/geront/gnt148

Stevenson, D. G. (2006). Nursing home consumer complaints and quality of care: A national view. *Medical Care Research and Review, 63*(3), 347–368. https://doi.org/10.1177/1077558706287043

Takeda, M., Tanaka, T., Okochi, M., & Kazui, H. (2012). Non-pharmacological intervention for dementia patients. *Psychiatry and Clinical Neurosciences, 66*(1), 1–7. https://doi.org/10.1111/j.1440-1819.2011.02304.x

Tinetti, M. E., Fried, T. R., & Boyd, C. M. (2012). Designing health care for the most common chronic condition--multimorbidity. *JAMA, 307*(23), 2493–2494. https://doi.org/10.1001/jama.2012.5265

Troyer, J. L., & Sause, W. L. (2011). Complaints against nursing homes: Comparing two sources of complaint information and predictors of complaints. *The Gerontologist, 51*(4), 516–529. https://doi.org/10.1093/geront/gnr023

Troyer, J. L., & Sause, W. (2013). Association between traditional nursing home quality measures and two sources of nursing home complaints. *Health Services Research, 48*(4), 1256–1278. https://doi.org/10.1111/1475-6773.12021

United States Government Accountability Office. (2003). *Nursing home quality: Prevalence of serious problems, while declining, reinforces importance of enhanced oversight*. Retrieved December 22, 2020, from https://www.gao.gov/new.items/d03561.pdf.

United States Government Accountability Office. (2011). *Nursing homes: More reliable data and consistent guidance would improve CMS oversight of state complaint investigations*. Retrieved December 22, 2020, from https://www.gao.gov/new.items/d11280.pdf.

United States Government Accountability Office. (2015). *Nursing home quality: CMS should continue to improve data and oversight*. Retrieved December 22, 2020, from https://www.gao.gov/assets/680/673480.pdf.

Walshe, K. (2001). Regulating U.S. nursing homes: Are we learning from experience? *Health Affairs, 20*(6), 128–144. https://doi.org/10.1377/hlthaff.20.6.128

Walshe, K., & Harrington, C. (2002). Regulation of nursing facilities in the United States: An analysis of resources and performance of state survey agencies. *The Gerontologist, 42*(4), 475–487. https://doi.org/10.1093/geront/42.4.475

Williams, A., Straker, J. K., & Applebaum, R. (2016). The nursing home five-star rating: How does it compare to resident and family views of care? *The Gerontologist, 56*(2), 234–242. https://doi.org/10.1093/geront/gnu043

Zimmerman, S., Carder, P., Schwartz, L., Silbersack, J., Temkin-Greener, H., Thomas, K. S., Ward, K., Jenkens, R., Jensen, L., Johnson, A. C., Johnson, J., Johnston, T., Kaes, L., Katz, P., Klinger, J. H., Lieblich, C., Mace, B., O'Neil, K., Pace, D. D., Scales, K., et al. (2022). The imperative to reimagine assisted living. *Journal of the American Medical Directors Association, 23*(2), 225–234. https://doi.org/10.1016/j.jamda.2021.12.004

Zimmerman, S., Stone, R., Carder, P., & Thomas, K. (2024). Does assisted living provide assistance and promote living? *Health affairs (Project Hope), 43*(5), 674–681. https://doi.org/10.1377/hlthaff.2023.00972

Chapter 3
Cognitive Decline and Polypharmacy in Long-Term Care

Mia E. Lussier and Gail B. Rattinger

Introduction

Cognitive impairment is a deficit in any of the domains of cognition, including attention, memory, planning, judgment, and language, amongst others. Cognitive decline can be short or long-term and may be a manifestation of underlying health conditions, vitamin deficiency, substance misuse, or a neurocognitive disorder as defined by the DSM-5 criteria. Notably, cognitive decline is a common and well-documented feature of the aging process. As life expectancies increase and the overall proportion of older adults increases, understanding both modifiable and non-modifiable risk factors, as well as appropriate care management and treatment strategies for cognitive impairment, is essential for providing optimal patient-centered health outcomes.

Cognitive Impairment and Associated Risk Factors

Risk factors for cognitive impairment/decline include aging, specific genetic factors, and lower education level, as well as a variety of clinical conditions, including cerebrovascular disease, stroke, diabetes, thyroid disorders, sleep disorders, depression, substance misuse, brain disorders, neurologic diseases such as Parkinson's disease and history of head injuries or traumatic brain injuries. Moreover, for the aging population, a further contributing factor for cognitive decline includes medications, often used in aging populations for the treatment of chronic conditions.

M. E. Lussier (✉) · G. B. Rattinger
School of Pharmacy and Pharmaceutical Sciences, Binghamton University, Binghamton, NY, USA
e-mail: mlussier@binghamton.edu; gratting@binghamton.edu

K. K. Bhattacharyya (ed.), *Health Promotion in Long-Term Care Facilities*,
https://doi.org/10.1007/978-3-031-91038-8_3

The single largest risk factor for cognitive decline is aging. For community-dwelling older adults, the prevalence of cognitive impairment is estimated to be approximately 22%, while in nursing home residents, the prevalence is thought to be as high as 70% (Pais et al., 2020). Common age-related cognitive changes often include disruptions to the activities or independent activities of daily living. These can include confusion about appointments, difficulty remembering names or sometimes having difficulty finding the right word or words, occasionally making mistakes with household finances, "losing" or misplacing common items, and feeling more comfortable with established ways of doing things or routines (Alzheimer's Association, 2024).

Depending on the etiology, symptoms of cognitive decline may be modified through interventions such as disease management, medication optimization, or lifestyle interventions. Improvements in cardiovascular health and metabolic control, along with diet and exercise, have been shown to improve or at least slow cognitive decline in some cases (Puri et al., 2023). Dietary modifications have been shown to have benefits, including the Mediterranean diet, DASH diet, and MIND diet (Box 3.1) (Puri et al., 2023). In cases of hypothyroidism or some vitamin B deficiencies, cognitive decline can be reversed with treatment for the thyroid disorder or the vitamin deficiency. Also, dehydration can be a source of cognitive decline, which can be reversed with proper hydration.

Box 3.1 Diet and Cognition

Traditionally, the Mediterranean diet had been known for reducing cardiovascular risk; however, the Mediterranean diet has also been shown to lower the risk of mild cognitive impairment by 25% (Fu et al., 2022). This diet emphasizes the consumption of plant-based foods and healthy fats. The Mediterranean diet encourages daily intake of fruits, vegetables, whole grains, and extra virgin olive oil while limiting the intake of red meats and sweets (high sugar content foods) to one serving per week.

The Dietary Approach to Stop Hypertension (DASH) diet is another diet focused primarily on improving cardiovascular health which is also associated with a 28% lower risk of mild cognitive impairment (van den Brink et al., 2019). The DASH diet emphasizes the consumption of fruits, vegetables, whole grains, fat-free/low-fat dairy, fish, poultry, nuts, beans, and vegetables. This diet also limits intake of high-saturated fat foods and sugar-sweetened foods and beverages.

The Mediterranean-DASH Diet Intervention for Neurodegenerative Delay (MIND) diet combined many of the components of the Mediterranean and DASH diets while also specifically incorporating brain healthy foods such as those high in folate, vitamin E, and flavonoids. This brain health specific diet was found to lower risk of developing Alzheimer's disease by 53% (van den Brink et al., 2019).

However, it is estimated that 30–50% of older adults with mild cognitive impairment will progress to some form of major cognitive disorder within 5 years (Jones et al., 2024). Of particular note, cognitive decline can also progress to Alzheimer's disease or other dementias (ADRD) including vascular dementias (Campbell et al., 2013). This occurs when the process of cognitive decline is accelerated beyond that associated with normal aging and typically follows a clinical pathway from preclinical to severe dementia (UC Irvine Institute for Memory Impairments and Neurological Disorders [UC MIND], 2024). In the preclinical phase, brain changes have begun to occur, and patients or family members may notice cognitive changes, but they are not yet identifiable by widely used cognitive testing such as the Mini-Mental State Exam (Tombaugh & McIntyre, 1992; UC MIND, 2024). Patients can progress to mild cognitive impairment (MCI), which includes more extensive cognitive changes yet remain independent in performing their basic activities of daily living (ADLs) (bathing, dressing, eating, and toileting) (UC MIND, 2024). When a patient is no longer able to perform their basic ADLs due to cognitive impairment, a patient can be diagnosed with dementia ranging from mild-to-severe (UC MIND, 2024).

Many risk factors have been identified that contribute to the progression of mild cognitive impairment to dementia. Risk factors can either be non-modifiable, such as genetics, or modifiable, such as other chronic disease states and neuropsychiatric symptoms. The major risk factors for Alzheimer's disease in those 65 years or older (late-onset dementia) are age, genetics, and a family history of Alzheimer's disease, with age being the strongest of the three risk factors (Alzheimer's Association, 2024). Researchers have identified the APOE e4 allele as the most consistent genetic predictor of dementia, with carriers of at least one e4 allele being twice as likely to progress from MCI to dementia and homozygous e4 carriers being four times as likely to progress from MCI to dementia (Campbell et al., 2013). This allele was also found to be a predictor of more rapid disease progression with a hazard ratio of 1.77. Another genetic risk factor has been found to be the clusterin T-allele, which confers a lower risk of disease progression.

Medications, Polypharmacy, and Cognition

Medication use in older adults (65 years of age and older) is highly prevalent, with nearly 90% of older adults currently taking at least one prescription medication (Kirzinger et al., 2019). The proportion of patients taking at least one medication in long-term care facilities, such as nursing homes, is higher than the proportion of community-dwelling older adults taking at least one medication (95.4% vs. 81.8%) (Simoni-Wastila et al., 2007). For those residing in long-term care facilities, the odds of having at least one potentially inappropriate medication were found to be 1.84 times higher compared to community-dwelling older adults (Lee et al., 2022). Further estimates suggest that over 1 in 4 nursing home residents are taking at least one potentially inappropriate medication in their current medication regimen (Morin et al., 2016). Medications can be considered potentially inappropriate if the risk–benefit ratio favors risk and/or safer or more effective alternatives are available (Beers et al., 1991). Two of the most commonly cited sources of identifying potentially inappropriate medications include the American Geriatric Society Beers Criteria® and the STOPP/START criteria (Box 3.2) (American Geriatrics Society, 2023; O'Mahony et al., 2023; Tian et al., 2023).

Box 3.2 Commonly Used Tools to Identify Potentially Inappropriate Medications in Older Adults

The American Geriatric Society Beers Criteria® was initially published in 1991 and includes a list of medications that are potentially inappropriate for older adults. The list is updated and published every 3 years with the most recent update in 2023. The Beer's Criteria® contains four sections on medications to avoid in certain patient populations and medications to use at low doses or avoid in patients with renal impairment. The lists of medications to avoid are categorized; list categories include the following: use in patients 65 years of age or older; use in patients with specified health conditions such as cardiovascular disease and central nervous system disorders; medications with drug–drug interactions; and medications whose harms outweigh their benefits (American Geriatrics Society, 2023).

The START (Screening Tool to Alert to Right Treatment)/STOPP (Screening Tool of Older Persons' Prescriptions) was initially published in 2008 and is used to identify not only potentially inappropriate medications in older adults but also to screen for potential gaps in prescribing (i.e., underprescribing). Currently (2024), the third iteration of the STOPP/START criteria are in use. The START criteria outlines span six system domains including the cardiovascular, respiratory, central nervous, gastrointestinal, musculoskeletal, and endocrine systems. The STOPP criteria specifically outlines criteria across 10 domains including the cardiovascular, central nervous, gastrointestinal, musculoskeletal, respiratory, urogenital, and endocrine systems as well as drugs that adversely affect fallers (patients with a prior history of falling), analgesic medications and use of duplicative drug classes (O'Mahony et al., 2023).

In addition to often being prescribed potentially inappropriate medications, residents of long-term care facilities often have medication regimens with multiple medications, largely for the treatment of multiple comorbidities. It is estimated that long-term care facility residents have, on average, more than 12 chronic health conditions, many requiring management through medication use (National Investment Center, 2022). Taking multiple medications is known as polypharmacy (Box 3.3). For long-term care residents, the mean number of medications per resident is between 3.8 and 16.6, and the median number of medications per resident is between 4 and 14 (Jokanovic et al., 2015). A positive association with polypharmacy was found in patients with higher Charlson Comorbidity Index scores (a measure of the number of health problems) and in patients receiving care from a greater number of prescribers, whereas a negative association with polypharmacy was found in patients with cognitive impairment. Interestingly, despite the medication regimens of patients with cognitive impairment being less likely to meet polypharmacy levels, polypharmacy has been found to be associated with poorer cognitive function (Yu et al., 2024).

Box 3.3 Polypharmacy
The definition of polypharmacy is variable with some researchers and clinicians using numerical definitions, descriptive definitions, or a combination of both (Masnoon et al., 2017). Most commonly, polypharmacy is defined as the use of 5 or more medications but based on a particular definition can range anywhere from 2 or more medications to more than 11 medications and some definitions also include duration of medication use.

While specific medication classes can contribute to cognitive impairment, polypharmacy is an independent risk factor for cognitive decline (Yu et al., 2024). Polypharmacy, in some situations, may be appropriate if multiple chronic conditions are being adequately treated. Unfortunately, despite the potential appropriateness of utilizing multiple medications in some situations, as the number of regularly used medications in patient treatment increases, the likelihood of drug–drug or drug–disease interactions increases, each of which can contribute to cognitive decline (Nguyen et al., 2006). This increased risk is more common amongst older adults being treated by multiple providers, particularly when coordination of care amongst the health care team is sub-optimal. In care that is poorly coordinated, a prescriber may not be aware of a patient's full medication regimen from other prescribers or a patient's complete health history and, therefore, may prescribe new medications that interact with a patient's current medications or may be treating a side effect of another (other) medication(s) or be duplicative to an already existing medication. These situations further perpetuate or potentiate polypharmacy through what is often described as a "prescribing cascade."

In particular, certain medications or medication classes (described below) are known to contribute to cognitive impairment. In older adults, the cognitive side effects of medications are more common, often due to normal age-related changes in the body's systems. For example, normal decline in renal function may cause decreased clearance of water-soluble medications. Those with chronic kidney disease and severely reduced renal function are at even higher risk of decreased medication clearance; this is why renal dose reductions are common for many medications. Notably, since renal function declines with age, long-term medications used for chronic conditions may need to be checked for dose adjustments periodically. Unfortunately, inappropriate or lack of renal dose adjustments has been found to occur in approximately 34% of nursing home residents (AlQashqri, 2023).

Additionally, changes in body-fat composition can increase the amount of lipophilic medications that are absorbed into the body (Turnheim, 2003). Further, though not as routinely documented, changes in hepatic function can impact medication effects through reduced metabolism in the body and reduced clearance from the body.

Medications/medication classes that can contribute to cognitive impairment in older adults include agents across multiple medication classes with anticholinergic properties (including diphenhydramine and other antihistamines, oxybutynin and other urinary incontinence medications, and benztropine most commonly used in Parkinson's disease), glucocorticoids, opioids, antiepileptics, dopaminergic agents, benzodiazepines, and antipsychotics. Much of the research in this space is focused on anticholinergic agents or medications that were not developed as anticholinergics yet have anticholinergic side effects due to blocking activity on acetylcholine receptors, which can cause cognitive impairment through blocking the action of acetylcholine, which is necessary for proper learning and memory (Hasselmo, 2006; Naseri et al., 2023). Many anticholinergic scales have been developed in an attempt to quantify the anticholinergic burden of individual medications and a patient's overall medication regimen (Lisibach et al., 2021). A 2021 systematic review found a 1.2-fold increased risk of all-cause dementia in patients taking anticholinergic medications (Zheng et al., 2021). Additionally, they found the relationship between anticholinergic medications and dementia to be dose-dependent. Unfortunately, despite this evidence, current estimates suggest that nearly 25% of long-term care residents use at least one medication with high anticholinergic activity (Malagaris et al., 2020).

Opioids are another medication class that can impact cognition. The mechanism by which opioids affect cognitive impairment is multifactorial and includes causing delirium, hallucinations, and sedation, affecting learning and memory, reducing the respiratory rate and thus oxygen supply to the brain, and disrupting neurotransmitters in the brain, such as gamma-aminobutyric acid (GABA). Overall, studies of the effects of opioids on cognition have been mixed, suggesting both a possible protective effect and a possible detrimental effect on cognition. There are many confounding factors that could be contributing to the impact of opioid use on cognition, such as chronic pain, depression, and disability (Pask et al., 2020; Whitlock et al., 2017). Given the possible association of opioids with reduced cognition, it is concerning to see that over 30% of long-term care patients are prescribed opioids, and half of those are prescribed opioids for long-term use (≥90 days) (Hunnicutt et al., 2018; Mehta et al., 2021).

Benzodiazepines have a variety of uses, including anxiety and seizure management, sleep, and sedation. However, they are often harmful as they can be habit-forming and, particularly in older adults, increase fall risk as well as impact cognition. Benzodiazepines can cause cognitive impairment in several domains, including visuospatial ability, speed of processing, and verbal learning. The mechanism by which benzodiazepines can cause cognitive impairment is through the release of gamma-aminobutyric acid (GABA), which slows the nervous system. Studies have shown that older adults who use benzodiazepines have significantly reduced cognitive processing speeds and that people who misuse benzodiazepines have lower Mini-Mental Status Exam scores (Liu et al., 2020). Additionally, studies have also shown that the cognitive effects of benzodiazepines can be seen for as long as 6 months after medication discontinuation (Baker et al., 2004). Despite the cognitive effects of benzodiazepines, over 10% of nursing home residents have been prescribed a short-acting benzodiazepine, and approximately 4% have been prescribed a long-acting benzodiazepine (Malagaris et al., 2022).

Antipsychotic agents are another common class of medications that can contribute to cognitive decline in older adults. Antipsychotic agents are commonly used to treat mental health and behavioral disorders, including schizophrenia. Antipsychotic agents have been shown to negatively affect cognition, including verbal learning, memory, and composite functioning, and may affect cognition through modulation of excitatory, inhibitory, and anticholinergic systems (Allott et al., 2024). The prevalence of antipsychotic use in older adults ranges from 1.36% to 2.09%, increases with age, and is more common in men. As well, nearly 50% of antipsychotic users are long-term users of these medications (Olfson et al., 2015).

Antipsychotics in Long-Term Care

Antipsychotics are often prescribed for patients residing in long-term care facilities to treat the behavioral and psychological symptoms of dementia (BPSD), which occur in nearly 90% of persons with dementia (PWD) (Cerejeira et al., 2012). These symptoms may include delusions, hallucinations, apathy, anxiety, depression, or disinhibition. BPSD can be an important reason/motivator for the movement of PWD from residing in the community to a long-term care facility (Toot et al., 2017). The practice of treating BPSD with antipsychotics has come into question, given their modest efficacy in treating dementia-related psychosis as well as their significant adverse event profile. As early as 2003, antipsychotics were given a warning for increasing the risk of cerebrovascular events (two times greater relative risk), and since that time, antipsychotics have received a black box warning for increasing mortality risk in patients with dementia (Meeks & Jeste, 2008). More recently, additional risks have been identified for patients with dementia taking antipsychotics, which include increased risk of cerebrovascular and cardiovascular events, pneumonia, fractures, and acute kidney injury (Mok et al., 2024). Given the significant imbalance in the risk–benefit profile of antipsychotic use in patients with dementia, these agents should be reserved for use in patients with severe BPSD symptoms who have failed both non-pharmacologic and alternative pharmacologic therapy (Box 3.4).

Box 3.4 Treatment of Behavioral and Psychological Symptoms of Dementia (BPSD)

Using medications to treat Behavioral and Psychological Symptoms of Dementia (BPSD) should generally be reserved for situations in which the patient with dementia is at risk of harming themselves or others. Antipsychotics have the best evidence amongst the different medication classes used to treat BPSD, yet the effect of these agents remains modest while the risks remain high. Other medication classes such as anticonvulsants and antidepressants have shown modest effects in treating BPSD, and medications to treat cognition, such as memantine and cholinesterase inhibitors, have shown no benefit for behavioral and psychological symptom management.

Best practices, therefore, recommend non-medication related strategies to treat BPSD starting with addressing all reversible causes such as dehydration, malnutrition, constipation, hearing impairment, visual impairment, and pain. Additionally, behavioral and environmental interventions have been found to be more effective and safer than medication management and include the use of structured activities, music therapy, and problem-solving as well as training and support for trained caregivers. Unfortunately, these interventions are often time and resource intensive and patients often need individualized plans—these resources are limited which has contributed to the over-use of antipsychotics compared to these other proven strategies.

Despite the known risks of using antipsychotics, their use remains prevalent in the long-term care setting. At the end of 2021, estimates from the Centers for Medicare and Medicaid Services (CMS) suggest a 14.5% risk-adjusted rate for long-term care residents using antipsychotics, with rates higher in those with dementia diagnoses compared to similar individuals without dementia (Centers for Medicare & Medicaid Services [CMS], 2022). Multiple predictors of antipsychotic medication use have been established in the literature, including patients with psychosis, delirium, anxiety or depression, posttraumatic stress disorder, wandering, and those with fewer registered nurse hours (Phillips et al., 2018; Travers et al., 2024).

Even though antipsychotic agents have moderate efficacy and a high-risk profile, long-term care staff have been found to generally have positive beliefs about the effectiveness of antipsychotics and find this class of medications to be an appropriate strategy to manage BPSD symptoms (Raza et al., 2023). Staff reported time being a major barrier to managing BPSD and antipsychotics being one strategy to address this constraint (Raza et al., 2023). Additionally, staff felt they did not have appropriate knowledge on other non-pharmacologic measures that can be used to treat BPSD symptoms (Raza et al., 2023).

Given that not all predictors of antipsychotic use are patient-specific, the ethics regarding the use of antipsychotics in long-term care residents with BPSD has come under question. The use of antipsychotics in long-term care residents is considered a chemical restraint (Robins et al., 2021), often being considered an easier solution than using appropriate non-pharmacologic therapy for the treatment of BPSD symptoms. This explains why facilities with lower staffing and fewer registered nurse hours are more likely to have residents using antipsychotics.

There may be an argument that these non-clinical uses of antipsychotics are ethically justified by citing the lesser evil justification. The lesser evil justification argues that the risks to other residents by limiting the time staff can care for these residents by caring for residents with BPSD are higher than the risk to the single resident being given an antipsychotic. However, this argument has come under scrutiny in a 2023 paper published in the *Journal of Medical Ethics,* which calls into question whether the use of antipsychotics in long-term care residents is an applicable situation under which to use the lesser evil justification (Soofi, 2023). The approach and ethical justification of using antipsychotics as a chemical constraint conflict with the idea of dementia citizenship in which persons with dementia are seen as active agents with existing rights, further providing an argument against their frequent use.

Centers for Medicare and Medicaid Services (CMS) Requirements Related to Antipsychotics

As the evidence has grown to suggest a greater risk than benefit for antipsychotic use in older adults in long-term care facilities, policymakers have stepped in to intervene. Between 2012 and 2013, the CMS initiated three strategies to improve the use of antipsychotics in long-term care facilities (Lucas & Bowblis, 2017). The first of these strategies was implemented in March 2012 with the launch of the National Partnership to Improve Dementia Care (see Fig. 3.1). This intervention focused on increasing research, obtaining buy-in, and increasing public awareness of issues regarding antipsychotic use in long-term care facilities. Four months later, in July 2012, CMS required reporting of antipsychotic use and considered this to be one of the quality measures for nursing homes. This increased transparency for potential residents when choosing long-term care facilities. Finally, in May 2013, unnecessary antipsychotic use was added as a consideration for surveyors in hopes of changing the behaviors of clinicians at long-term care facilities related to their use of antipsychotics in clinical practice (Lucas & Bowblis, 2017).

Together, these strategies were found to decrease the prevalence of antipsychotic use from 25.11% in 2009 to 22.67% in 2015, with higher reductions in facilities with a higher prevalence of patients with dementia compared to those with a lower prevalence of patients with dementia (Lucas & Bowblis, 2017). Additionally, it was found that states with higher baseline levels of antipsychotic drug use had a higher percent change (reduction) in use compared to low-use states (−2.09% vs. -1.72%).

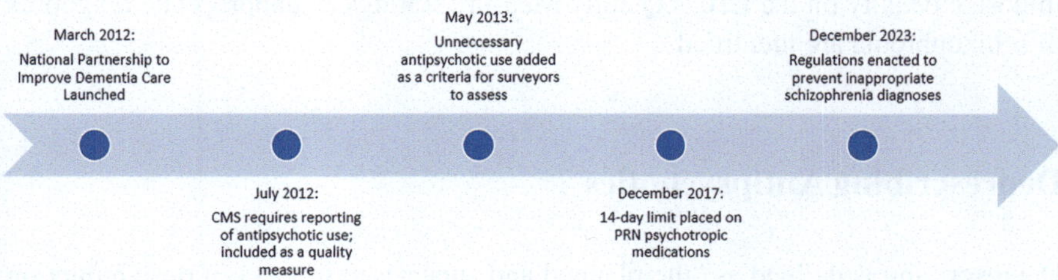

Fig. 3.1 Timeline of Centers for Medicare and Medicaid Services Regulations Related to Antipsychotics (2013–2023) (Sources: Lucas & Bowblis, 2017; CMS, 2017; CMS, 2024)

Overall, the impact of these policy changes on antipsychotic use was found to be modest, but estimates suggest this may have resulted in up to 655 saved lives per year. Unfortunately, these policies may have resulted in unintended consequences such as increasing the use rates of other psychotropic medications (i.e., anticonvulsants) and increasing the number of unsupported schizophrenia diagnoses (Grimm, 2022).

As evidence suggested that psychotropic medication use continued at a high rate, CMS passed and implemented additional regulations related to psychotropic medication use in 2017 (CMS, 2017). Included in these regulations was an expansion from including only antipsychotic psychotropic medications to include other therapeutic classes of psychotropic medications such as antidepressants, antianxiety medications, and sedative-hypnotics as these therapeutic classes all affect brain activity. A 14-day limit was also placed on all as needed (PRN) orders for psychotropic medications. This limit could only be extended if the prescriber believed extended use was appropriate, the clinical rationale was documented, and a specific duration of use was included in the updated order.

In the case of the use of antipsychotic agents, these updated regulations were even more stringent (CMS, 2017); orders could not be extended beyond the initial 14-days duration without a new order. Additionally, a new order was only allowable if the prescriber directly examined the resident and provided documentation of the clinical rationale for further use of antipsychotic medications. The clinical rationale was required to include the benefits of the medication to the resident as well as how the use of antipsychotics had improved the resident's expression, indications, or distress levels. Of note, these restrictions were not applicable to residents with diagnoses of schizophrenia, Huntington's disease, or Tourette's.

Most recently, in January 2023, CMS placed additional regulations to prevent the misuse of antipsychotics in long-term care residents by attempting to identify inaccurate schizophrenia diagnoses. Inappropriate schizophrenia reporting/diagnosing is one way to circumvent the 2017 regulations related to "as needed antipsychotic use". A study of Medicare claims linked to the Minimum Data Set (MDS) found both underreporting of antipsychotic use in facility reports compared to claims and also found an overreporting of qualifying conditions (i.e., a reported diagnosis without a claim), which ranged from 46.5% for Tourette's to 54.8% for schizophrenia to 72.4% for Huntington's disease, far exceeding expected prevalence rates (Chen & Grabowski, 2023). This 2023 regulation allows CMS to audit nursing homes and impose a penalty on the LTC's Quality Measure Ratings if inappropriate diagnoses of schizophrenia are identified.

Deprescribing Antipsychotics

Deprescribing is defined as "the planned and supervised process of dose reduction or stopping of medication that might be causing harm, or no longer be of benefit" (Canadian Medication Appropriateness and Deprescribing Network, 2024) Scott and colleagues have suggested a framework for deprescribing (Box 3.5), which is commonly referenced in the deprescribing literature (Scott et al., 2015).

Box 3.5 Deprescribing Framework

1. Ascertain all drugs patient is currently taking and the reasons/indication for each one.
2. Consider overall risk of drug-induced harm in individual patients and determine the required deprescribing interventions.
3. Assess each drug in regard to its current or future benefit potential compared with current or future harm/burden potential.
4. Prioritize drugs for discontinuation that have the lowest benefit–harm ratio and lowest likelihood of adverse withdrawal reaction or disease rebound syndromes.
5. Implement a discontinuation regimen and monitor patients closely for improvement in outcomes or onset of adverse effects.

An algorithm for deprescribing antipsychotics was created by a panel of experts (including physicians, geriatricians, and pharmacists) in October 2016, and it suggests two different deprescribing approaches based on indication (Bjerre et al., 2018). For patients using antipsychotics for insomnia, direct discontinuation is recommended, and consideration of other causes of insomnia, non-pharmacological approaches, or the use of other safer medications for insomnia is suggested. Alternatively, for patients being treated for BPSD, the recommendation is to decrease the antipsychotic dose by 25%–50% every 1–2 weeks, with monitoring occurring during this same interval for both benefits and withdrawal symptoms. Recommendations for treating relapse of BPSD include non-pharmacologic approaches, re-trialing antipsychotics at the lowest possible dose for 3 months, or considering alternative medications.

Despite the known risk of using antipsychotics in older adults and long-term care residents, there is mixed evidence for deprescribing antipsychotics in this population. A Cochrane systematic review from 2013 looked to evaluate the effects of deprescribing antipsychotics on successful withdrawal and the impact on neuropsychiatric symptoms in patients with Alzheimer's dementia. Overall, it was determined that discontinuation was possible without negative consequences on behavioral symptoms; however, they were unable to assess the effects on cognition. They noted that many of the trials included were underpowered to detect any clinically meaningful difference(s) in outcomes.

More recently, a multi-center study occurring from April 2014 to October 2016 across 23 nursing homes found no improvement in BPSD symptoms for patients who were deprescribed antipsychotics, suggesting that discontinuing antipsychotics does not worsen the BPSD symptoms which they are being used to treat (Brodaty et al., 2018). There was also no change in adverse effects such as falls and hospitalizations or on cognition, which may suggest that deprescribing antipsychotics as an intervention for long-term care patients does not have the intended positive effects that would be anticipated. Additionally, the study found that 19% of participants were re-prescribed an antipsychotic or were never able to completely discontinue their antipsychotic, suggesting that deprescribing interventions may only result in short-term changes in antipsychotic use. Other studies evaluating the deprescribing of antipsychotics are ongoing (Benthien et al., 2023).

Conclusion

As the population of older adults increases due to longer life expectancy, there is an increasing prevalence of age-related cognitive decline, including Alzheimer's disease and related dementias. Multiple risk factors for these cognition-related disorders exist, including both non-modifiable and modifiable risk factors. One such modifiable risk factor is medication use. Older adults in long-term care facilities are at increased risk of polypharmacy and inappropriate medication use, including the use of antipsychotic medications, which has a risk–benefit imbalance that leans toward increased risk. Due to this and the rising use of antipsychotics in long-term care, the CMS has enacted multiple policies from 2012 to 2023 to address antipsychotic use, which have seen modest levels of success. Algorithms to help deprescribe antipsychotics have been published, but the evidence related to deprescribing these medications is mixed, and a beneficial effect of deprescribing on cognition has yet to be established. However, many current studies in this area are underpowered to find a clinically meaningful difference, and additional high-quality research is needed in this area.

References

Allott, K., Chopra, S., Rogers, J., Dauvermann, M. R., & Clark, S. R. (2024). Advancing understanding of the mechanisms of antipsychotic-associated cognitive impairment to minimise harm: A call to action. *Molecular Psychiatry, 29*(8), 2571–2574. https://doi.org/10.1038/s41380-024-02503-x

AlQashqri, H. (2023). Renally inappropriate medications in the old population: Prevalence, risk factors, adverse outcomes, and potential interventions. *Cureus, 15*(11), e49111. https://doi.org/10.7759/cureus.49111

Alzheimer's Association. (2024). Alzheimer's disease facts and figures. *Alzheimer's & dementia: the journal of the Alzheimer's Association, 20*(5), 3708–3821. https://doi.org/10.1002/alz.13809

American Geriatrics Society. (2023). By the 2023 American Geriatrics Society Beers Criteria® Update Expert Panel. American Geriatrics Society 2023 updated AGS Beers Criteria® for potentially inappropriate medication use in older adults. *Journal of the American Geriatrics Society, 71*(7), 2052–2081. https://doi.org/10.1111/jgs.18372

Barker, M. J., Greenwood, K. M., Jackson, M., & Crowe, S. F. (2004). Persistence of cognitive effects after withdrawal from long-term benzodiazepine use: A meta-analysis. *Archives of Clinical Neuropsychology, 19*(3), 437–454. https://doi.org/10.1016/S0887-6177(03)00096-9

Beers, M. H., Ouslander, J. G., Rollingher, I., Reuben, D. B., Brooks, J., & Beck, J. C. (1991). Explicit criteria for determining inappropriate medication use in nursing home residents. UCLA division of geriatric medicine. *Archives of Internal Medicine, 151*(9), 1825–1832.

Benthien, K. S., Lech, L. V. J., Birke, H., Jørgensen, S. M., Andersen, T., Hansen, S. V., Andersen, J. T., Karstoft, K., Schiøtz, M., & Vermehren, C. (2023). Protocol for DEprescribing and care to reduce antipsychotics in dementia (DECADE)-a hybrid effectiveness-implementation pilot study. *PLoS One, 18*(11), e0294024. https://doi.org/10.1371/journal.pone.0294024

Bjerre, L. M., Farrell, B., Hogel, M., Graham, L., Lemay, G., McCarthy, L., Raman-Wilms, L., Rojas-Fernandez, C., Sinha, S., Thompson, W., Welch, V., & Wiens, A. (2018). Deprescribing antipsychotics for behavioural and psychological symptoms of dementia and insomnia: Evidence-based clinical practice guideline. *Canadian family physician Medecin de famille canadien, 64*(1), 17–27.

Brodaty, H., Aerts, L., Harrison, F., Jessop, T., Cations, M., Chenoweth, L., Shell, A., Popovic, G. C., Heffernan, M., Hilmer, S., Sachdev, P. S., & Draper, B. (2018). Antipsychotic deprescription for older adults in long-term care: The HALT study. *Journal of the American Medical Directors Association, 19*(7), 592–600.e7. https://doi.org/10.1016/j.jamda.2018.05.002

Campbell, N. L., Unverzagt, F., LaMantia, M. A., Khan, B. A., & Boustani, M. A. (2013). Risk factors for the progression of mild cognitive impairment to dementia. *Clinics in Geriatric Medicine, 29*(4), 873–893. https://doi.org/10.1016/j.cger.2013.07.009

Canadian Medication Appropriateness and Deprescribing Network. (2024). *What is deprescribing?* Accessed October 2023 from https://deprescribing.org/what-is-deprescribing/.

Centers for Medicare & Medicaid Services [CMS]. (2017). Revision to State Operations Manual (SOM) appendix PP for phase 2, F-tag revision and related issues, Section F757. Accessed October 2023 from https://www.cms.gov/medicare/provider-enrollment-and-certification/surveycertificationgeninfo/policy-and-memos-to-states-and-regions-items/survey-and-cert-letter-17-36.

Centers for Medicare & Medicaid Services [CMS]. (2022). National Partnership to Improve Dementia Care in Nursing Homes: Antipsychotic Medication Use Data Report (April 2022). Accessed October 2023 from https://www.cms.gov/files/document/antipsychotic-medication-use-data-report-2021q4-updated-07292022.pdf

Centers for Medicare & Medicaid Services [CMS]. (2024). Revised long-term care (LTC) surveyor guidance: Significant revisions to enhance quality and oversight of the LTC survey process. Assessed on March 8, 2025, from: https://www.cms.gov/files/document/revised-long-term-care-ltc-surveyor-guidance-significant-revisions-enhance-quality-and-oversight-ltc.pdf.

Cerejeira, J., Lagarto, L., & Mukaetova-Ladinska, E. B. (2012). Behavioral and psychological symptoms of dementia. *Frontiers in Neurology, 3*, 73. https://doi.org/10.3389/fneur.2012.00073

Chen, A. C., & Grabowski, D. C. (2023). Nursing homes underreport antipsychotic use but Overreport diagnoses qualifying for appropriate use. *Health Affairs Scholar, 1*(2), qxad022. https://doi.org/10.1093/haschl/qxad022

Fu, J., Tan, L. J., Lee, J. E., & Shin, S. (2022). Association between the mediterranean diet and cognitive health among healthy adults: A systematic review and meta-analysis. *Frontiers in Nutrition, 9*, 946361. https://doi.org/10.3389/fnut.2022.946361

Grimm, C. A. (2022). *Long-Term Trends of Psychotropic Drug use in Nursing Homes*. Accessed October 2023 from https://oig.hhs.gov/reports/all/2022/long-term-trends-of-psychotropic-drug-use-in-nursing-homes/.

Hasselmo, M. E. (2006). The role of acetylcholine in learning and memory. *Current Opinion in Neurobiology, 16*(6), 710–715. https://doi.org/10.1016/j.conb.2006.09.002

Hunnicutt, J. N., Chrysanthopoulou, S. A., Ulbricht, C. M., Hume, A. L., Tjia, J., & Lapane, K. L. (2018). Prevalence of long-term opioid use in long-stay nursing home residents. *Journal of the American Geriatrics Society, 66*(1), 48–55. https://doi.org/10.1111/jgs.15080

Jokanovic, N., Tan, E. C., Dooley, M. J., Kirkpatrick, C. M., & Bell, J. S. (2015). Prevalence and factors associated with polypharmacy in long-term care facilities: A systematic review. *Journal of the American Medical Directors Association, 16*(6), 535.e1–535.12. https://doi.org/10.1016/j.jamda.2015.03.003

Jones, A., Ali, M. U., Kenny, M., Mayhew, A., Mokashi, V., He, H., Lin, S., Yavari, E., Paik, K., Subramanian, D., Dydynsky, R., Aryal, K., Correia, R. H., Dash, D., Manis, D. R., O'Connell, M., Liu-Ambrose, T., Taler, V., McMillan, J. M., Hogan, D. B., et al. (2024). Potentially modifiable risk factors for dementia and mild cognitive impairment: An umbrella review and meta-analysis. *Dementia and Geriatric Cognitive Disorders, 53*(2), 91–106. https://doi.org/10.1159/000536643

Kirzinger, A., Neuman, T., Cubanski, J., & Brodie, M. (2019). Data note: prescription drugs and older adults. Accessed October 9, 2023 from https://www.kff.org/affordable-care-act/issue-brief/data-note-prescription-drugs-and-older-adults/.

Lee, Y., Jang, S., Kang, H. J., & Jang, S. (2022). Comparative analysis of potentially inappropriate medication use in long-term care facility residents and community-dwelling elders: A matched cohort study. *Medicine, 101*(49), e31739. https://doi.org/10.1097/MD.0000000000031739

Lisibach, A., Benelli, V., Ceppi, M. G., Waldner-Knogler, K., Csajka, C., & Lutters, M. (2021). Quality of anticholinergic burden scales and their impact on clinical outcomes: A systematic review. *European Journal of Clinical Pharmacology, 77*(2), 147–162. https://doi.org/10.1007/s00228-020-02994-x

Liu, L., Jia, L., Jian, P., Zhou, Y., Zhou, J., Wu, F., & Tang, Y. (2020). The effects of benzodiazepine use and abuse on cognition in the elders: A systematic review and meta-analysis of comparative studies. *Frontiers in Psychiatry, 11*, 00755. https://doi.org/10.3389/fpsyt.2020.00755

Lucas, J. A., & Bowblis, J. R. (2017). CMS strategies to reduce antipsychotic drug use in nursing home patients with dementia show some progress. *Health Affairs (Project Hope), 36*(7), 1299–1308. https://doi.org/10.1377/hlthaff.2016.1439

Malagaris, I., Mehta, H. B., & Goodwin, J. S. (2022). Trends and variation in benzodiazepine use in nursing homes in the USA. *European Journal of Clinical Pharmacology, 78*(3), 489–496. https://doi.org/10.1007/s00228-021-03244-4

Malagaris, I., Mehta, H. B., Li, S., & Goodwin, J. S. (2020). Decrease of anticholinergic drug use in nursing home residents in the United States, 2009 to 2017. *Journal of the American Geriatrics Society, 68*(12), 2797–2804. https://doi.org/10.1111/jgs.16776

Masnoon, N., Shakib, S., Kalisch-Ellett, L., & Caughey, G. E. (2017). What is polypharmacy? A systematic review of definitions. *BMC Geriatrics, 17*(1), 230. https://doi.org/10.1186/s12877-017-0621-2

Meeks, T. W., & Jeste, D. V. (2008). Beyond the black box: What is the role for antipsychotics in dementia? *Current Psychiatry, 7*(6), 50–65.

Mehta, H. B., Kuo, Y. F., Raji, M. A., Westra, J., Boyd, C., Alexander, G. C., & Goodwin, J. S. (2021). State variation in chronic opioid use in long-term care nursing home residents. *Journal of the American Medical Directors Association, 22*(12), 2593–2599.e4. https://doi.org/10.1016/j.jamda.2021.04.016

Mok, P. L. H., Carr, M. J., Guthrie, B., Morales, D. R., Sheikh, A., Elliott, R. A., Camacho, E. M., van Staa, T., Avery, A. J., & Ashcroft, D. M. (2024). Multiple adverse outcomes associated with antipsychotic use in people with dementia: Population based matched cohort study. *BMJ (Clinical Research Ed.), 385*, e076268. https://doi.org/10.1136/bmj-2023-076268

Morin, L., Laroche, M. L., Texier, G., & Johnell, K. (2016). Prevalence of potentially inappropriate medication use in older adults living in nursing homes: A systematic review. *Journal of the American Medical Directors Association, 17*(9), 862.e1–862.e8629. https://doi.org/10.1016/j.jamda.2016.06.011

Naseri, A., Sadigh-Eteghad, S., Seyedi-Sahebari, S., Hosseini, M. S., Hajebrahimi, S., & Salehi-Pourmehr, H. (2023). Cognitive effects of individual anticholinergic drugs: A systematic review and meta-analysis. *Dementia & Neuropsychologia, 17*, e20220053. https://doi.org/10.1590/1980-5764-DN-2022-0053

National Investment Center. (2022). Understanding the health need and spending of senior housing residents. NORC at the University of Chicago. Accessed October 2023 from https://www.nic.org/blog/understanding-the-healthcare-needs-and-spending-of-senior-housing-and-nursing-home-residents/.

Nguyen, J. K., Fouts, M. M., Kotabe, S. E., & Lo, E. (2006). Polypharmacy as a risk factor for adverse drug reactions in geriatric nursing home residents. *The American Journal of Geriatric Pharmacotherapy, 4*(1), 36–41. https://doi.org/10.1016/j.amjopharm.2006.03.002

O'Mahony, D., Cherubini, A., Guiteras, A. R., Denkinger, M., Beuscart, J. B., Onder, G., Gudmundsson, A., Cruz-Jentoft, A. J., Knol, W., Bahat, G., van der Velde, N., Petrovic, M., & Curtin, D. (2023). STOPP/START criteria for potentially inappropriate prescribing in older people: Version 3. *European Geriatric Medicine, 14*(4), 625–632. https://doi.org/10.1007/s41999-023-00777-y

Olfson, M., King, M., & Schoenbaum, M. (2015). Antipsychotic treatment of adults in the United States. *The Journal of Clinical Psychiatry, 76*(10), 1346–1353. https://doi.org/10.4088/JCP.15m09863

Pais, R., Ruano, L., Carvalho, P., & O., & Barros, H. (2020). Global cognitive impairment prevalence and incidence in community dwelling older adults-a systematic review. *Geriatrics (Basel, Switzerland), 5*(4), 84. https://doi.org/10.3390/geriatrics5040084

Pask, S., Dell'Olio, M., Murtagh, F. E. M., & Boland, J. W. (2020). The effects of opioids on cognition in older adults with cancer and chronic noncancer pain: A systematic review. *Journal of Pain and Symptom Management, 59*(4), 871–893.e1. https://doi.org/10.1016/j.jpainsymman.2019.10.022

Phillips, L. J., Birtley, N. M., Petroski, G. F., Siem, C., & Rantz, M. (2018). An observational study of antipsychotic medication use among long-stay nursing home residents without qualifying diagnoses. *Journal of Psychiatric and Mental Health Nursing, 25*(8), 463–474. https://doi.org/10.1111/jpm.12488

Puri, S., Shaheen, M., & Grover, B. (2023). Nutrition and cognitive health: A life course approach. *Frontiers in Public Health, 11*, 1023907. https://doi.org/10.3389/fpubh.2023.1023907

Raza, A., Piekarz, H., Jawad, S., Langran, T., & Donyai, P. (2023). A systematic review of quantitative studies exploring staff views on antipsychotic use in residents with dementia in care homes. *International Journal of Clinical Pharmacy, 45*(5), 1050–1061. https://doi.org/10.1007/s11096-023-01645-2

Robins, L. M., Lee, D. A., Bell, J. S., Srikanth, V., Möhler, R., Hill, K. D., & Haines, T. P. (2021). Definition and measurement of physical and chemical restraint in long-term care: A systematic review. *International Journal of Environmental Research and Public Health, 18*(7), 3639. https://doi.org/10.3390/ijerph18073639

Scott, I. A., Hilmer, S. N., Reeve, E., Potter, K., Le Couteur, D., Rigby, D., Gnjidic, D., Del Mar, C. B., Roughead, E. E., Page, A., Jansen, J., & Martin, J. H. (2015). Reducing inappropriate polypharmacy: The process of deprescribing. *JAMA Internal Medicine, 175*(5), 827–834. https://doi.org/10.1001/jamainternmed.2015.0324

Simoni-Wastila, L., Shaffer, T., & Stuart, B. (2007). A national comparison of prescription drug expenditures by Medicare beneficiaries living in the community and long-term care facility settings. Accessed October 2023 from https://aspe.hhs.gov/sites/default/files/migrated_legacy_files//42411/pdnatcom.pdf.

Soofi, H. (2023). Non-clinical uses of antipsychotics in resource-constrained long-term care facilities: Ethically justifiable as lesser of two evils? *Journal of Medical Ethics, 49*(10), 694–698. https://doi.org/10.1136/jme-2022-108639

Tian, F., Chen, Z., Zeng, Y., Feng, Q., & Chen, X. (2023). Prevalence of use of potentially inappropriate medications among older adults worldwide: A systematic review and meta-analysis. *JAMA Network Open, 6*(8), e2326910. https://doi.org/10.1001/jamanetworkopen.2023.26910

Tombaugh, T. N., & McIntyre, N. J. (1992). The mini-mental state examination: A comprehensive review. *Journal of the American Geriatrics Society, 40*(9), 922–935. https://doi.org/10.1111/j.1532-5415.1992.tb01992.x

Toot, S., Swinson, T., Devine, M., Challis, D., & Orrell, M. (2017). Causes of nursing home placement for older people with dementia: A systematic review and meta-analysis. *International Psychogeriatrics, 29*(2), 195–208. https://doi.org/10.1017/S1041610216001654

Travers, J. L., Hade, E. M., Friedman, S., Raval, A., Hadson, K., & Falvey, J. R. (2024). Staffing and antipsychotic medication use in nursing homes and neighborhood deprivation. *JAMA Network Open, 7*(4), e248322. https://doi.org/10.1001/jamanetworkopen.2024.8322

Turnheim, K. (2003). When drug therapy gets old: Pharmacokinetics and pharmacodynamics in the elderly. *Experimental Gerontology, 38*(8), 843–853. https://doi.org/10.1016/s0531-5565(03)00133-5

van den Brink, A. C., Brouwer-Brolsma, E. M., Berendsen, A. A. M., & van de Rest, O. (2019). The Mediterranean, dietary approaches to stop hypertension (DASH), and Mediterranean-DASH intervention for neurodegenerative delay (MIND) diets are associated with less cognitive decline and a lower risk of Alzheimer's disease-a review. *Advances in Nutrition (Bethesda, MD), 10*(6), 1040–1065. https://doi.org/10.1093/advances/nmz054

UC Irvine Institute for Memory Impairments and Neurological Disorders. (2024). *Mild cognitive impairment*. Accessed October 2024 from https://mind.uci.edu/dementia/mild-cognitive-impairment/

Whitlock, E. L., Diaz-Ramirez, L. G., Glymour, M. M., Boscardin, W. J., Covinsky, K. E., & Smith, A. K. (2017). Association between persistent pain and memory decline and dementia in a longitudinal cohort of elders. *JAMA Internal Medicine, 177*(8), 1146–1153. https://doi.org/10.1001/jamainternmed.2017.1622

Yu, X., Qian, Y., Zhang, Y., Chen, Y., & Wang, M. (2024). Association between polypharmacy and cognitive impairment in older adults: A systematic review and meta-analysis. Geriatric Nursing, 59, 330–337. https://doi.org/10.1016/j.gerinurse.2024.07.005.

Zheng, Y. B., Shi, L., Zhu, X. M., Bao, Y. P., Bai, L. J., Li, J. Q., Liu, J. J., Han, Y., Shi, J., & Lu, L. (2021). Anticholinergic drugs and the risk of dementia: A systematic review and meta-analysis. *Neuroscience and Biobehavioral Reviews, 127*, 296–306. https://doi.org/10.1016/j.neubiorev.2021.04.031

Chapter 4
Dementia Citizenship in Mitigating Global Challenges of Polypharmacy in Long-Term Care

Panagiota Tragantzopoulou and Vaitsa Giannouli

Introduction

Cognitive ability refers to the skills required for tasks involving perception, learning, memory, reasoning, language, and other mental functions (Tragantzopoulou & Giannouli, 2024). As people age, they become more vulnerable to cognitive decline, which can range from mild impairment to more severe conditions like dementia (Pais et al., 2020). Cognitive decline is a leading factor for admission into nursing homes, resulting in a growing number of older adults residing in these facilities. The increasing number of elderly individuals presents a major challenge for healthcare systems, particularly due to the rise of age-related conditions (Carvalho et al., 2014). Notably, as life expectancy increases, so does the prevalence of multiple health conditions, leading to the need for more medications. However, with an increase in the number of medications comes a higher likelihood of drug–drug and drug–disease interactions, along with a greater risk of adverse effects (Gallagher & O'Mahony, 2008). The number of medications prescribed to older adults is steadily rising, and prescribing for this population is becoming more complicated. Research among old people with dementia indicates that 18.8% of acute hospital admissions are linked to adverse drug reactions (Gustafsson et al., 2016). Given the increasing complexity of healthcare for older adults, implementing effective strategies to manage polypharmacy is essential in reducing the risks associated with multiple medications and improving the overall quality of care in long-term care settings. This chapter will focus on the challenges of polypharmacy in long-term care, with a

P. Tragantzopoulou
School of Social Sciences, University of Westminster, London, UK
e-mail: g.tragantzopoulou@westminster.ac.uk

V. Giannouli (✉)
School of Medicine, Aristotle University of Thessaloniki, Thessaloniki, Greece
e-mail: giannouli.vaitsa@ac.eap.gr

K. K. Bhattacharyya (ed.), *Health Promotion in Long-Term Care Facilities*,
https://doi.org/10.1007/978-3-031-91038-8_4

particular emphasis on older individuals and the increasing prevalence of cognitive decline. It will examine how cognitive impairment exacerbates the complexity of medication management, contributing to adverse drug reactions and hospital admissions. Furthermore, the chapter will explore strategies and interventions, including multidisciplinary approaches, to mitigate the risks of polypharmacy and improve medication management for elderly individuals in long-term care settings.

Impact of Polypharmacy on the Quality of Life of Long-Term Care Residents

Many long-term care settings are struggling to keep up with the demands of aging populations and the rising incidence of dementia. It has been acknowledged globally that these systems have significant weaknesses, including concerns about the misuse of medications (Harrison et al., 2020; Jokanovic et al., 2016). This issue is not isolated to specific regions, as healthcare systems worldwide face similar challenges in managing polypharmacy and ensuring appropriate medication use, particularly in residential care settings. Polypharmacy is widespread in residential care settings, where the use of potentially inappropriate medications (PIMs) is also common and may be associated with the length of nursing home stay (Sönnerstam et al., 2022). A study analyzing medication prescribing patterns in 720 residents of residential aged care facilities (RACFs) found that cognitively intact residents were prescribed significantly more medications than those with cognitive impairments (Shafiee Hanjani et al., 2021). While 82% of all residents received at least one anticholinergic or sedative medication, and 26.9% were exposed to PIMs, there were no significant differences across cognitive groups in their use of these drugs (Shafiee Hanjani et al., 2021). This raises important ethical questions about whether such practices truly prioritize the well-being of residents or whether they reflect systemic inefficiencies, including understaffing and lack of proper training.

Psychotropic drugs are frequently prescribed to individuals with dementia, particularly soon after they enter a care facility, a period of transition and adaptation to the facility that may involve challenges in adjusting to the new environment (Toot et al., 2017). These medications are sometimes used to manage challenging behaviors associated with dementia, such as hallucinations or agitation. While this practice may appear to address immediate behavioral concerns or multiple comorbidities, it often bypasses the opportunity to explore non-pharmacological interventions that could be equally or more effective in the long term. The risk of inappropriate polypharmacy is particularly high in individuals with cognitive impairment or dementia, as they may experience greater sensitivity to the adverse reactions of medications when compared to those with normal cognitive function (Reeve et al., 2017). However, given the significant risks, including drug interaction, frailty, strokes, and mortality, guidelines recommend that antipsychotics be used for a limited time, with non-drug approaches like behavioral therapies being preferred (Gutiérrez-Valencia et al., 2018; Tampi et al., 2016). The continued high rates of psychotropic prescriptions, despite these known risks and guidelines, suggest that barriers to change remain deeply entrenched in aged care practices. Whether these barriers stem from cultural norms within care facilities, financial incentives, or the need for more robust regulatory oversight is worth questioning.

The Movement to Reduce Antipsychotic Use in Long-Term Care

The growing concern over the excessive use of medications in long-term care settings has prompted various initiatives aimed to reduce inappropriate prescribing practices, improve patient outcomes, and enhance the quality of care. These initiatives reflect a global recognition of the need to address polypharmacy and improve medication management in aging populations, with healthcare systems around the world dealing with similar challenges related to prescribing practices and medication safety. Tamura et al. (2011) investigated the effects of a geriatrician-led intervention on polypharmacy in a long-term care facility, focusing on 74 residents prescribed nine or more medications. Geriatric medicine fellows and faculty reviewed medication regimens, identifying high-risk drugs using the Beers Criteria and potential drug–drug interactions. They recommended whether to continue, taper, or discontinue medications, which were discussed with the residents' primary care physicians (PCPs) for final decisions. A subsequent chart review confirmed the implementation of these recommendations. The intervention resulted in significant reductions in the average number of total medications (from 16.64 to 15.54), as well as decreases in scheduled, PRN, high-risk, contraindicated medications, and those with potential drug interactions or lacking indications. These findings underscore the effectiveness of systematic medication reviews in mitigating polypharmacy in nursing homes and highlight the intervention's dual role as a training tool for geriatric medicine fellows.

Based on the Beers Criteria, a nurse-led intervention was implemented in Switzerland, aiming to reduce inappropriate medication (IM) prescriptions in a nursing home setting (Blozik et al., 2010). The intervention involved four key components. First, the Beers Criteria were adapted to the Swiss context by removing unavailable or essential medications without alternatives. Second, an IM identification system was implemented, where nursing staff compared residents' medication lists to a tailored IM list and were notified of any inappropriate prescriptions. Third, a discontinuation process was established, with nursing staff recommending discontinuation to prescribing physicians during ward rounds and providing follow-up reminders if no action was taken. Lastly, one-hour training sessions were conducted for nursing leaders and staff to ensure proper implementation of the IM identification and discontinuation processes. This collaborative approach showed a significant reduction in IM prescriptions, decreasing from 14.5% pre-intervention to 2.8%

post-intervention. Although there was a non-significant increase at the 1-year follow-up, the intervention was considered feasible and effective, highlighting the role of nursing staff in managing medication in long-term care.

In an additional study aimed at enhancing the appropriateness of drug prescribing in nursing homes, a targeted educational intervention was implemented for both physicians and residents across 20 nursing homes in Belgrade, Serbia (Ilic et al., 2015). This intervention comprised structured lectures and accompanying brochures focused on the pharmacokinetics and pharmacodynamics of medications in older adult residents, as well as the utilization of established prescribing criteria such as Beers, START, and STOPP. The results demonstrated a significant reduction in inappropriate prescriptions, with the number of drugs deemed unsuitable according to the Beers Criteria decreasing from 349 to 37 and those classified by the STOPP criteria dropping from 70 to 20. Additionally, there was a notable improvement in the omission of necessary medications, highlighting the effectiveness of the educational initiative in optimizing pharmacotherapy for older adults in nursing care settings.

Furthermore, an intervention was implemented using a multidisciplinary team (MDT) approach to optimize medication use among 422 residents in 20 care homes, with pharmacists conducting detailed medication reviews and presenting findings to care home nurses and general practitioners (Campbell et al., 2015). The team assessed the necessity and appropriateness of each medication while ensuring residents were consulted about their treatment preferences. As a result, 1346 interventions were made, leading to the discontinuation of 704 medications in 298 residents, averaging 1.7 medications stopped per resident and achieving a 17.4% reduction in prescribed medications. The primary reasons for stopping medications included lack of current indication, safety concerns, and resident preferences. The initiative was safe, with only nine minor adverse events reported, and resulted in substantial savings of approximately €99,340, or €235 per resident reviewed. By minimizing exposure to unnecessary or harmful medications, individuals are less likely to experience adverse effects, which can also lead to direct cost savings for the healthcare system.

The Sicherheit der Medikamentherapie bei AltenheimbewohnerInnen, Safety of medication therapy in NHRs (SiMbA study), conducted between 2016 and 2018 in Austrian nursing homes, aimed to improve medication appropriateness through an interprofessional intervention involving general practitioners, nurses, and pharmacists (Dellinger et al., 2020). The intervention included a comprehensive three-step educational program, integration of a Health Information Technology (HIT) tool for better communication and data access, and a structured therapy check process. Participants underwent both online and face-to-face training, and a mobile-enabled HIT tool facilitated access to patient records and medication monitoring. Results showed that the intervention group experienced a significant reduction in Medication Appropriateness Index (MAI) scores, with a mean change of −3.35 points compared to −1.45 in the control group, indicating improved medication appropriateness. Notably, among participants with higher baseline MAI scores (≥23), the intervention group saw a mean reduction of −10.31 points, suggesting that the intervention was particularly effective for those most at risk of inappropriate medication use. Despite overall differences in baseline characteristics, such as age and comorbidity, the intervention's structured approach and collaborative framework yielded promising results in optimizing medication therapy for nursing home residents.

The studies reviewed illustrate that engaging multidisciplinary teams—including pharmacists, nurses, and general practitioners—can significantly improve prescribing practices and enhance patient outcomes. These global efforts highlight the importance of collaborative, systematic approaches in addressing medication management challenges in long-term care settings. Each intervention demonstrates a consistent trend toward reducing inappropriate medications while prioritizing the safety and preferences of residents. However, while the results are promising, ongoing challenges remain in sustaining these improvements over time, particularly with the observed non-significant increases in inappropriate medication prescriptions at follow-up. Therefore, it is essential to continue advocating for education, training, and ongoing evaluation of prescribing practices to ensure that the momentum generated by these initiatives leads to long-lasting changes in medication management for vulnerable populations in nursing homes.

The Concept of "Dementia Citizenship" and Future Directions

Historically, and even in recent times, dementia has often been conceptualized through a deficit-oriented biomedical framework, which emphasizes deficiencies and defines individuals primarily by neurocognitive decline and other negative terms (O'Connor et al., 2022). However, this reductionist view overlooks the concept of personhood, reducing individuals to their diagnosis and presumed incapacity without acknowledging them as whole persons in their social environments. It fails to account for their personal interactions and relationships, thereby perpetuating the stigma and discrimination placed on them due to the narrow focus on cognitive impairment. In response to the limitations of the deficit-oriented framework, Bartlett & O'Connor (2007) introduced the term social citizenship, advocating for a more socio-political approach to understanding dementia. They define social citizenship as the rights and status that should be afforded to individuals with dementia, ensuring they are free from discrimination and given opportunities to actively participate in society (Bartlett & O'Connor, 2007). This concept emphasizes that people with dementia should not only be treated with justice and recognition of their personal worth but also have their rights respected. Additionally, they should have some degree of responsibility and agency in shaping decisions at both personal and societal levels. The framework of social citizenship provides a foundation for advancing research and practice in dementia care, shifting the focus toward rights-based approaches and social inclusion. It moves beyond viewing dementia solely through a medical lens, addressing broader issues of justice, dignity, and participation in the lives of individuals with dementia.

In countries across Europe, such as Italy, Spain, and France, polypharmacy rates are alarmingly high, particularly among those with multiple chronic conditions, which is common in dementia patients (Bennie et al., 2024). The variation in polypharmacy management strategies between European countries, compounded by differences in healthcare systems, reimbursement policies, and prescribing practices, underscores the need for a unified, rights-based approach to medication management. As we move forward in addressing the issue of polypharmacy in long-term care, it is essential to adopt an integrated approach that combines ethical considerations, policy reforms, and the principles of dementia citizenship. Future strategies should prioritize the creation of comprehensive guidelines that not only advocate for the reduction of unnecessary medications but also promote the inclusion of individuals with cognitive decline and their families in discussions about their care and treatment options. This shift emphasizes the importance of respecting individuals' rights and recognizing their personhood, ensuring that they are active participants in their healthcare decisions (Goossens et al., 2019). Ethical implications arise when considering the balance between necessary medical interventions and the autonomy of residents, particularly in terms of informed consent and shared decision-making (Varkey, 2021). Policies should support the training of healthcare providers in person-centered care practices, emphasizing the value of communication and collaboration with patients and their families. Furthermore, fostering a culture of dementia citizenship entails advocating for systemic changes that reduce stigma and discrimination, empowering individuals with dementia to reclaim their agency and engage meaningfully in their communities. By addressing these ethical and policy dimensions, we can create a supportive environment that not only mitigates the risks associated with polypharmacy but also honors the dignity and rights of those living with dementia.

Conclusion

This chapter explored the critical issue of polypharmacy in long-term care settings, particularly in the context of aging populations and increasing rates of cognitive impairment. We discussed how cognitive decline contributes to the complexity of medication management, leading to a higher prevalence of inappropriate prescribing practices that can result in adverse drug reactions and hospital admissions. The chapter highlighted various interventions aimed at reducing polypharmacy, including multidisciplinary approaches that involve pharmacists, nurses, and general practitioners. These initiatives demonstrated promising results in optimizing medication use and improving patient outcomes while underscoring the importance of addressing systemic inefficiencies within long-term care facilities. As we look to the future, it is essential to continue advocating for innovative strategies that prioritize the principles of dementia citizenship. This involves shifting the focus from a deficit-oriented biomedical model to a rights-based approach that recognizes individuals with dementia as active participants in their care. By fostering a culture of inclusion and support, we can mitigate the risks associated with polypharmacy and enhance the overall quality of care for vulnerable populations in long-term care settings. Moving forward, collaborative efforts must be sustained to ensure that the lessons learned from successful interventions lead to lasting changes in medication management and the treatment of individuals with cognitive decline.

References

Bartlett, R., & O'Connor, D. (2007). From personhood to citizenship: Broadening the lens for dementia practice and research. *Journal of Aging Studies, 21*(2), 107–118. https://doi.org/10.1016/j.jaging.2006.09.002

Bennie, M., Santa-Ana-Tellez, Y., Galistiani, G. F., Trehony, J., Despres, J., Jouaville, L. S., Poluzzi, E., Morin, L., Schubert, I., MacBride-Stewart, S., Elseviers, M., Nasuti, P., & Taxis, K. (2024). The prevalence of polypharmacy in older Europeans: A multi-national database study of general practitioner prescribing. *British Journal of Clinical Pharmacology, 90*(9), 2124–2136. https://doi.org/10.1111/bcp.16113

Blozik, E., Born, A. M., Stuck, A. E., Benninger, U., Gillmann, G., & Clough-Gorr, K. M. (2010). Reduction of inappropriate medications among older nursing-home residents: A nurse-led, pre/post-design, intervention study. *Drugs & Aging, 27*(12), 1009–1017. https://doi.org/10.2165/11584770-000000000-00000

Campbell, D., Baqir, W., Barrett, S., Desai, N., Hughes, J., Copeland, R., Laverty, A., & Mackintosh, J. (2015). CP-008 a clinico-ethical framework for multidisciplinary medicines review in nursing homes: A health foundation shine project. *European Journal of Hospital Pharmacy. Science and Practice, 22*(Suppl 1), A3–A4. https://doi.org/10.1136/ejhpharm-2015-000639.8

Carvalho, A., Rea, I. M., Parimon, T., & Cusack, B. J. (2014). Physical activity and cognitive function in individuals over 60 years of age: A systematic review. *Clinical Interventions in Aging, 9*, 661–682. https://doi.org/10.2147/cia.s55520

Dellinger, J. K., Pitzer, S., Schaffler-Schaden, D., Schreier, M. M., Fährmann, L. S., Hempel, G., Likar, R., Osterbrink, J., & Flamm, M. (2020). Improving medication appropriateness in nursing homes via structured interprofessional medication-review supported by health information technology: A non-randomized controlled study. *BMC Geriatrics, 20*(1), 506–506. https://doi.org/10.1186/s12877-020-01895-z

Gallagher, P., & O'Mahony, D. (2008). STOPP (screening tool of older persons' potentially inappropriate prescriptions): Application to acutely ill elderly patients and comparison with beers' criteria. *Age and Ageing, 37*(6), 673–679. https://doi.org/10.1093/ageing/afn197

Goossens, B., Sevenants, A., Declercq, A., & Van Audenhove, C. (2019). "We DECide optimized"—training nursing home staff in shared decision-making skills for advance care planning conversations in dementia care: Protocol of a pretest-posttest cluster randomized trial. *BMC Geriatrics, 19*(1), 33–33. https://doi.org/10.1186/s12877-019-1044-z

Gustafsson, M., Sjölander, M., Pfister, B., Jonsson, J., Schneede, J., & Lövheim, H. (2016). Drug-related hospital admissions among old people with dementia. *European Journal of Clinical Pharmacology, 72*(9), 1143–1153. https://doi.org/10.1007/s00228-016-2084-3

Gutiérrez-Valencia, M., Izquierdo, M., Cesari, M., Casas-Herrero, Á., Inzitari, M., & Martínez-Velilla, N. (2018). The relationship between frailty and polypharmacy in older people: A systematic review. *British Journal of Clinical Pharmacology, 84*(7), 1432–1444. https://doi.org/10.1111/bcp.13590

Harrison, S. L., Sluggett, J. K., Lang, C., Whitehead, C., Crotty, M., Corlis, M., Wesselingh, S. L., & Inacio, M. C. (2020). The dispensing of psychotropic medicines to older people before and after they enter residential aged care. *Medical Journal of Australia, 212*(7), 309–313. https://doi.org/10.5694/mja2.50501

Ilic, D., Bukumiric, Z., & Jankovic, S. (2015). Impact of educational intervention on prescribing inappropriate medication to elderly nursing homes residents. *Srpski Arhiv za Celokupno Lekarstvo, 143*(3–4), 174–179. https://doi.org/10.2298/SARH1504174I

Jokanovic, N., Tan, E. C. K., Dooley, M. J., Kirkpatrick, C. M., Elliott, R. A., & Bell, J. S. (2016). Why is polypharmacy increasing in aged care facilities? The views of Australian health care professionals. *Journal of Evaluation in Clinical Practice, 22*(5), 677–682. https://doi.org/10.1111/jep.12514

O'Connor, D., Sakamoto, M., Seetharaman, K., Chaudhury, H., & Phinney, A. (2022). Conceptualizing citizenship in dementia: A scoping review of the literature. *Dementia, 21*(7), 2310–2350. https://doi.org/10.1177/14713012221111014

Pais, R., Ruano, L., Moreira, C., Carvalho, O. P., & Barros, H. (2020). Prevalence and incidence of cognitive impairment in an elder Portuguese population (65-85 years old). *BMC Geriatrics, 20*(1), 470–410. https://doi.org/10.1186/s12877-020-01863-7

Reeve, E., Trenaman, S., Rockwood, K., & Hilmer, S. (2017). Pharmacokinetic and pharmacodynamic alterations in older people with dementia. *Expert Opinion on Drug Metabolism & Toxicology, 13*(6), 651–668. https://doi.org/10.1080/17425255.2017.1325873

Shafiee Hanjani, L., Hubbard, R. E., Freeman, C. R., Gray, L. C., Scott, I. A., & Peel, N. M. (2021). Medication use and cognitive impairment among residents of aged care facilities. *Internal Medicine Journal, 51*(4), 520–532. https://doi.org/10.1111/imj.14804

Sönnerstam, E., Gustafsson, M., & Lövheim, H. (2022). Potentially inappropriate medications in relation to length of nursing home stay among older adults. *BMC Geriatrics, 22*(1), 70–70. https://doi.org/10.1186/s12877-021-02639-3

Tampi, R. R., Tampi, D. J., Balachandran, S., & Srinivasan, S. (2016). Antipsychotic use in dementia: A systematic review of benefits and risks from meta-analyses. *Therapeutic Advances in Chronic Disease, 7*(5), 229–245. https://doi.org/10.1177/2040622316658463

Tamura, B. K., Bell, C. L., Lubimir, K., Iwasaki, W. N., Ziegler, L. A., & Masaki, K. H. (2011). Physician intervention for medication reduction in a nursing home: The polypharmacy outcomes project. *Journal of the American Medical Directors Association, 12*(5), 326–330. https://doi.org/10.1016/j.jamda.2010.08.013

Toot, S., Swinson, T., Devine, M., Challis, D., & Orrell, M. (2017). Causes of nursing home placement for older people with dementia: A systematic review and meta-analysis. *International Psychogeriatrics, 29*(2), 195–208. https://doi.org/10.1017/S1041610216001654

Tragantzopoulou, P., & Giannouli, V. (2024). Spatial orientation assessment in the elderly: A comprehensive review of current tests. *Brain Sciences, 14*(9), 898. https://doi.org/10.3390/brainsci14090898

Varkey, B. (2021). Principles of clinical ethics and their application to practice. *Medical Principles and Practice, 30*(1), 17–28. https://doi.org/10.1159/000509119

Chapter 5
Health Promotion in Long-Term Care Services and Supports: Increasing the Numbers and Extending the Capacity of Direct Care Workers

Alfred Boakye and Jennifer Craft Morgan

The World Health Organization encourages health systems to be modified to ensure affordable access to evidence-based medical care to meet older adults' healthcare needs. Most older adults want to age in place in the community but need constellations of paid and unpaid care to manage such a feat. Aging in place and maintaining or improving one's health require instrumental and affective support of and access to health promotion supports such as rehabilitative services, exercise, high-quality food, and social support. The essential role of direct care workers in helping older adults across long-term care services and supports (LTSS) in practicing various health promotional activities is already evidenced. In order for direct care workers to support health promotion, systemic issues related to staffing, recruitment, retention, workload, consistent assignment, and career advancement need to be put in place. Recruitment, retention, and training of individuals in staff roles are vital to providing good quality care to residents. Services and support organizations have been experiencing widespread shortages and instability in the direct care workforce and this issue was exacerbated by the COVID-19 pandemic. This chapter will discuss the current outlook and how increasing the number, capacity (e.g., through technologies), and the availability of direct care workers to support high-quality person-centered care which includes health promotion, meaningful engagement, and person-directed activities is vital.

A. Boakye (✉)
Division of Gerontology, School of Medicine, University of Maryland, Baltimore, MD, USA
e-mail: Alfred.boakye@som.umaryland.edu

J. C. Morgan
Jennifer Craft Morgan, Gerontology Institute, Georgia State University, Atlanta, GA, USA
e-mail: jmorgan39@gsu.edu

K. K. Bhattacharyya (ed.), *Health Promotion in Long-Term Care Facilities*,
https://doi.org/10.1007/978-3-031-91038-8_5

The Direct Care Workforce Outlook

By 2034, the number of older adults will outnumber people under age 18 (U.S. Census Bureau, 2022). This societal shift has social and economic policy implications for the USA, older adults, families, and paid and unpaid caregivers. The population of adults aged 65 and older is projected to increase from 57.8 million to 88.8 million between 2022 and 2060 (Paraprofessional Health Institute (PHI), 2024). Older adults and people with disabilities will need a growing number of care partners, which include a growing number of paid direct care workers across long-term care services and supports. Approximately five million direct care workers, up from 3.5 million workers in 2014, provide care to older adults and people with disabilities in various long-term care settings: residential care homes, home care, assisted living communities, and nursing homes (U.S. Bureau of Labor Statistics, 2024). Between 2022 and 2032, about 860,000 new jobs are expected to be added to the direct care workforce compared to any single profession nationwide (U.S. Bureau of Labor Statistics, 2023). The term "direct care worker" usually includes workers in the following Bureau of Labor Statistical (BLS) occupational categories: home health aides, nursing assistants, and personal care aides. Personal and home care/health aides work in private homes, assisted living communities, and residential care homes, and nursing assistants work in nursing homes and also in hospitals (PHI, 2024). Although their occupation titles vary from state to state, direct care workers provide care and support to older adults and people with disabilities who find it difficult to manage their activities of daily living (including bathing, dressing, and grooming) and instrumental activities of daily living (including grocery shopping, medication management, and food preparation). The direct care workforce is disproportionally Black, Indigenous, and People of Color (BIPOC), women, and immigrants who have some form of education and experience occupational inequalities while providing care. A total of 58% work in home care settings making up the highest proportion of the direct care workforce. Direct care workers in other sectors, such as hospitals, comprise 20% of the direct care workforce, 13% in residential care settings, and 9% in nursing homes (BLS Occupational Employment and Wage Statistics (OEWS), 2024). About 84% and 16% of home care workers are females and males, respectively. With a median age of 47, about 67% of home care workers are people of color. Thirty-two percent of home care workers are immigrants, 34% have at least one child under 18, about 29% provide unpaid care to an older adult family member, and 46% have attained at least a high school degree. Home care aides have an annual median income of $21,889, 12% do not have health insurance, 40% live in low-income households, and 58% rely on some form of public assistance (BLS OEWS, 2024; PHI, 2024; Ruggles et al., 2024).

Similar to home care aides, residential care aides are predominantly women (84%), have a median age of 40 years, are predominately people of color (61%), are often immigrants (24%), and have at least one child under 18 years (34%). A total of 31% of residential care aides provide unpaid care to an older adult family member. More than 50% of residential care aides have attained at least a high school degree, receive some form of public assistance (45%), earn an annual median income of $28,142 (slightly above home care aides), and about 51% who receive health insurance through their employer or union (BLS OEWS, 2024; Flood et al., 2023; PHI, 2024; Ruggles et al., 2024).

The demographics of nursing assistants generally mirror that of home care and residential care aides. Although nursing assistants make up the lowest percentage of the direct care workforce (9%), most are women (89%). The median age is 39, and nursing assistants constitute 59% of all nursing home staff. Twenty-one percent of nursing assistants are immigrants, 18% care for an older adult family, have at least one child under age 18 (36%), and have attained a high school degree (44%). While 74% work full-time, 89% have some form of health insurance through their employer, union, or spouse, receive a median annual income of $29,185, and rely on some form of assistance from the government (39%) (BLS OEWS, 2024; Centers for Medicare & Medicaid Services (CMS), 2024; PHI, 2024; Ruggles et al., 2024).

The quality of the work combined with the multiple social vulnerabilities of workers poses physical and emotional risks to direct care workers compared to other health and non-healthcare settings (Stone, 2010; Kelly et al., 2020). Direct care workers strive to provide care to older adults, those with a disability, and those living with dementia and derive high intrinsic rewards from developing meaningful relationships with clients/residents and "giving back" to older adults and people with disabilities (Morgan et al., 2013). Direct care workers face workplace challenges that impede their ability to provide optimal levels of care. Most of these challenges include but are not limited to heavy workloads, low compensation, limited training and career opportunities, no paid time off, and stifled staff-supervisor relationships. These challenges are discussed in detail in the next section of this chapter. Figure 5.1 provides a comprehensive summary of the profile of direct care workers across long-term care settings in the United States. All the data are displayed in percentages for easy comprehension.

Challenges and the Impact of the COVID-19 Pandemic

Direct care workers form the backbone of the long-term care system in the USA and continue to face challenges threatening their health, well-being, quality of life, and the overall quality of care provided to care recipients. The long-standing shortage of direct care workers has impacted millions of older adults, limiting access to quality healthcare (Harootunian et al., 2023). The challenges include but are not limited to job demands (which often include heavy workloads, low or uncertain staffing), emotional and physical demands, economic (low wages, little to no paid time off, and few benefits), very limited career opportunities (no training and upward mobility opportunities), and work environment (unsafe working conditions such as physical injury). Adding to the demanding and stressful nature of the care work, these workers are often underappreciated or unrecognized. In providing care, direct care workers feel alienated. At the same time, they offer comprehensive physical and

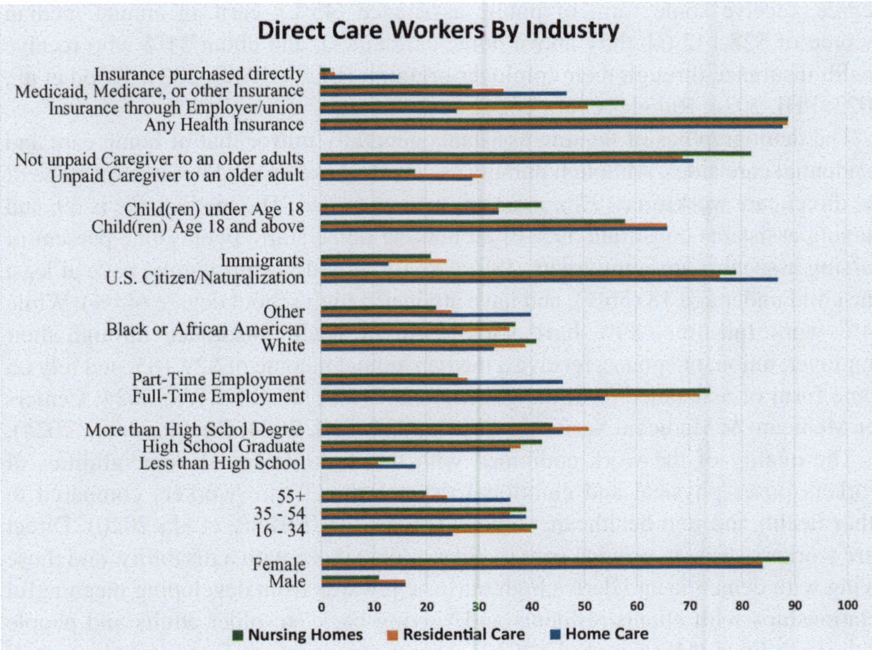

Fig. 5.1 Percentages of combined data sources on the demographic profiles of direct care workers by industry. Note: All data (2022) except unpaid family caregiving status was pooled by Ruggles et al. (2024). Unpaid family caregiving status (2021) was pooled by Flood et al. (2023). All the data presented here were analyzed by PHI (June 2023; 2024)

emotional care to residents and clients who may be living with dementia or other chronic health conditions. Care workers are tasked to juggle the constraints and mundane nature of the job, which go unrecognized and often unappreciated. In return, they occasionally receive various forms of abuse, such as physically resisting care, constant screaming, physical violence, and even aggression (Hilton et al., 2021; Rodrigues et al., 2020).

The relationship between workplace challenges and turnover has been substantially documented by researchers across different settings (see Kelly et al., 2020; Scales & Lepore, 2020). Nursing homes have reported the highest turnover rates (over 90%) and 65% for home care workers (Gandhi et al., 2020; Holly, 2021). Adding to the shortage and turnover rates, over 25% of referred patients have been turned away by home healthcare providers, and 44% of nursing homes have limited new resident admissions (Harootunian et al., 2023). As the USA experiences a demographic shift by 2050, the number of older adults will increase. The change in demography underscores the prevalence of workplace disparities for direct care workers and profound implications for those who benefit from the services of these workers. In the face of these challenges, several organizations, interest groups, and the government have engaged in collaborative initiatives to improve recruitment, training, professional development, and retention and explore frameworks or models to grow the direct care workforce. An example is a recent report from the White House where the Biden-Harris administration has taken steps to strengthen the work of the direct care workforce by partnering with states to find the best ways to support direct care workers to increase access to high-quality care (U.S. Department of Health and Human Services, 2024). This partnership is spearheaded by the Association of Community Living (ACL) in collaboration with the U.S. Department of Health and Human Services and twenty (20) other states to improve recruitment, retention, and development of the direct care workforce.

One of the world's major public health emergencies was the Coronavirus disease 2019 (COVID-19) and its impact on healthcare systems worldwide (Fukuti et al., 2020)). Long-term care challenges were exacerbated during the COVID-19 pandemic and continue to pose an extra layer of vulnerability among direct care workers compared to other jobs (Morgan et al., 2023; Shen et al., 2022; White et al., 2021). Compared to other countries, the United States lost between 40% and 60% of direct care workers during COVID-19. For example, in 2020, an estimated 420,000 nursing home workers left the workforce, and two-thirds of states closed at least one Medicaid home and community-based service (HCBS) provider, limiting access to care resources (National Conference of State Legislatures 2023). Relational care, which was supposed to be a reward for caregiving, turned into emotional exhaustion during COVID-19, which provided little choice and autonomy between workers, residents, and resident's families, a catalyst for person-centered care implementation (Bhattacharyya et al., 2022). Direct care workers were tasked to provide additional services mainly out of their job descriptions, either in nursing homes, assisted living communities, or private homes. Workers had to cope with feelings of hopelessness and uncertainties amid work overload and role conflicts, leading to increased rates of burnout, much higher than in other healthcare settings (Boamah et al., 2022; Mo & Shi, 2020; White et al., 2021). The fear of infection and infecting household members of direct care workers was of great concern. This created mixed emotional effects, anxiety, depression, and emotional exhaustion exacerbated by COVID-19.

Other Organization for Economic Co-operation and Development (OECD) countries, such as Canada, have also reported increasing staff shortages within their long-term care sector. Like the USA, Canada has experienced several challenges before, during, and after the COVID-19 pandemic. These include high absenteeism, increased overtime hours, poor technology, high stress and mental health problems, depressive symptoms, and panic attacks, which were exacerbated during COVID-19 (Langins et al., 2020; Clarke, 2021).

The mismatch between the demands of care work and the rewards of care has created consequences that ripple across and undermine the effectiveness of the long-term care system. The implications of this mismatch does not affect direct care workers alone but also the access of older adults and people with disabilities to the care and support they require to maximize health promotion and quality of life. Another implication of this mismatch is that it increases recruitment and training costs, strains long-term care employers' already limited healthcare budgets, and shifts the burden on unpaid family caregivers. As we expand on performance and care outcomes connected with direct care workers' demographic profiles and challenges, the authors will share some best practices, including the benefits of incorporating technology in long-term care settings.

Incorporating Technology into Direct Care Work

The emergence and expansion of technology in various settings have received considerable attention. Long-term care settings have been included in their utilization, although significant barriers such as awareness, access, and technology adoption seem prevalent. Whether in the home, assisted living community, or nursing home, residents and direct care workers have shown optimism for adopting technology to help navigate physical, cognitive, and social challenges (Chapman et al., 2023). Technology has been found to support older adults in accessing health care and communication and improving social engagement and mobility (Task Force on Research and Development for Technology to Support Aging Adults, 2019). Due to the increase in dementia and disability, the high demand for specialized care, and the shortage of direct care workers, technology is more than a valuable tool with the potential to support the aging population. While evidence supports the use of technology among older adults (see Tak et al., 2010), that is not the focus of this discussion. This chapter explores the impact of technological advances among direct care workers as a mitigating strategy for the workforce shortage and care demands and how these technologies can improve work efficiency. We will also draw on a global strategy for using technology to enhance work outcomes, workers' quality of life, and the quality of care for residents. The hope here is to increase the capacity of direct care workers without replacing the valuable connections between older adults and their care partners and while increasing the time available for person-centered care. We intend to provide evidence on how technology can strengthen the direct care workforce through innovation and improve the care experience for the direct care workers and those they care for.

Electronic health records (EHRs), sensors, and assistive technologies such as robots to prevent falls and transfer patients to reduce strain on care workers have been extensively documented. For example, by activating sensors or robotics, care workers can transfer residents from one bed to another, to and from a chair, or move from one place to another. In more sophisticated nursing homes, sensors attached to resident beds send signals to the nurse's station anytime a resident falls out of bed. Other technologies installed in the lighting systems provide residents' health information in real-time. Electronic health records offer a one-stop shop for a patient's medical history, usually maintained over time by a care provider. This tool helps to automate and streamline workflow and enables direct care workers to access patient information to provide evidence-based decision support and report outcomes (Kruse et al., 2017). In the home, assisted living, or nursing home, care staff can easily access health information to make decisions and provide more person-centered care to their care recipients. They can integrate the medical history and care needs into organizing, administering, reporting, and evaluating care interventions. EHRs are accessible through mobile phones, computers, and personal digital assistants (PDAs), which store and send information to care partners. Aside from reducing strain, using technology among direct care workers can save time and costs for physical and emotional injuries, enhance collaboration and communication, improve the quality of care outcomes through monitoring and management, and enhance the effectiveness and efficiency of care workers. We focus on three countries that have adopted different forms of technology to support the direct care workforce—Japan, Denmark, and Sweden.

Japan has invested several billions of dollars (excess of $300 million) in research and development of emerging technologies over the past two decades to improve the care trajectories of older adults (Wright, 2023). The investment in research and development has translated into building devices such as care robots to monitor physical activities and grooming, lift older people if they cannot do that themselves, and efficiently manage residents living with dementia. For example, in nursing homes such as Nerima Garden in Tokyo, caregivers, through their smartphones, can monitor residents to know when they are sleeping, awake, or moving. Retirement homes managed by Hitowa Care Services have installed sensors under resident beds to report when they are in bed, report their heartbeat, and send data to the nursing station. Any unusual data triggers an alarm signal for the staff to run to the aid of the resident. This saves the staff time to focus on other care needs beyond the machine's ability (Kolling, 2022). With support from policymakers, Japanese robotics companies believe that robots are the answer to the workforce shortage and an answer to relieve care burdens on workers, which led to the publication of a book by Nakayama (2006) titled "Robots Will Save *Japan.*" However, this has received reactions from researchers such as Wright (2023), who, through his work *"Robots Won't Save Japan—An Ethnography of Eldercare Automation,"* reveals the likely transformation of ethics, meaning, and practices of caregiving to undermine human relationships which are pivotal to cultivating good care.

Denmark has built technologies to innovate health and assistive care. With an increasing number of older adults, estimated to be about 300,000 by 2050, a shortage of 14,500 care workers is expected by 2035. Mette Kierkgaard and Sophie Løhde, who serve as the Minister for Senior Citizens and Minister for the Interior and Health, respectively, (at the time of writing this chapter) have pointed out the benefits of incorporating technology into Denmark's healthcare system to support direct care workers. This includes improved quality of life and freedom, optimized work conditions for care workers, optimized resource allocation, personalized treatments, access to care, and enhanced diagnostic precision to transform and alleviate strain on the healthcare system. Healthcare Denmark, a public–private partnership for promoting expertise and innovation in Danish healthcare and life science, has shared a comprehensive report on the utilization of assistive technology in the Danish healthcare system (Health Care Denmark, 2023). An example is how AI-based sensors have been utilized to streamline tasks, boost care, document medical history, and analyze patients' sleep–wake cycles. The AI-based technology platform converts visual data into figures for staff use through computer vision. The technology platform alleviates staff burden and burnout so they can focus on patient care and improve patient-quality health outcomes. Another example is the adoption of virtual visits in-home care in the Viborg municipality in the Central Denmark region. Virtual visits offers alternatives to traditional home visits (more useful post-COVID to reduce infection) while maintaining the importance of human interactions through complimented visits. In 2020, 32% of nursing homes and 30% of private homes incorporated virtual visits. As of 2022, virtual visits had doubled (60% in nursing homes and 52% in home care) (Momentum, 2023).

Similar to Japan and Denmark, Sweden integrates technology in care settings to provide meaningful support to older adults. The integration revolves around a complex socio-technical system. Despite advances in technology, care staff are still mandated to invest considerable time in routinized activities such as documentation and following up on daily activities (Persson et al., 2023). Known as "welfare technology," Sweden has incorporated technologies such as social alarms, door sensors, robot pets, and video communication for three reasons. One, to promote self-reliant and independent living among older adults and people with disability; two, to strengthen the work of long-term care staff; and finally, to respond to the workforce shortages in various care settings. These technologies enhance the privacy and safety of older adults while promoting person-centered and person-directed care among care workers. For example, social alarms are wearable devices connected to an alarm button that send signals in the form of beeps to a receiver. In nursing and private home settings, care workers who wear these social alarms are just a button away when residents require immediate care. Due to the increased need for the security and safety of older people, Sweden has high expectations of welfare technologies and are clearly described in e-health policies (Nilsson et al., 2022). Following the population aging trajectories of Japan and Denmark, Sweden has invented robots such as Evondos to support the administration of medications; Bestic, to aid eating; Hybrid Assistive Limb, an exoskeleton that supports physical capabilities; Poseidon, a robot to aid showers; and JustoCat, a robot that supports persons with dementia. These welfare technologies are intended to reduce the workload of care workers. Despite the acceptance and use of modern technologies in care settings, its expansion has been rather slow due to financial challenges, ethical issues, the lack of technical know-how of users, and the fear of taking away the jobs of care workers (Johansson-Pajala & Gustafsson, 2020).

Conclusion

Direct care workers face many work-related challenges and also experience multiple layers of vulnerabilities due to their social position. In order to improve recruitment, retention, training, and job quality, policy and industry efforts need to address the multiple challenges that direct care workers face. These efforts must raise job quality and improve career advancement and professionalization in order to improve the trajectory of these vital workers. One of these multiple strategies includes how to increase the capacity of direct care workers and unpaid care partners as they support older adults and people with disabilities. Technology has the potential to increase the capacity of care partners so that older adults and people with disabilities can have person-centered care that helps to maximize quality of life and meaningful engagement. Older adults and people with disabilities need instrumental and affective support to engage successfully in health promotion activities. Aging in place and maintaining or improving health for today's older adults and people with disabilities are reliant on both an increased number and improved capacity of both direct care workers and unpaid family/friend care partners. Systemic changes are critically needed to improve access to and support of these key players in LTSS.

References

Bhattacharyya, K. K., Morgan, J. C., & Burgess, E. O. (2022). Person-centered care in nursing homes: Potential of complementary and alternative approaches and their challenges. *Journal of Applied Gerontology, 41*(3), 817–825.

Boamah, S. A., Weldrick, R., Havaei, F., Irshad, A., & Hutchinson, A. (2022). Experiences of healthcare workers in long-term care during COVID-19: A scoping review. *Journal of Applied Gerontology, 42*(5), 118–1136.

Centers for Medicare & Medicaid Services. (2024). Medicaid Program; Ensuring Access to Medicaid Services. Federal Register, 89 Fed. Reg. 40542 (May 10, 2024). https://www.federalregister.gov/documents/2024/05/10/2024-08363/medicaid-program-ensuring-access-to-medicaid-services.

Chapman, S. A., Miller, J. R., & Spetz, J. (2023). Emerging health technologies in long-term care and suppliers' views on their potential to assist and support the workforce. *Medical Care Research and Review, 80*(6), 619–630.

Clarke, J. (2021). Impacts of the COVID-19 pandemic in nursing and residential care facilities in Canada [research report]. https://www.150.statcan.gc.ca/n1/pub/45-28-0001/2021001/article/00025-eng.htm.

Flood, S. M., Miriam, K., Renae, R., Steven, R. J., Warren, R., & Westberry, M. (2023). Current Population Survey, 2022. IPUMS USA: Version 9.0. https://doi.org/10.18128/D030.V10.0; analysis by PHI (June 2023).

Fukuti, P., Uchôa, C. L. M., Mazzoco, M. F., Corchs, F., Kamitsuji, C. S., Rossi, L., Rios, I. C., Lancman, S., Bonfa, E., Barros-Filho, T. E. P., & Miguel, E. C. (2020). How institutions can protect the mental health and psychosocial well-being of their healthcare workers in the current COVID-19 pandemic. *Clinics (São Paulo, Brazil), 3*(75), 1963.

Gandhi, A., Yu, H., & Grabowski, D. C. (2020). High nursing staff turnover in nursing homes offers important quality information. *Health Affairs, 40*(3), 384.

Harootunian, L., Perry, K., Buffett, A., Serafini, M. W., O'Gara, B., & Hoagland, G. W. (2023). Addressing the direct care workforce shortage: A bipartisan call to action. Health Report. Bipartisan Policy Center.

Healthcare Denmark. (2023). Innovating health and assistive care in Denmark. A publication in the Triple-I paper series: Denmark Informs—Inspires—Invites. Editors: Ida Hvitved, Signe Dilling-Larsen, and Ari Vigur Hansen. November 2023.

Hilton, N. Z., Ham, E., Rodrigues, N. C., Kirsh, B., Chapovalov, O., & Seto, M. C. (2021). Contribution of critical events and chronic stressors to PTSD symptoms among psychiatric workers. *Psychiatric Services, 71*(3), 221–227. https://doi.org/10.1176/appi.ps.201900226

Holly, R. (2021). Home health care news. May 19, 2021. https://homehealthcarenews.com/2021/05/a-huge-victory-home-care-turnover-remains-stable-at-65-2/, "'A Huge Victory': Home Care Turnover Remains Stable at 65.2%," As of April 22, 2022.

Johansson-Pajala, R. M., & Gustafsson, C. (2020). Significant challenges when introducing care robots in Swedish elder care. *Disability and Rehabilitation: Assistive Technology, 17*(2), 166–176. https://doi.org/10.1080/17483107.2020.1773549

Kelly, C., Morgan, J. C., Kemp, C., & Deichert, J. (2020). A profile of the assisted living direct care workforce in the United States. *Journal of Applied Gerontology, 39*(1), 16–27.

Kolling, M. (2022). When rooms take care of their inhabitants: How Japan is countering the aging of its population with technology. The Neue Zurcher Zeitung. Retrieved from https://www.nzz.ch/english/how-japan-is-using-technology-to-care-for-its-aging-population-ld.1713444.

Kruse, C. S., Mileski, M., Vijaykumar, A. G., Viswanathan, S. V., Suskandla, U., & Chidambaram, Y. (2017). Impact of electronic health records on long-term care facilities: Systematic review. *JMIR Medical Informatics, 5*(3).

Langins, M., Curry, N., Lorenz-Dant, K., Comas-Herrera, A., & Rajan, S. (2020). The COVID-19 pandemic and long-term care: What can we learn from the first wave about how to protect care homes. *Eurohealth, 26*(2), 77–82.

Mo, S., & Shi, J. (2020). The psychological consequences of the COVID-19 on residents and staff in nursing homes. *Work, Aging and Retirement, 6*(4), 254–259.

Momentum. (2023). Screen visits in the care sector are gaining ground in more and more municipalities. Located November 1, 2023 at: https://www.kl.dk/momentum/arkiv/2023/15-skaermbesoeg-i-plejesektoren-vinder-frem-i-flere-og-flere-kommuner.

Morgan, J. C., Ahmad, W., Chen, Y.-Z., & Burgess, E. O. (2023). The impact of COVID-19 on the person-centered care practices in nursing homes. *Journal of Applied Gerontology, 42*(7), 1582–1587.

Morgan, J. C., Dill, J., & Kalleberg, A. L. (2013). The quality of healthcare jobs: Can intrinsic rewards compensate for low extrinsic rewards? *Work, Employment and Society, 27*(5), 802–822.

Nakayama, S. (2006). Robotto ga nihon o suku'u [Robots Will Save Japan]. Tokyo: Tōyō Keizai Shinpōsha.

Nilsson, M., Andersson, S., Magnusson, L., & Hanson, E. (2022). Keeping the older population and their informal carers healthy and independent using digital technology: A discourse analysis of local policy. *Ageing & Society*, 1–31.

Paraprofessional Health Institute (PHI). (2024). Direct care workers in the United States. *Key Facts*, 2024.

Persson, J., Larsson, R., Erlingsdottir, G., & Rydenfält, C. (2023). How digital systems are used in Swedish home care nursing practice: A qualitative interview study to identify challenges and opportunities. *Computers, Informatics, Nursing, 41*(8), 586–594.

Rodrigues, N. C., Ham, E., Hilton, N. Z., & Seto, M. C. (2020). Workplace characteristics of forensic and non-forensic psychiatric units associated with PTSD symptoms. *Psychological Services*, Advance online publication. https://doi.org/10.1037/ser0000405

Ruggles, S., Flood, S., Sobek, M., Backman, D., Chen, A., Cooper, G., Richards, S., Rodgers, R., & Schouweiler, M. (2024). *IPUMS USA: Version 15.0 American community survey, 2022*. IPUMS. https://doi.org/10.18128/D010.V15.0. Analysis by PHI March 2024.

Scales, K., & Lepore, M. J. (2020). Always essential: Valuing direct care workers in long-term care. *The public policy and aging report.* https://doi.org/10.1093/ppar/praa022

Shen, K., McGarry, B. E., Grabowski, D. C., Gruber, J., & Gandhi, A. D. (2022). Staffing patterns in US nursing homes during COVID-19 outbreaks. *JAMA Health Forum, 3*(7).

Stone, R. I. (2010). Direct care workers in long-term care and implications for assisted living. In M. M. Ball, M. M. Perkins, C. Hollingsworth, & C. L. Kemp (Eds.), *Frontline workers in assisted living (Chapter 1)* (pp. 20–22). Johns Hopkins University Press.

Tak, S. H., Benefield, L. E., & Mahoney, D. F. (2010). Technology for long-term care. *Research in Gerontological Nursing, 3*(1), 61–72.

Task Force on Research and Development for Technology to Support Aging Adults. (2019). *Emerging technologies to support an aging population.* Committee on Technology of the National Science & Technology Council.

U.S. Bureau of Labor Statistics. (2024). Division of Occupational Employment and Wage Statistics (OEWS). 2024. *May 2014 to May 23 National Occupational Employment and Wage Estimates*. https://www.bls.gov/oes/current/oessrci.html; analysis by PHI (June 2024).

U.S. Bureau of Labor Statistics (BLS), Employment Projections Program (EPP). (2023). *National employment matrix—industry*. https://data.bls.gov/projections/nationalMatrixHome?ioType=i; analysis by PHI (June 2023).

U.S. Census Bureau. (2022). 2020 Census will help policymakers prepare for the incoming wave of aging boomers. Census.gov. Retrieved on September 9, 2024, from https://www.census.gov/library/stories/2019/12/by-2030-all-baby-boomers-will-be-age-65-or-older.html.

White, E. M., Wetle, T. F., Reddy, A., & Baier, R. R. (2021). Front-line nursing home staff experiences during the COVID-19 pandemic. *Journal of the American Medical Directors Association, 22*(1), 199–203.

Wright, J. (2023). *Robots won't save Japan. An ethnography of eldercare automation*. ILR Press.

Chapter 6
Impact of Disasters and Pandemics on Residents' Behavioral Health in Long-Term Care: Implications for Health Promotion

Lisa M. Lind and Lisa M. Brown

Use of Health Promotion During Disasters and Pandemics

A strong and growing body of evidence indicates that health promotion is effective across settings and ages. According to the World Health Organization, "Health promotion enables people to increase control over their own health. It covers a wide range of social and environmental interventions that are designed to benefit and protect individual people's health and quality of life by addressing and preventing the root causes of ill health, not just focusing on treatment and cure" (WHO, 2024). Health promotion initiatives are particularly important for older people receiving long-term care services because many have complex health needs and weakened immune systems, making them more susceptible to physical and mental illnesses and complications during crises. Long-term care services and health promotion programs are offered in a range of settings, from community home-based care to residential facilities, such as assisted living and skilled nursing. However, standard health promotion approaches used by clinicians to enhance the physical and mental well-being of long-term care (LTC) residents may be insufficient during disasters and pandemics. This is problematic because in the United States, the number of LTC residents is expected to grow during the coming decade. Current numbers show that approximately 1.2 million people live in nursing homes and nearly one million live in assisted living facilities (Statista, 2024a, 2024b). As the intensity of disasters continues to evolve and the number of people living into late life steadily

L. M. Lind (✉)
Deer Oaks Behavioral Health, San Antonio, TX, USA
e-mail: llindphd@deeroaks.com

L. M. Brown
Palo Alto University, Palo Alto, CA, USA
e-mail: lbrown@paloaltou.edu

K. K. Bhattacharyya (ed.), *Health Promotion in Long-Term Care Facilities*,
https://doi.org/10.1007/978-3-031-91038-8_6

increases, effective health promotion programs are needed to enhance resilience and outcomes for residents during emergencies.

Different Types of Disasters and Pandemics and Preparedness, Response, and Recovery Concerns for LTC Residents

During a pandemic, existing health promotion efforts will need to be extended to include disease prevention and health protections that are focused on maintaining positive states of well-being, curtailing the spread and transmission of disease, reducing the development and severity of diseases, and averting specific morbidities. Health promotion initiatives such as vaccination campaigns and hygiene practices can significantly reduce the risk of infectious diseases spread within long-term care facilities. Moreover, disasters often result in environmental changes that make pandemics more likely to occur. For example, displacement of people coupled with the disruption of health care and sanitation practices, zoonotic disease transmission resulting from animals living in closer proximity to humans, and supply chain disruptions all foster conditions that are conducive to the spread of disease. Empowering long-term care residents to take an active role in their personal health care can enhance compliance with various safety and hygiene protocols.

To achieve these goals, especially when tangible and human resources may be stressed and limited, outside support and assistance will be needed from various governmental agencies and healthcare systems to identify, mitigate, and prevent disease spread and deaths. However, the recent pandemic revealed that a subgroup of the population supported individual liberties and opposed mass restrictive actions, other than for the select protection of high-risk older adults. In this instance, disease prevention efforts were complicated as some people felt the restrictive measures were unfair to less vulnerable individuals. Notably, the Office of the Inspector General reported that in 2020, virtually all nursing homes had COVID-19-infected residents, with approximately 1300 nursing homes reaching an infection rate of 75% or more during the first year of the COVID-19 pandemic (HHS, 2023). Regardless of their personal beliefs, long-term care staff need to understand that they have a duty to adhere to facility guidelines and protect the residents in their care.

The COVID-19 pandemic also made evident the challenge of dealing with misinformation and disinformation. A trusted authority who can effectively educate and communicate with residents and their families can potentially offset some of the damaging misinformation that poses a risk to physical well-being. Although various efforts were made to stop the erosion of trust in health authorities during the COVID-19 pandemic, local providers who are known to staff and residents may be perceived as more credible in the guidance they offer. Taking steps to ensure a coordinated response that addresses each person's unique needs enhances communication among healthcare providers, families, and residents, fosters a sense of community support, builds overall morale, and enhances social connectedness.

During disasters such as hurricanes, earthquakes, fires, and human-caused events such as violence, terrorism, and technological accidents, the emphasis is typically on mitigation, preparation, response, and recovery. Recently, there has been a growing recognition that hypercomplex emergencies are becoming the norm rather than the exception. Historically, disaster planners have approached emergencies as single, large-scale, geographically limited incidents. Hypercomplex emergencies have simultaneous co-occurring events and cascading consequences. For example, Hurricane Sandy affected a vast geographical region and displaced people with varying levels of vulnerability. The existing emergency response system was overwhelmed by storm surge, wind, heavy rainfall and flooding, snow, power outages, and significant structural damage. The resulting downed power lines, damaged gas lines, and multiple fires complicated evacuation and efforts to conduct rescues and provide aid.

Staff training and advance preparation are the keys to safeguarding long-term care residents and staff's physical and mental health for both pandemics and catastrophic events. It is beneficial for health promotion programs that might be implemented during crisis events be shared before an occurrence. Moreover, it is beneficial to prepare and conduct drills using intended practices on a regular basis (Brown et al., 2012).

Mental and Behavioral Health Responses of Residents to Disasters and Pandemics

The emotional impact of pandemics and disasters encompasses anticipatory emotional responses, coping with the event in real time, and subsequent effects after the event has concluded. Since the COVID-19 pandemic, the impact of pandemics and major disasters on the mental health of long-term care residents has been more fully appreciated. The nature of this pandemic, with its uncertainty, multiple waves of disease transmission, new variants, and local and global impacts, has provided opportunities for researchers to examine its influence on subgroups of the population living in diverse settings. In the general population, it has been suggested that there have likely been multiple peaks of emotional impact, with the first peak of emotional symptoms associated with events leading up to and surrounding the event, such as lack of information, misinformation, and a rapid increase in COVID-19 cases (Ho et al., 2020; Lima et al., 2020; Ransing et al., 2020). The earliest stages of the COVID-19 pandemic were associated with increased levels of depression and anxiety symptoms in the general population (Manchia et al., 2022). The trajectory of emotional symptoms in long-term care (LTC) residents during the pandemic revealed that residents were more anxious at the onset of the COVID-19 pandemic than prior to the presence of COVID-19 illness and death (Rose et al., 2023).

A second peak of mental health symptoms was also observed as deaths rose, and social and economic disruption was witnessed, contributing to anxiety, grief, loss, post-traumatic stress reactions, depression, and exacerbation of pre-existing mental health conditions (Neria et al., 2008; Ransing et al., 2020). Specific to LTC settings, mental health providers working in LTC settings during the first 7 months of the pandemic reported observing a negative impact on residents' emotional, behavioral, and cognitive functioning, loneliness, and quality of life, with emotional status and loneliness most significantly affected (Lind et al., 2023). During previous major public health emergencies, more than half of the population developed mental health problems, and recent studies suggest a high probability of an increase in the burden of mental health issues in the post-COVID pandemic era (Ransing et al., 2020; Ren & Guo, 2020; Taylor & Asmundson, 2020; Vadivel et al., 2021). In a study of LTC residents, so far, we have seen that post-COVID levels of anxiety and depression have been higher for residents with higher levels of pre-COVID anxiety and depression and that residents showed higher levels of post-pandemic initial anxiety compared to pre-pandemic anxiety with a slow decline in severity over time (Ward et al., 2024).

Although many LTC residents may be emotionally affected by major disasters and pandemics, some residents may not manifest a change in emotional or behavioral functioning. Resiliency, the capacity to cope with difficult situations, is a characteristic of human nature, and most people can adapt over time following a major disaster or pandemic. Longitudinal follow-up has shown signs of resilience in the general population and has suggested resilience even from unexpected groups, such as older adults who are more vulnerable to the physical effects of COVID-19 (Gambin et al., 2021; Klaiber et al., 2021; Manchia et al., 2022). Although older adults may experience distress, overall, they are resilient if sufficient social support, adaptive coping, and technology are in place (Moye, 2022). Resilience is more likely to occur when an individual has good social support and adequate coping skills. Therefore, facility staff must ensure that residents can access supportive interventions and ongoing mental health resources. Addressing these challenges will be crucial in fostering resilience and well-being in this vulnerable population moving forward. Health promotion efforts to enhance mental health and foster safe connections with others can promote resilience and improve overall well-being for people of all ages.

Residents in LTC settings may or may not be cognizant of the emotional impact that a major disaster or pandemic is having on them, depending on their level of awareness, cognitive status, and insight. Therefore, LTC staff should watch for signs and symptoms of emotional reactions that include distress, agitation, isolation, irritability, fear, shock, confusion, eating less, anxiety, sleep disturbance, changes in cognitive status, substance use, stress, depression, behavioral changes, and suicidal thoughts. Keep in mind that not every individual will be impacted to the same degree or in the same way as others. Individuals who have a pre-existing psychiatric disorder, who are older, or who have chronic diseases are among the groups who may be at greater risk for exhibiting emotional symptoms (Vadivel et al., 2021). In addition, having a history of prior trauma exposure can also influence an individual's emotional response following a major stressor, such as a natural disaster or pandemic. A large percentage of residents in LTC settings make up these vulnerable groups, as approximately 30% of residents have been noted to have a psychiatric diagnosis (Fashaw et al., 2020), most older adults (50%–90%) will have been exposed to at least one traumatic event in their lifetime (Forman-Hoffman et al., 2012; Monson et al., 2016) prior to the pandemic, and the majority of LTC residents have one or more chronic illnesses, making them more vulnerable to being emotionally impacted during a major disaster or pandemic. Staff training on recognizing the signs and symptoms of emotional conditions will be essential to health promotion.

Avoiding Disruption of Emotional Support: Lessons Learned from the COVID-19 Pandemic

The psychological impact of quarantine in previous disease outbreaks, such as SARS, Ebola, the H1N1 influenza pandemic, and Middle East respiratory syndrome, has been associated with depression, anxiety, and post-traumatic stress. Symptoms may include confusion, anger, irritability, insomnia, poor concentration, indecisiveness, stress, fear, and alcohol use (Brooks et al., 2020; Hawryluck et al., 2004). During the COVID-19 pandemic, quarantine took on an unprecedented form in that residents did not have to be COVID-positive to experience quarantine and isolation protocols. The fact that someone resided in an LTC setting resulted in their being quarantined from the outside world due to the unprecedented decision by the government to mandate the restriction of visitors in nursing homes during the COVID-19 pandemic. Although this may have made sense from a virus prevention strategy, the potential impact on emotional health was a drastic oversight. Residents' access to their support system was limited to telephone or video calls and looking through glass windows as their loved ones stood outside looking in. During a time of heightened anxiety, watching the news about mass casualties constantly, awareness of frequent deaths within the LTC, being physically moved to an isolation room if infected, and restricting access to residents' support system seems counterintuitive.

Both disasters and pandemics can break down social support and lead to increased anxiety and social isolation. Given that we know that social connectedness is essential for adaptive coping during times of stress and crises, it is understandable that mandatory visitor restrictions and other quarantining procedures may negatively impact residents' emotional functioning by resulting in loneliness, agitation, anxiety, and depression, decreased quality of life, a decline in cognitive functioning, failure to thrive, and behavioral changes (Coe et al., 2023; Hugelius et al., 2021; Levere et al., 2021; Lind et al., 2023; Koszalinski & Olmos, 2022; Plangger et al., 2022; Van der Roest et al., 2020; Wammes et al., 2020). Mandatory visitor restrictions also can contribute to the psychological distress of family caregivers who reported stress, emotional instability, difficulty with communication, and feelings of guilt (Honda et al., 2024).

In addition to family members and friends not being allowed to enter LTC facilities because of mandatory visitor restrictions, many mental health providers were also not allowed entry into LTC facilities. The fact that the government had not formally designated mental health providers as essential healthcare workers at the time created a situation where facilities had to individually decide whether they would allow clinicians to enter. A survey of clinicians providing psychological and psychiatric services in LTC settings 7 months into the pandemic indicated that 71% of providers reported not being allowed access to their patients in-person or via telehealth, resulting in disruption of mental health services, with some reporting that their patients had not received mental health services at all during that period (Lind et al., 2023). Although in other settings, telehealth was able to expand quickly and successfully to offer access to mental health services during the pandemic, similar attempts to deliver mental health services via telehealth in LTC settings were often challenging and replete with technological and personnel barriers (Lind et al., 2023).

An important lesson has hopefully been learned from the COVID-19 pandemic. Implementing infection control procedures should not occur at the expense of the residents' mental health. Facilitating continued communication between residents and their informal and formal support systems should be encouraged and supported. As suggested by others, facilities should collaborate with family members on how best to support residents' needs, engage in context-specific, timely, and consistent communication, and allow for visits between residents and family members while upholding infection control protocol. Facilities should provide residents access to external services relevant to their comprehensive care needs and offer mental health support (Lam et al., 2024; Wammes et al., 2020). Integrating mental health plans into emergency preparedness will ensure that staff have guidance during stressful times.

Trauma-Informed Care

Individual trauma "results from an event, series of events, or set of circumstances that is experienced by an individual as physically or emotionally harmful or life-threatening and that has lasting adverse effects on the individual's functioning and mental, physical, social, emotional, or spiritual wellbeing" (SAMHSA, 2014, p. 7). Before the COVID-19 pandemic, it was estimated that nearly 90% of the population had been exposed to a traumatic event during their lifetime (Kilpatrick et al., 2013). The pervasiveness of trauma and its association with physical and behavioral health and well-being has been well established, with links to conditions such as cardiovascular disease, diabetes, autoimmune disorders, depression, anxiety, and substance use. Awareness of the prevalence and potential sequelae of trauma has led to a growing number of organizations and service systems at state and federal levels exploring ways to make their services more responsive to people who have experienced trauma.

Several months before the COVID-19 pandemic, CMS added a provision related to Trauma-Informed Care (F699) into federal regulations with the intent to ensure that long-term care (LTC) facilities deliver care and services which, in addition to meeting professional standards, are delivered using approaches which are culturally sensitive and account for the experiences and preferences of the resident in order to eliminate or mitigate triggers that may cause re-traumatization. Re-traumatization, or when an individual re-experiences or relives their traumatic experience, can inadvertently occur in healthcare settings and organizations. For example, if a resident has a history of being trapped in a fire, the sound of the facility fire alarm during a fire drill could trigger symptoms that are related to the earlier trauma. Symptoms may be evident as increased agitation, panic, yelling, or trying to flee from the perceived danger. Specific to major disasters and pandemics, possible triggers could include news media coverage, weather warnings, use of personal protective equipment (PPE), being placed in isolation because of an infection or illness, and having an ambulance arrive at the facility.

The takeaway is to keep in mind that residents' interpretation of any situation may result in a freeze, fight, or flight response that may not always be viewed as rational by others. In addition, anything in one's surroundings can be a potential trigger to potential re-traumatization. This is why it is essential to know a resident's trauma history. In addition, it is crucial to be aware that facility staff may also have a trauma history. Universal precautions (considering that residents and staff most likely have encountered past traumas) and taking trauma-specific precautions (having an understanding of a person's trauma history and using this information to protect against potential triggers) are considered best practices (Ganzel et al., 2024).

The timing of the implementation of trauma-informed care (TIC) was beneficial in the sense that LTC staff were likely more aware of the signs, symptoms, and impact of trauma, and efforts were underway prior to the pandemic to improve the quality of care for LTC residents with trauma histories. Underlying the ability to provide person-centered trauma-informed care is knowing each resident's trauma history. Taking a sensitive and caring approach to gathering this information is essential, as when trust is formed, individuals may be more open to disclosing such private information. It is beneficial to normalize the screening process by informing residents that everyone is asked about their prior trauma exposure. For example, letting residents know that many people have been exposed to an event that was physically or emotionally harmful, and when something reminds us of the event (whether it is a sound, touch, or smell), it might trigger a stress response. Staff members want to ensure that we do everything possible to prevent re-traumatization. Explaining that the information they share is to help inform pertinent care team members on how to best work with them and that this information is not shared with other residents. Let residents know that you have a set of standard questions to ask to help gather this information, and depending on what is shared, you can work together to identify ways that staff can incorporate person-centered strategies into their care plan to ensure that they feel safe and empowered. For detailed guidance on direct and indirect trauma screening instruments and trauma assessment, refer to Ganzel et al. (2024).

Fundamental principles of TIC that are particularly important during disasters or pandemics include safety, trustworthiness, peer support, collaboration, and empowerment. The ideal situation is that the key components are in place before such an event so that when environmental and human resources are stressed, an underlying foundation is already in place. For example, if residents and staff perceive the facility environment as an emotionally safe place, they will hopefully be in a better position to ensure that residents feel secure and protected during disasters or pandemics. Building trust between residents and staff through consistent and reliable care daily will contribute to residents feeling that staff are trustworthy in meeting their needs during a major disaster. If peer support opportunities are in place pre-disaster or pandemic, residents will have established outlets for support to connect with during stressful times. If residents feel empowered because of existing collaboration with staff and members of their interdisciplinary team (IDT), they may fare better during times when their control is diminished by circumstances resulting from a disaster or pandemic. Empowerment can help residents gain and maintain a sense of autonomy and control by focusing on their strengths and resiliency.

Integrating trauma-informed care in LTC facilities before, during, and after disasters is vital for promoting resilience and recovery among residents. Nursing homes can better support their residents' mental and emotional well-being by prioritizing safety, trust, and empowerment in challenging times. Offering preparedness training to staff on TIC principles helps them recognize the signs and symptoms of trauma and be proactive in preventing exacerbation while also being able to respond appropriately. Engaging in psychological first aid immediately following a disaster to provide emotional support and resources will be imperative. They are providing person-centered care by recognizing that each resident comes with their own lived experiences and will have individualized responses to emotional support, practical help, and times of stress to adapt interventions to address their unique needs. Keeping timely and consistent communication open between administration, line staff, families, and residents about updates is essential to maintaining trust and promoting safety by reducing anxiety and fostering security. Finally, post-disaster recovery should include ongoing support, monitoring residents for signs and symptoms of trauma, and ensuring continued access to mental health professionals. For a review of TIC as it relates to LTC, the reader is referred to Ganzel et al. (2024).

Psychological First Aid

Psychological first aid (PFA) is a set of evidence-informed foundational skills within the TIC framework which assist individuals in the immediate aftermath of a disaster. Both PFA and TIC are designed to promote healing and well-being among those affected by trauma and to prevent re-traumatization by implementing supportive and respectful environments. The use of PFA techniques is an appropriate first response to a traumatic stressor by reducing initial distress and fostering short- and long-term adaptive functioning and coping. Similar to medical first aid techniques that offer immediate care after a physical injury, PFA seeks to stabilize a person after a traumatic event to prevent or mitigate future psychological problems or to keep the person safe until more intensive and formal treatment becomes available. Typically, first aid programs can be learned by attending a training workshop and do not require formal, advanced education and licensure. The goals of PFA are to prevent further harm and to promote adaptive coping. Key components of most PFA programs include active listening, assessment of needs, providing reassurance, crisis management, and referrals to professional help if needed (Brown et al., 2009; McCabe et al., 2014).

Therapy, Assessment, and Treatment

Using PFA techniques during an unfolding and evolving crisis does not require assessing the resident to determine the appropriateness of the intervention. However, the provider should consider if the traumatized person is oriented to person, place, and time, able to follow directions, and not a danger to self or others. If there are any concerns, seeking an evaluation by a well-trained clinician is advantageous. A small but significant number of people will require more than PFA to help them recover from exposure to a traumatic stressor. It is not uncommon for people who have experienced a traumatic stressor to attribute their symptoms to the disaster or pandemic and not readily seek care for the resulting mental health issues.

A solid working alliance between the clinician and the resident is necessary when assessing mental health problems and developing treatment goals. This is especially true when assessing for trauma-related disorders because the symptoms of PTSD are often challenging to identify, as they can be masked or exacerbated by other disorders such as traumatic brain injury, depression, substance use, or anxiety disorder (Lupesko-Persky & Brown, 2019). In addition, people may not realize they have PTSD because they view their symptoms as a sign that they are having difficulty coping with the disaster or pandemic (Ellis & Zaretsky, 2018). When appropriate, and with the resident's informed consent, it can be helpful to obtain information from collateral sources such as family members, partners, or close friends, as they can shed light on the residents' behavior and current concerns. In addition to conducting a structured or semi-structured clinical interview, there are a variety of trauma and stressor-related disorder self-report measures that can be used to identify the presence of symptoms, rate their onset and severity, as well as monitor if the treatment is working (Lupesko-Persky & Brown, 2019).

It is worth noting that culture informs the psychological processes of both assessment and treatment. Culture is complex and multi-faceted and encompasses race, sex, age, religion, social status, education, financial resources, and veterans' status. Cultural identities influence a person's comprehension, understanding, and presentation of their mental health symptoms, treatment processes, and outcomes. PFA is available in multiple languages, and programs can be tailored to address unique cultural or population-specific needs.

Using Technology to Offset the Adverse Mental Health Consequences During Disasters

Technology can be leveraged at various stages of major disasters and pandemics to assist with offsetting adverse mental health consequences. From a disaster preparedness standpoint, simulation technology can be used for training on various disaster scenarios and to practice mental health crisis management. Training scenarios can include de-escalating heightened anxiety, recognizing and preventing trauma responses, practicing supportive communication, and identifying signs and symptoms of emotional distress. Using mobile apps can allow for staff engagement in learning on demand and allowing for review of information as needed. In addition, utilizing virtual or augmented reality can create immersive training experiences that allow staff to experience high-demand scenarios in a controlled environment. Immediately prior to and during a disaster or pandemic, technology can be utilized to communicate effective, clear, and concise messaging to inform staff, families, and residents of pertinent information related to the situation. Sending auditory or video messaging may help ensure that messaging is sent in a compassionate and understanding manner, hopefully contributing to decreased anxiety for its recipients. Training staff on how to use nonviolent communication methods to assure residents and families during a crisis is advantageous. It can include using messaging apps for updates and reassurance. It is essential to have devices available to allow for video visits between residents and their primary social support contacts.

Ensuring that psychological and psychiatric services are made available at all stages of a major event is imperative. Due to the policy changes enacted during the COVID-19 public health emergency, the adoption of telehealth services to deliver mental health care became more acceptable. If in-person mental health services are not feasible due to infection control guidelines, allocating and designating staff to support telehealth facilitation is vital. Facilities investing in multiple devices that could be used for telehealth and providing technology training to patients who are capable of independently engaging in telehealth may foster increased independence for patients and result in less reliance on staff for technical assistance (Lind et al., 2023). In a study that examined clinical data from residents in LTC settings who had been receiving psychological services prior to and during the COVID-19 pandemic, it was revealed that telehealth appeared to mitigate anxiety during the pandemic for residents with higher pre-COVID anxiety (Ward et al., 2024).

Given that disasters and pandemics can be anxiety-provoking for most people, it highlights the importance of making telehealth available to ensure continued access to medically necessary mental health services for residents. It is essential to have a prepared plan for telehealth facilitation, with an equal importance placed on mental health services. Awareness of local agencies that can offer assistance or resources during poor Wi-Fi coverage or other environmental barriers will be essential to implementing a facility telehealth plan.

Focusing on social connectedness will be an important aspect of enhancing residents' well-being during disasters and pandemics. At times when physical contact could potentially have an adverse medical outcome, reliance on virtual or remote group activities, video conferencing with family and friends, and access to online support groups and resources will be critical. In the event of not having access to the Internet or online resources, it will be essential to have prepared activities for residents. Focusing on anxiety and stress reduction will be an integral part of health promotion during a disaster or pandemic. This could include using apps that teach mindfulness, relaxation, and stress reduction. If available, streaming music, movies, or listening to audiobooks can serve as distractions during stressful events. Those with access to virtual reality apps or platforms can provide a mental escape from stressful situations to virtual calming environments or virtual travel to national parks or vacation locations. Of course, many of these activities will require ensuring reliable Internet access and necessary apps and devices. In addition to using technology to enhance health, we summarize key health promotion strategies that should be considered for use during disasters and pandemics in Box 6.1.

Box 6.1 Key Health Promotion Strategies During Disasters and Pandemics

- Communicate, in a timely manner, current facts, expectations, and upcoming changes related to the event to staff, residents, and family members to proactively prevent an increased anticipatory anxiety response.
- Create and maintain a physically and emotionally safe environment that encompasses the fundamental components of trauma-informed care.
- Integrating mental health plans into emergency preparedness will ensure that staff have guidance during stressful times.
- Provide reassurance and calmness in order to minimize anticipatory anxiety.
- Have a plan in place to mitigate potential triggers to trauma.
- Engage in universal precaution.
- Implementation of infection control procedures should not occur at the expense of resident mental health.
- Identify which residents may be at greater risk of being emotionally impacted by the event. This may include those with a prior psychiatric history, lack of social support, dementia, or history of trauma.
- Periodically and routinely assess mental health needs, being cognizant of signs and symptoms of anxiety, depression, and trauma reactions.
- Provide informal, ongoing emotional support to all residents while ensuring that those who are exhibiting signs of emotional symptoms or have a prior mental health condition or history of trauma have access to formal mental health support.

- Informal support (family, friends) and formal (mental health services) should not be disrupted. Always allow residents access to their support systems if possible.
- Recognize that mental health services are always essential, especially during stressful and traumatic events.
- Ensure resources are available for telehealth to be provided when in-person access to mental health providers is limited.
- Teach, model, and practice relaxation and mindfulness strategies with residents during times of stress.
- Provide activities that can serve as a distraction, preferably activities that involve social connection.
- Foster continued social connections between residents and their family and friends by allowing access to video conferencing.
- When quarantine is deemed necessary, social and emotional needs should continue to be met. Provide communication and rationale for the length of isolation needed.
- Attempt to re-establish prior routines as soon as possible.
- Engage in psychological first aid immediately following a disaster to provide emotional support and resources to residents and staff.

References

Brooks, S. K., Webster, R. K., Smith, L. E., Woodland, L., Wessely, S., Greenberg, N., & Rubin, G. J. (2020). The psychological impact of quarantine and how to reduce it: Rapid review of the evidence. *Lancet, 395*(10227), 912–920. https://doi.org/10.1016/S0140-6736(20)30460-8

Brown, L. M., Bruce, M. L., Hyer, K., Mills, W. L., Vongxaiburana, E., & Polivka-West, L. (2009). A pilot study evaluating the feasibility of psychological first aid for nursing home residents. *Clinical Gerontologist, 32*(3), 293–308. https://doi.org/10.1080/07317110902895317

Brown, L. M., Dosa, D. M., Thomas, K., Hyer, K., Feng, Z., & Mor, V. (2012). The effects of evacuation on nursing home residents with dementia. *American Journal of Alzheimer's Disease and Other Dementias, 27*(6), 406–412. https://doi.org/10.1177/1533317512454709

Coe, A. B., Montoya, A., Chang, C.-H., Park, P. S., Bynum, J. P. W., Shireman, T. I., Zhang, T., McCreedy, E. M., & Gerlach, L. B. (2023). Behavioral symptoms, depression symptoms, and medication use in Michigan nursing home residents with dementia during COVID-19. *Journal of the American Geriatrics Society, 71*(2), 414–422. https://doi.org/10.1111/jgs.18116

Ellis, J., & Zaretsky, A. (2018). Assessment and management of posttraumatic stress disorder. *Continuum, 24*(3), 873–892. https://doi.org/10.1212/CON.0000000000000610

Fashaw, S. A., Thomas, K. S., McCreedy, E., & Mor, V. (2020). Thirty-year trends in nursing home composition and quality since the passage of the omnibus reconciliation act. *Journal of the American Medical Directors Association, 21*(2), 233–239. https://doi.org/10.1016/j.jamda.2019.07.004

Forman-Hoffman, V. L., Bose, J., Batts, K. R., Glasheen, C., Hirsch, E., Karg, R. S., Huang, L. N., & Hedden, S. L. (2012). Correlates of lifetime exposure to one or more potentially traumatic events and subsequent posttraumatic stress among adults in the United States: Results from the Mental Health Surveillance Study, 2008–2012. In CBHSQ data review. Substance Abuse and Mental Health Services Administration (US).

Gambin, M., Sękowski, M., Woźniak-Prus, M., Wnuk, A., Oleksy, T., Cudo, A., et al. (2021). Generalized anxiety and depressive symptoms in various age groups during the COVID-19 lockdown in Poland. Specific predictors and differences in symptoms severity. *Comprehensive Psychiatry, 105*, 152222. https://doi.org/10.1016/j.comppsych.2020.152222

Ganzel, B., Kusmaul, N., Cheatham, C., Hector, P., Clarke, D., & Perley, R. (2024). Trauma informed care. In R. Perley (Ed.), *Managing the long-term care facility: Practical approaches to providing quality care* (2nd ed.) Jossey-Bass/Wiley.

HHS (2023). Office of Inspector General Data Brief: More than a thousand nursing homes reached infection rates of 75 percent or more in the first year of the COVID-19 pandemic; better protections are needed for future emergencies. Accessed November 4, 2024.

Hawryluck, L., Gold, W. L., Robinson, S., Pogorski, S., Galea, S., & Styra, R. (2004). SARS control and psychological effects of quarantine, Toronto, Canada. *Emerging Infectious Diseases, 10*(7), 1206–1212. https://doi.org/10.3201/eid1007.030703

Ho, C. S., Chee, C. Y., & Ho, R. C. (2020). Mental health strategies to combat the psychological impact of coronavirus disease 2019 (COVID-19) beyond paranoia and panic. *Annals of the Academy of Medicine, Singapore, 49*(3), 155–160.

Honda, A., Liu, Y., Ono, M., Nishida, T., Tsukigi, T., Fauth, E. B., & Honda, S. (2024). Impact of visitation restrictions on the mental health of family caregivers during the COVID-19 pandemic: A mixed methods study. *Journal of Advanced Nursing, 80*, 1652–1665. https://doi.org/10.1111/jan.15918

Hugelius, K., Harada, N., & Marutani, M. (2021). Consequences of visiting restrictions during the COVID-19 pandemic: An integrative review. *International Journal of Nursing Studies, 121*, 104000. https://doi.org/10.1016/j.ijnurstu.2021.104000

Kilpatrick, D. G., Resnick, H. S., Milanak, M. E., Miller, M. W., Keyes, K. M., & Friedman, M. J. (2013). National estimates of exposure to traumatic events and PTSD prevalence using DSM-IV and DSM-5 criteria. *Journal of Traumatic Stress, 26*(5), 537–547. https://doi.org/10.1002/jts.21848

Klaiber, P., Wen, J. H., DeLongis, A., & Sin, N. L. (2021). The ups and downs of daily life during COVID-19: Age differences in affect, stress, and positive events. *The Journals of Gerontology: Series B, 76*(2), e30–e37. https://doi.org/10.1093/geronb/gbaa096

Koszalinski, R. S., & Olmos, B. (2022). Communication challenges in social isolation, subjective cognitive decline, and mental health status in older adults: A scoping review (2019–2021). *Perspectives in Psychiatric Care*. Advance online publication. https://doi.org/10.1111/ppc.13115

Lam, M. C. H., Egan, M. Y., & Durocher, E. (2024). Recommendations related to visitor and movement restrictions in long-term care and retirement homes in Ontario during the COVID-19 pandemic: Perspectives of residents, families, and staff. *Canadian Journal on Aging / La Revue canadienne du vieillissement*. https://doi.org/10.1017/S0714980823000715

Levere, M., Rowan, P., & Wysocki, A. (2021). The adverse effects of the COVID-19 pandemic on nursing home resident well-being. *Journal of the American Medical Directors Association, 22*(5), 948–954.e2. https://doi.org/10.1016/j.jamda.2021.03.010

Lima, C. K. T., Carvalho, P. M. M., Lima, I. A. A. S., Nunes, J. V. A. O., Saraiva, J. S., de Souza, R. I., da Silva, C. G. L., & Neto, M. L. R. (2020). The emotional impact of coronavirus 2019-nCoV (new coronavirus disease). *Psychiatry Research, 287*, 112915. https://doi.org/10.1016/j.psychres.2020.112915

Lind, L. M., Ward, R. N., Rose, S. G., & Brown, L. M. (2023). The impact of the COVID-19 pandemic on psychological service provision, mental health practitioners, and patients in long-term care settings: Results from a rapid response survey. *Professional Psychology: Research and Practice, 54*(1), 93–102. https://doi.org/10.1037/pro0000486

Lupesko-Persky, O., & Brown, L. M. (2019). Trauma and stressor-related disorders. *Diagnostic Interviewing*, 179–211.

Manchia, M., Gathier, A. W., Yapici-Eser, H., Schmidt, M. V., de Quervain, D., van Amelsvoort, T., Bisson, J. I., Cryan, J. F., Howes, O. D., Pinto, L., van der Wee, N. J., Domschke, K., Branchi,

I., & Vinkers, C. H. (2022). The impact of the prolonged COVID-19 pandemic on stress resilience and mental health: A critical review across waves. *European Neuropsychopharmacology: The Journal of the European College of Neuropsychopharmacology, 55*, 22–83. https://doi.org/10.1016/j.euroneuro.2021.10.864

McCabe, O. L., Everly, G. S., Brown, L. M., Wendelboe, A. M., Hamid, N. H., Tallchief, V. L., & Links, J. (2014). Psychological first aid: A consensus-derived, empirically-supported, competency-based training model. *American Journal of Public Health, 104*(4), 621–628. https://doi.org/10.2105/AJPH.2013.301219

Monson, E., Lonergan, M., Caron, J., & Brunet, A. (2016). Assessing trauma and posttraumatic stress disorder: Single, open-ended question versus list-based inventory. *Psychological Assessment, 28*(8), 1001–1008. https://doi.org/10.1037/pas0000223

Moye, J. (2022). Mental health in older adults during COVID: Creative approaches and adaptive coping. *Clinical Gerontologist, 45*(1), 1–3. https://doi.org/10.1080/07317115.2021.2011181

Neria, Y., Nandi, A., & Galea, S. (2008). Post-traumatic stress disorder following disasters: A systematic review. *Psychological Medicine, 38*(4), 467–480. https://doi.org/10.1017/S0033291707001353

Plangger, B., Unterrainer, C., Kreh, A., Gatterer, G., & Juen, B. (2022). Psychological effects of social isolation during the COVID-19 pandemic 2020. *GeroPsych: The Journal of Gerontopsychology and Geriatric Psychiatry, 35*(1), 17–29. https://doi.org/10.1024/1662-9647/a000283

Ransing, R., Adiukwu, F., Pereira-Sanchez, V., Ramalho, R., Orsolini, L., Teixeira, A. L. S., Gonzalez-Diaz, J. M., Pinto da Costa, M., Soler-Vidal, J., Bytyçi, D. G., El Hayek, S., Larnaout, A., Shalbafan, M., Syarif, Z., Nofal, M., & Kundadak, G. K. (2020). Mental health interventions during the COVID-19 pandemic: A conceptual framework by early career psychiatrists. *Asian Journal of Psychiatry, 51*, 102085. https://doi.org/10.1016/j.ajp.2020.102085

Ren, F. F., & Guo, R. J. (2020). Public mental health in post-COVID-19 era. *Psychiatria Danubina, 32*(2), 251–255. https://doi.org/10.24869/psyd.2020.251

Rose, S. G., Ward, R. N., Lind, L. M., & Brown, L. M. (2023). Effects of the COVID-19 pandemic on anxiety symptoms in long-term care residents: A multilevel growth curve analysis. *Journal of the American Medical Directors Association, 24*(6), 862–867.e1. https://doi.org/10.1016/j.jamda.2023.03.029

Statista. (2024a). Number of residents in certified nursing facilities in the United States as of 2023, by state. Accessed November 4, 2024. https://www.statista.com/statistics/1168843/number-residents-certified-nursing-facilities-state/.

Statista. (2024b). Number of residents in assisted living communities in the U.S. 2016–2022. Accessed on: November 4, 2024. https://www.statista.com/statistics/1490559/number-of-adults-in-assisted-living-communities-us/#statisticContainer.

Substance Abuse and Mental Health Services Administration (SAMHSA). (2014). *SAMHSA's concept of trauma and guidance for a trauma-informed approach. HHS publication no. (SMA) 14-4884*. Substance Abuse and Mental Health Services Administration.

Taylor, S., & Asmundson, G. J. G. (2020). Life in a post-pandemic world: What to expect of anxiety-related conditions and their treatment. *Journal of Anxiety Disorders, 72*, 102231. https://doi.org/10.1016/j.janxdis.2020.102231

Vadivel, R., Shoib, S., El Halabi, S., El Hayek, S., Essam, L., Gashi Bytyçi, D., Karaliuniene, R., Schuh Teixeira, A. L., Nagendrappa, S., Ramalho, R., Ransing, R., Pereira-Sanchez, V., Jatchavala, C., Adiukwu, F. N., & Kudva Kundadak, G. (2021). Mental health in the post-COVID-19 era: Challenges and the way forward. *General Psychiatry, 34*(1), e100424. https://doi.org/10.1136/gpsych-2020-100424

Van der Roest, H. G., Prins, M., van der Velden, C., Steinmetz, S., Stolte, E., van Tilburg, T. G., & de Vries, D. H. (2020). The impact of COVID-19 measures on well-being of older long-term care facility residents in the Netherlands. *Journal of the American Medical Directors Association, 21*(11), 1569–1570. https://doi.org/10.1016/j.jamda.2020.09.007. Epub 2020 Sep 10.

Wammes, J. D., Kolk, D., van den Besselaar, J. H., MacNeil-Vroomen, J. L., Buurmanvan, B. M., & van Rijn, M. (2020). Evaluating perspectives of relatives of nursing home residents on the nursing home visiting restrictions during the COVID-19 crisis: A Dutch cross-sectional survey study. *Journal of the American Medical Directors Association, 21*(12), 1746–1750.e3. https://doi.org/10.1016/j.jamda.2020.09.031

Ward, R. N., Lind, L. M., Rose, S. G., & Brown, L. M. (2024). Depression and anxiety in long-term care residents during the COVID-19 pandemic: The influence of telehealth availability, cognitive status, and trauma history. *Clinical Gerontologist*, 1–10. Advance online publication. https://doi.org/10.1080/07317115.2024.2305876

World Health Organization (WHO). Health Promotion. https://www.who.int/news-room/questions-and-answers/item/health-promotion Accessed September 22, 2024.

Chapter 7
Critical Staffing Issues and the Impact of COVID-19 on Long-Term Care Workforce Management

Jessica Vanderwerf and Lindsay J. Peterson

Introduction

Long-standing issues in the long-term care sector came sharply to light during the COVID-19 pandemic. Understaffing, high employee turnover, inefficient retention strategies, and other pre-existing problems worsened as the virus spread into nursing homes and assisted living communities, even with masking, lockdown orders, and other infection control efforts (Beltran et al., 2024; Gasdaska et al., 2022). Despite offering higher wages, bonuses, internal promotions, training programs, and other incentives, nearly all of the nursing homes surveyed in 2024 reported having trouble hiring new staff, with more than two-thirds of those surveyed citing a lack of interested or qualified candidates (American Health Care Association/National Center for Assisted Living, 2024).

COVID-19, with its multiple variants, came in waves through 2020, 2021, and 2022. Social distancing measures and personal protective equipment (PPE) were essential for infection control, but they also intensified social isolation, increasing the vulnerability of this population. Public health emergency measures were finally lifted in the USA in May 2023, with vaccinations, testing, and treatment becoming readily available. Through the prolonged emergency, however, the long-term care industry experienced severe employee attrition, particularly among direct care workers who were physically and emotionally exhausted by their struggles to

[1] Reprinted from *Journal of the American Medical Directors Association*, Vol 21(7), Katherine S. McGilton et al., Uncovering the Devaluation of Nursing Home Staff During COVID-19: Are We Fuelling the Next Health Care Crisis?, Table 1, p. 4, Copyright 2020, with permission from Elsevier.

J. Vanderwerf · L. J. Peterson (✉)
School of Aging Studies, University of South Florida, Tampa, FL, USA
e-mail: vanderwerf@usf.edu; ljpeterson@usf.edu

K. K. Bhattacharyya (ed.), *Health Promotion in Long-Term Care Facilities*,
https://doi.org/10.1007/978-3-031-91038-8_7

protect and save the older adults in their care. Many care homes turned to agencies or increased their agency use to fill their open direct care positions (Stepick et al., 2024) despite earlier research about the risks of using temporary workers (Castle & Engberg, 2007).

These challenges notwithstanding, many who worked in long-term care demonstrated resilience, developing team-based peer support and other programs to help navigate the unprecedented pressures of the pandemic and stabilize staffing (Boamah et al., 2023; Martin et al., 2023).

The Critical Role of Direct Care Staff in Long-Term Care Health Promotion

About 1.4 million people receive daily care in nearly 27,000 nursing homes across the USA. They depend on a direct care workforce of certified nursing assistants (CNAs), licensed practical nurses (LPNs), and registered nurses (RNs) who operate in an increasingly complex long-term care environment. As care alternatives have increased over the past two decades (e.g., home-and-community-based services), nursing homes have become the primary site of care for people with significant needs who are unable to live independently (Siskind et al., 2024). Today's nursing homes provide services such as IV therapy, rehabilitation and care for dementia, severe mental illness, and other chronic and disabling health conditions that impair one's ability to bathe, dress, move from a bed to a chair, or walk independently. Resident acuity is also rising among the more than 800,000 people in assisted living in the USA (Regan, 2022; Zimmerman et al., 2022).

Direct Care Staffing and Quality

As the need for residential long-term care has grown, so have the staffing challenges. Staffing levels and composition are crucial factors influencing resident health and safety. Key considerations include the number of staff relative to residents, the availability of specialized personnel, and the experience and qualifications of the staff, as well as the retention of qualified staff. Dozens of peer-reviewed studies going back two decades have examined the relationship between direct care staffing and the quality of the care residents receive (e.g., Jutkowitz et al., 2023).

Researchers found associations between higher nurse aide staffing and fewer deficiencies on regulatory surveys (Boscart et al., 2018; Chen & Grabowski, 2015; Hyer et al., 2011; Lerner et al., 2014). Other research linked higher CNA/nurse aide staffing levels and lower use of antipsychotic medication (Mukamel et al., 2024), fewer pressure sores, and reduced use of physical restraints and catheters (Castle & Anderson, 2011). Importantly, Castle and Engberg (2007) highlighted that higher

CNA staffing was more effective in nursing homes that depended less on contract staffing agencies and used higher proportions of RNs in their staffing mix.

In a study conducted in 2008 that presaged the issues to emerge during the COVID-19 pandemic, Hutt et al. (2008) found that nurse and CNA staffing affected adherence to treatment guidelines for pneumonia. They concluded that staffing, as well as turnover, influenced multiple aspects of the process, including vaccination, treatment, and communication with attending physicians. While CNAs provide the majority of the hands-on care that residents receive, RNs supervise the direct care staff, assess residents' conditions, manage and coordinate their care, and may provide specialized care to meet specific needs. RNs have higher levels of education and training than nurse aides, and research has found strong and consistent relationships between higher numbers of RNs and fewer regulatory deficiencies (Kim et al., 2009; Lerner et al., 2014; Lin, 2014). RN staffing has also been associated with fewer pressure ulcers (Lee et al., 2014; Lin, 2014; Orth et al., 2021) and urinary tract infections (Konetzka et al., 2008).

While a great deal of research has linked staffing and the quality of care, results are sometimes mixed because of the complexity of the variables that affect nursing home staffing and quality (e.g., Armijo-Olivio et al., 2020). The National Academies of Sciences, Engineering, and Medicine (NASEM) assessed the state of nursing home care in its *National Imperative to Improve Nursing Home Quality* (2022). Concerning staffing, the NASEM found that research evidence was strongest for the positive effect of higher RN staffing, though it also found merit in the research linking CNA staffing to better quality.

Staff Retention, Turnover, and Quality of Care Many researchers and policy analysts contend that staffing numbers provide only part of the story, citing staff retention and turnover as key aspects of how care is delivered in long-term care. Retention of CNAs and RNs is associated with better overall quality of care (Lerner et al., 2014), while higher staff turnover is associated with worse outcomes for residents, such as increased rehospitalizations and higher numbers of regulatory deficiencies (Castle et al., 2007; Thomas et al., 2013; Shen et al., 2023), including infection control deficiencies (Loomer et al., 2022). Turnover may even be more important than staffing numbers in explaining resident outcomes (Trinkoff et al., 2013). The reason is that aides and nurses who come and go are not likely to form relationships that enable them to perceive, understand, and respond to residents' specific needs, making it more difficult for them to provide consistent and appropriate care.

Researchers and policy analysts cite low wages and poor management to explain low retention and high turnover (Espinoza, 2020; Bryant et al., 2023). However, low staffing itself may be a prime contributor to the extent that it increases the daily workload and burden for direct care staff, causing many to leave their jobs and making nursing homes an unattractive work environment for prospective employees. In one qualitative study with nursing home CNAs, Krein et al. (2022) reported that while some discussed their pay, many others complained about staffing levels, saying the demands it placed on their time prevented them from delivering the personalized care they felt was important. They also expressed a need for more support and training, including time for training. As one respondent said, *"I've seen the worst, people overworked, you've got managers that (are) always on the floors, so they can't do their other jobs, the CNAs are overwhelmed, and the residents are not getting the care they need, and it's just not a good thing all across the board"* (p. 1180).

Mukamel et al. (2024) discussed the critical factor of time in the delivery of care to explain their finding of a relationship between increased CNA staffing and lower use of antipsychotic medication in nursing homes. CNAs who can dedicate more time to each resident are better positioned to recognize residents' needs and may help prevent instances of agitation that can arise when those needs are not addressed. This is particularly true of residents with dementia who cannot clearly express their thoughts or preferences. The same idea could apply to long-tenured staff in a nursing home or an assisted living community, who are likely to be more able to anticipate residents' needs because they have had more time to get to know them.

The issues of time and tenure and turnover, as well as staff training and support, speak to an underlying issue in nursing home quality—that is, the well-being of those who work in long-term care is central to resident care. The intertwining of the lives and well-being of long-term care staff and residents became tragically evident during the COVID-19 pandemic.

The Effect of the COVID-19 Emergency on Long-Term Care Staff

Harvard medical school professor David Grabowski reported to a Congressional subcommittee in 2023 that more than 1.6 million cases of COVID-19 had occurred among nursing home residents in the USA alone, leading to roughly 176,000 deaths—the equivalent of 12% of all residents living in nursing homes at the start of the pandemic. Additional deaths occurred because of gaps in medical care and increased illness (U.S. House Committee on Oversight and Accountability, 2023). Based on research conducted early in the pandemic, increased mortality of assisted living residents was consistent with the mortality of nursing home residents (Thomas et al., 2021).

Even before the COVID-19 pandemic, long-term care homes often failed to maintain staffing levels considered to be adequate (Geng et al., 2019). The reasons ranged from low wages to limited training and advancement options and difficult, disheartening working conditions. COVID-19 intensified existing challenges while creating new threats as it fell to aides, nurses, and managers to protect residents, and then, if an outbreak occurred, to provide hands-on care to residents as they battled the disease or succumbed to it.

Much of the early COVID-19 research focused on resident illness and death, but staff were also at substantial risk of contracting the disease. As of early 2022, more than 2300 nursing home staff were reported to have died from COVID-19 (Shen et al., 2022). Two years earlier, evidence of staff fatalities spurred researchers to write in a newspaper editorial that staff death rates could "more than double the rate of previous years' deadliest occupations, such as logging and commercial fishing." The writers continued: "Under normal circumstances, [long-term care staff] perform a physically and emotionally demanding job, providing an intimate level of care for some of our most vulnerable citizens often for low wages and limited benefits. The presence of COVID-19 in more than half of the roughly 15,000 U.S. nursing homes, combined with the heartbreakingly inadequate response from federal and state governments, has made going to work an act of bravery and selflessness" (McGarry et al., 2020).

Going into the pandemic, many nursing aides lacked paid sick leave, health insurance, and other benefits, making it difficult for them to seek health care (de Perio et al., 2023; PHI, 2021). When the pandemic struck, they similarly found themselves with insufficient personal protective equipment (PPE) and COVID-19 testing supplies and work environments (e.g., shared resident rooms) that increased the challenge of providing care (Boamah et al., 2023; Estabrooks et al., 2020; Lai et al., 2020). These circumstances increased workers' risk of becoming exposed and infecting other residents and their families (Lai et al., 2020; White et al., 2021). A 2020 US study found that half of long-term care workers were at increased risk of severe illness from COVID-19, including hospitalization and death (Gibson & Greene, 2020).

The Anxiety of Providing Care During COVID-19

Fear of COVID-19 was a top concern among long-term care staff. In interviews with care home staff in England, Cockshott et al. (2024) discussed staff members' shock at the rapid spread of the disease. As one said, "*it was horrific for us because obviously a lot of our people are very vulnerable... we unfortunately lost, I think it was 11 residents we lost, and one member of staff to COVID over a space of about three weeks*" (p. 5).

In a US study of assisted living administrators, one participant shared that, "*My workers thought it was a death sentence to work with COVID patients. Fear was constant...It was a tougher battle to convince workers to work than fighting the virus*" (Bahr et al., 2023, p. 4). Nursing home care staff described their personal fears in another study. "*You're not only worried about yourself and your residents, but you're worried about bringing it home as well*" (Snyder et al., 2021, p. 6).

Assisted living administrators in a US study discussed the emotional weight of managing care during the pandemic (Kyler-Yano et al., 2022, p. 193). "*The gravity, especially right now, how many souls I'm responsible for, especially with COVID, and the fact that the virus could rip through our building and kill half of our people and then infect our staff and they bring it home to their families. Those are things that keep me awake at night.*"

The fear and stigma associated with contracting and transmitting the virus caused many workers to isolate themselves from friends and family. In a multi-national study conducted in Spain, Italy, Peru, and Mexico, a geriatric nurse said, *"I am terrified to think that I have it without knowing, and that I am infecting the residents"* (Sarabia-Cobo et al., 2021, p. 872). Fear of the virus was especially prominent in memory care, where it was a struggle to maintain precautions among residents who did not comprehend the danger of exposure (Vogel et al., 2024).

The Stress of Meeting Residents' Needs Amid Stringent, Changing Pandemic Precautions

Mandated social restrictions increased the strains of providing long-term care in the USA (Beltran et al., 2024; Hackett et al., 2023) and across the globe. Sweeney and colleagues (2021) reported on the stress that care home staff in Ireland experienced as they dealt with multiple changing guidelines and tried to manage the effect on residents who were afraid and isolated. A care home nurse in a study in England and Scotland described the persistent stress and discouragement: *"The pressure has been there throughout from the minute we were preparing, just in case we had a COVID case, to even now, we are constantly testing, constantly aware. My emotions are, we have been hung out to dry and totally forgotten"* (Birt et al., 2023, p. 230). A Spanish nursing home worker put it more plainly. *"There has been no foresight, we are abandoned, exhausted…We fight alone"* (Sarabia-Cobo et al., 2021, p. 873).

Widespread Loss of Staff and Effects on Residents

As the pandemic measures continued, amid rising infection rates among residents and nursing home staff, staffing shortages became more extreme. In interviews with nursing home leaders (e.g., administrators and directors of nursing), Leland et al. (2024) described the widespread loss of staff, including front office employees, housekeeping, laundry, maintenance, and dietary services. Among direct care staff, participants described shortages in rehabilitation, nursing, social services, and activities. Considering the effect of staff losses, Ramanan et al. (2024) reported that over 22% of daily care tasks went uncompleted due to staffing shortages during the pandemic, resulting in increased hospitalizations and mortality rates from non-COVID-19-related conditions.

Staffing shortages significantly affected Black and Latino residents in nursing homes, especially in socioeconomically challenged areas that served a higher percentage of Medicaid patients, leading to elevated levels of staff burnout in these facilities (Lakon & Hipp, 2024) Residents from these populations were already facing elevated rates of COVID-19 infections and fatalities, and low staffing further limited their access to essential care and safety protocols.

Moral Distress

Several studies addressed the "moral distress" that long-term care staff members experienced during the pandemic (Boamah et al., 2023; Brit et al., 2023; Dohmen et al., 2022). Moral distress arises when someone acts in a way that is contrary to their moral or ethical values, often because of external pressures, such as low staffing, limiting the ability of existing staff to meet residents' needs during the pandemic.

In the research by Cockshott et al. (2024), staff discussed the effect of visitation restrictions on residents and their family members and the notable challenges of providing compassionate care at the end of life. As one related, "*When you've got a relative in the room and you're like, 'I'm sorry your time is up. You've got to go.' It's just an awful position to be in because who are we to say they can't say their goodbyes and for how long. That's the bit that I find difficult because I just think it's awful. It really is*" (p. 5).

Other researchers addressed the moral distress nursing staff experienced when they had to choose between their professional and personal obligations (Birt et al., 2023; Dohmen et al., 2022). As one said, "*I'm also a key-worker and the main care-worker for my granddad. During those two weeks [with COVID-19 in the care-home] I couldn't get to him. We had a service going in and looking after him*" (Birt et al., 2023, p. 230).

Birt et al. (2023) discussed the risk of moral distress worsening into moral injury or post-traumatic stress in the COVID-19 emergency and other extreme disasters. They highlighted the work of Gary & Berlinger (2020), who proposed that disaster recovery for care workers should be framed by an "ethic of care" in which safeguards apply to both those who receive care and those who provide it.

Stress, Worry, and Increasing Workloads Lead to Burnout

As job demands grew during 2020–2021 in long-term care homes, staff began to burnout. In scoping research by Boamah et al. (2023), more than a dozen studies reported chronic mental and physical fatigue, intensified exhaustion, fear, and anger. One British care home worker said, "*I burned out in the end. […] In hindsight, it was so draining because it was constant. And it was constant fear, and I think fear is the just the worst thing, the fear from getting ill and my actions making someone ill—or my lack of actions, I should say. That's a horrible thought to have*" (Bunn et al., 2021, p. 395).

Demands and distress were especially acute for staff who worked with residents living with dementia (Hackett et al., 2023; Holmes et al., 2024) who were confused and frightened by the radical change in procedures during the pandemic, including distancing, restrictions on family contact, and staff who kept their faces covered. Nursing homes and assisted living administrators in a US study described feeling afraid that the safeguards hastened residents' cognitive decline and death (Hackett et al., 2023, p. 1568). As one assisted living administrator said, *"I'm a firm believer, we did more damage isolating residents…All of it, not being able to see family, not being touched, the fear, all of that, did tremendous damage to their mental health. And I truly believe it killed quite a few of our residents because the depression was so severe."*

A study of staff in a nursing home memory care unit found the widespread perception that while they had received training in dementia care, they were not prepared for the realities of a pandemic (Holmes et al., 2024, p. 3). *"Not prepared at all? This was actually the first time in my whole career that I've had to deal with any kind of precautions that we've had to deal with, with COVID."* As caregivers left their jobs, those who remained faced increased workloads and pressure to maintain stringent infection control measures, and these factors contributed to heightened stress and burnout among caregivers in facilities worldwide who felt overextended and unsupported (Amblàs-Novellas et al., 2024; Battams & Martini, 2024; Brazier et al., 2023; Giebel et al., 2022; Holmes et al., 2024).

The COVID-19 pandemic emergency eased as vaccinations became available to long-term care residents and staff. However, the staffing crisis continued. The American Health Care Association/National Center for Assisted Living (2024) reported that nursing homes experienced the greatest loss of jobs of any health care sector during the pandemic, with 210,000 jobs lost from February 2020 to December 2022. Workforce levels were the lowest they had been in 30 years, and more than 80% of nursing homes were facing moderate to high levels of staffing shortages. More than half of providers reported having to limit new admissions due to staffing shortages. Nearly all reported asking current staff to work overtime/extra shifts, and more than 70% reported having to hire temporary agency staff to fill open positions.

Staffing Pressures Lead to More Use of Contract Workers

Research conducted by Stepick et al. (2024) found a sizable rise in the percentage of total CNA hours provided by contracted workers in nursing homes, increasing from 2% in 2017 to 11% in 2022. This work supported similar research that also found a jump in the percentage of nursing homes using agency staff, from 23% in 2018 to nearly 50% in 2022 (Bowblis et al., 2024), and further concluded that agency use patterns shifted during the pandemic. Rather than using staff to assist with a short-term need, as in the past, nursing homes were increasingly using agency staff to address chronic staffing shortages, making them more of a fixture in long-term care to the extent that staffing shortages continue.

While agency staff enable nursing homes to operate when they cannot fill open positions, there is a trade-off in quality. Although agency staff are expected to have the same level of skill and training as staff who are directly employed, they are unlikely to be familiar with individual residents, the facility's nursing team, and the facility's operations, making them less efficient and possibly less effective than directly employed staff. Research has found that agency staff are less likely to be consistently assigned to the same residents, possibly reducing the chances they will identify warning signs of health or safety issues in need of special attention (Kennedy & Bowblis, 2023). The analyses of Stepick et al. (2024) showed that higher proportions of contract (or agency) CNA hours were associated with worse Five-Star Quality Ratings, higher rates of extended use of catheters, urinary tract infections, and pressure sores, and lower rates of residents improving in function. The findings build on earlier research showing that increasing regularly employed CNA staffing leads to improved care quality outcomes, but the same positive association is not seen with increased contract CNA staffing levels (Castle & Engberg, 2007). Prior research also found that the use of contract licensed nurses was associated with more regulatory deficiencies, and the risks may be greater for facilities more dependent on Medicaid funding that do not attract competent staff but must spend their limited funds on agency services, further impairing their quality and ability to attract employees (Bourbonniere et al., 2006).

While further research is needed to more precisely understand agency use since the pandemic and the implications for the health promotion of residents, it is clear that this issue will become even more critical as the population of older adults grows, particularly the rapid growth of those who are 80 and older and most likely to require nursing home or assisted living care.

Key Recommendations that Emerged from COVID-19 Research

Since the COVID-19 pandemic emerged in an assisted living community in Washington state, a great volume of research has been conducted to assess and understand the effect on the long-term care workforce. The pandemic was unquestionably an upheaval that painfully demonstrated how much the health and well-being of residents depend on the health and well-being of the people who provide their care. The research described the terrible toll that long-term care workers paid globally, but within the research, there are numerous consistent recommendations, many of which reinforce prior research. The AARP consolidated a range of proposals to improve and stabilize the long-term care workforce, drawing on research and the 2022 NASEM recommendations (Travers et al., 2024). The AARP report and other research highlighted the following:

Staffing Levels

Research over the past two decades has left little question that higher staffing improves care, particularly nursing home RN staffing and CNA staffing, for particular tasks, such as assisting residents with dressing, bathing, movement, and other daily activities (Mukamel et al., 2024). The research concerning LPNs is more mixed, with some studies linking higher LPN staffing to lower quality (Castle & Engberg, 2007; Kim et al., 2009). This is believed to occur when RNs are replaced by LPNs, who typically have less training. Federal and state governments have a key role in determining how many nurses and aides are on hand every day in nursing homes. To arm the public with more information on nursing home quality, CMS posts staff turnover rates and weekend staffing levels in addition to weekday staffing (www.medicare.gov/care-compare). Less is known about assisted living. While the importance of staffing and staff training in assisted living has been established, more work is needed, particularly to understand residents' needs and establish acuity-based staffing recommendations (Zimmerman et al., 2022).

Wages

The issue of wages, particularly for nursing aides, has emerged again and again in research on the quality of nursing home care (Travers et al., 2024). Likewise, it was prominent in the research on COVID-19, with reports of nursing homes losing staff and not being able to find new workers because of low wages (Beltran et al., 2024; Leland et al., 2024). In 2023, CNAs earned a mean hourly wage of $18.33 (U.S. Bureau of Labor Statistics, 2024), less than $3200 per month before taxes, an insufficient amount to cover the rising costs of housing, food, and transportation. Resident care can suffer when frontline staff have to work multiple jobs, work overtime, and/or switch to working for an agency in order to cover every day needs, such as mortgage or rent, utilities, transportation, and childcare (Dill et al., 2022; Travers et al., 2024). The 2022 National Academies of Sciences, Engineering, and Medicine (NASEM) report on nursing home quality concluded that low direct care staff wages and benefits, combined with inadequate training, had made nursing homes undesirable places to work, a situation worsened by the pandemic (NASEM, 2022).

Correcting the undercompensation of direct care workers is one of the two workforce improvement priorities identified by the Moving Forward Coalition (Bonner & Longobardi, 2023). This national coalition was formed amid the COVID-19 pandemic, combining researchers, policy makers, and practitioners across the country to seek answers to the perennial question of how to improve nursing home quality, guided largely by the NASEM report. The coalition has proposed the creation of an evidence-informed guide to encourage state policymakers to use Medicaid incentive payment models, such as value-based payments to tie nursing home quality goals to payment increases (or decreases for goals not met). Few states have considered wage increases or other staffing metrics within their incentive payment programs (Bonner & Longobardi, 2023).

CNA Training, Advancement, and Empowerment

A second key focus of the Moving Forward Coalition is developing CNA career pathways, including programs that support CNAs who wish to advance into higher-paid leadership positions. It starts, however, with strong CNA training. Research has found that clinical and didactic training provided at CNAs' work sites increases their skills and efficiency (Mileski et al., 2016). One approach promoted by Moving Forward is the creation of apprenticeship programs to develop nationally recognized credentials to support CNA advancement (Bonner & Longobardi, 2023).

A study on how to keep CNAs from leaving their jobs identified a two-fold strategy that included strong wages but also involved empowering them (Kennedy et al., 2022). The study's "empowerment" measure considered staff teamwork, CNA involvement in quality improvement and hiring decisions, and having a clear career ladder for CNAs. Neither higher wages nor greater empowerment alone increased CNA retention. Both efforts were needed.

Mentoring and Leadership Development

Research during the pandemic found multiple examples of direct care workers, as well as managers, showing individual leadership and dedication to nursing home resident care during the most difficult days of the pandemic (Boamah et al., 2023; Dohmen et al., 2022). In their qualitative work, Cockshott et al. (2024) highlighted direct care staff who demonstrated strong teamwork and peer support, proactive problem-solving, and a sense of responsibility to their residents. In a study of direct care workers in general, Yip et al. (2024) described environments in which aides received substantial support from nurses. They established bonds through ongoing open interactions and collaboration, which helped to build self-efficacy among the aides.

Staff Satisfaction and Retention

The NASEM report (2022) identified the lack of respect and appreciation from supervisors as the top reason direct care workers leave their jobs, above inadequate pay and benefits. Research from the pandemic identified administrative leadership as critical to the management of the emergency (Berridge et al., 2020; Danesh et al., 2024; Johnston et al., 2021; Vogelsmeier et al., 2024). Martin et al. (2023) described the philosophies and practices of the leaders of nursing homes and assisted living communities considered to be exemplary by the Quality Improvement Program for Missouri (QIPMO). Each demonstrated a "transformational" leadership style characterized by team building, trust, and open communication with staff. As one of the administrators said, *"The only things I did differently were to have heart and flexibility...We educated, shared information timely, and didn't lose their trust"* (p. 22). Another said: *"There were no set rules. We made it work each day. We let people swap shifts to make it work. Staff saw our flexibility and effort and they stepped up"* (p. 23). Another described the charge nurse in the nursing home personally thanking each CNA at the end of the shifts.

Among their other practices were the creation of mentor and mentee incentives and encouraging staff to choose coworkers to receive recognition for their notable acts, enabling the chosen workers to receive some paid time off (Martin et al., 2023). Importantly, they went beyond infection control guidelines, providing additional education to all staff, demanding compliance, and being consistent in all communications while also supporting staff directly affected by COVID-19. One of them developed a practice of sending PPE and food to staff when a positive test result or illness prevented them from coming to work.

Many of these ideas and practices emerged in a list of staff-focused recommendations developed by an international group of long-term care researchers during the pandemic (McGilton et al., 2020; See Box 7.1). Their goal was to bring attention to the struggles of nursing home staff and the "devaluation" of their labor during the pandemic, but also to emphasize the need for leaders who understand that the health promotion of residents depends on staff stability. Many of the recommendations are pandemic-specific, but many others apply to the everyday operation of a nursing home.

Box 7.1 Supporting Staff in Nursing Homes During a Pandemic
Provide Clear Direction and Guidance

1. Promote daily huddles with staff to provide updates and address concerns.
2. Provide more 1:1 engagement between supervisors and staff with an emphasis on appreciation of the work being done.
3. Develop a leadership group that is available 24 h a day to communicate information and provide hands-on support to staff.
4. Consider the use of messaging platforms (e.g., a national and multiple regional WhatsApp group) to efficiently disseminate guidelines to managers and staff in a timely manner.
5. Encourage managers to prioritize ongoing communication with infection control officers.
6. Curate useful and clear resources for staff, residents, and their families; post them online in an easily accessible format; and broadly disseminate information.
7. Ensure at least 1 manager is physically present to address questions and concerns of staff on all shifts.

Keep Staff Healthy

8. Pay close attention to the emotional health and well-being of staff and offer stress management as well as grief support services without cost to staff.
9. Provide daily meals and snacks to staff, as well as open a "quick market" so staff can buy food before returning home.
10. Keep staff motivated and support staff morale by displaying letters of gratitude from families and the public.
11. Maintain weekly virtual rounds between medical care providers, consultants, and nursing home staff to discuss clinical care issues.
12. Assure staff of appropriate hours, including no overtime and provide rest periods to avoid burnout.

Implement Human Resource Policies

13. Optimize the use of health sciences students.
14. Implement hazard and sick leave pay and offer full-time employment and staffing flexibility.
15. Increase staffing by redeploying and educating staff from other health care facilities, such as hospitals, to work in nursing homes.

Implement New Clinical Practices Related to COVID-19

16. End-of-life care including advanced care planning, symptom relief, and postmortem care.
17. Human connectedness strategies to minimize resident isolation.
18. Policies regarding transfers of COVID-19 residents to and from hospitals.
19. Decision-making guidelines for developing infection control and isolation care plans (Ethical guidance for people who work in long-term care: What is the right thing to do in a pandemic? (https://bit.ly/dementiatoolkit). (Source: McGilton et al., 2020)).[1]

As another resource applying to everyday nursing home circumstances, the Centers for Medicare and Medicaid Services developed a toolkit (CMS, 2019) focusing on five areas: 1) job satisfaction, 2) team building and communication, 3) scheduling and staffing, 4) training, and 5) management and leadership—with each designed to help leadership to identify staff perceptions and develop workable plans to improve staff satisfaction and performance. Additional recommendations from Travers et al. (2024) include

- Ensuring all staff and managers are culturally competent
- Creating a retention specialist position, which could be part-time
- Conducting exit interviews to assess why staff leave
- Developing programs to increase workers' problem-solving skills
- Ensuring CNAs are included in interdisciplinary teams and resident care planning, as CMS requires.

Travers et al. (2024) underscored that supervisors have a powerful role in workers' lives, often having more influence than anyone else over whether a worker believes they have any value in the organization. This was especially true during the pandemic. In their report for the AARP, they quoted a nursing home supervisor who said, "Workers don't leave their jobs; they leave their supervisors."

Conclusion

Long-standing challenges in long-term care facilities, such as chronic understaffing, high turnover rates, and insufficient employee retention strategies, were exacerbated by the COVID-19 pandemic. Despite implementing measures like mask mandates and lockdowns, these facilities faced significant adverse/negative impacts from the infection. The significant staffing shortages, attributed to rising infection rates among residents and staff, highlight the urgent need for structural enhancements to better safeguard older adults and support the professionals who provide their care. During the COVID-19 pandemic, nursing homes experienced a significant increase in workloads, resulting in staff members feeling overextended and fatigued. Various studies indicated that employees experienced heightened levels of stress, anxiety, frustration, and chronic exhaustion. Many facilities struggled to maintain a steady workforce and often relied on contract or temporary staff to fill vacancies. To address these challenges and ensure the delivery of sustainable, high-quality care, it is essential to increase staffing levels, offer competitive compensation, empower employees, and foster a culture of teamwork.

References

American Health Care Association/National Center for Assisted Living. (2024). State of the nursing home sector: Survey of 441 nursing home providers highlights persistent staffing and economic crisis. https://www.ahcancal.org/News-and-Communications/Fact-Sheets/FactSheets/AHCA%20State%20of%20the%20Sector%202024.pdf.

Armijo-Olivo, S., Craig, R., Corabian, P., Guo, B., Souri, S., & Tjosvold, L. (2020). Nursing staff time and care quality in long-term care facilities: A systematic review. *The Gerontologist, 60*(3), e200–e217.

Amblàs-Novellas, J., Coll-Planas, L., Jerez-Roig, J., López, D., Martori, J. C., Ramon-Aribau, A., et al. (2024). Evaluation of the impact of the Covid-19 pandemic on people and organisations in long-term care facilities of Catalonia and proposals for improving the care model: The resicovid-19 project. *Journal of Long-Term Care*, 1–13.

Bahr, K. O., Bhavsar, G. P., & Zhao, D. (2023). "We are still tired": Staff and administrators' experiences during the COVID-19 pandemic within California residential care facilities for older adults. *BMC Geriatrics, 23*(1), 868–868. https://doi.org/10.1186/s12877-023-04537-2

Battams, S., & Martini, A. (2024). Impact of COVID-19 on the residential aged care workforce, and workers from culturally and linguistically diverse backgrounds: A rapid literature review. *Ageing International*, 1–36.

Beltran, S. J., Wagner, J., Dorris, L., & Miller, V. J. (2024). Navigating the storm: Challenges and career implications for nursing home administrators in the wake of COVID-19. *Journal of Gerontological Nursing, 50*(6), 17–24. https://doi.org/10.3928/00989134-20240502-04

Berridge, C., Lima, J., Schwartz, M., Bishop, C., & Miller, S. C. (2020). Leadership, staff empowerment, and the retention of nursing assistants: Findings from a survey of US nursing homes. *Journal of the American Medical Directors Association, 21*(9), 1254–1259.

Birt, L., Lane, K., Corner, J., Sanderson, K., & Bunn, D. (2023). Care-home nurses' responses to the COVID-19 pandemic: Managing ethical conundrums at personal cost. *Journal of Nursing Scholarship, 55*(1), 226–238. https://doi.org/10.1111/jnu.12855

Boamah, S. A., Weldrick, R., Havaei, F., Irshad, A., & Hutchinson, A. (2023). Experiences of healthcare workers in long-term care during COVID-19: A scoping review. *Journal of Applied Gerontology, 42*(5), 1118–1136.

Bonner, A., & Longobardi, I. (2023). Building a stronger direct care workforce: The moving forward nursing home quality coalition is taking action now. *Caring for the Ages, 24*(8), 19.

Boscart, V. M., Sidani, S., Poss, J., Davey, M., d'Avernas, J., Brown, P., & Costa, A. P. (2018). The associations between staffing hours and quality of care indicators in long-term care. *BMC Health Services Research, 18*, 1–7.

Bowblis, J. R., Brunt, C. S., Xu, H., Applebaum, R., & Grabowski, D. C. (2024). Nursing homes increasingly rely on staffing agencies for direct care nursing: Study examines nursing home staffing. *Health Affairs, 43*(3), 327–335. https://doi.org/10.1377/hlthaff.2023.01101

Bourbonniere, M., Feng, Z., Intrator, O., Angelelli, J., Mor, V., & Zinn, J. S. (2006). The use of contract licensed nursing staff in US nursing homes. *Medical Care Research and Review, 63*(1), 88–109.

Brazier, J. F., Geng, F., Meehan, A., White, E. M., McGarry, B. E., Shield, R. R., Grabowski, D. C., Rahman, M., Santostefano, C., & Gadbois, E. A. (2023). Examination of staffing shortages at US nursing homes during the COVID-19 pandemic. *JAMA Network Open, 6*(7), e2325993. https://doi.org/10.1001/jamanetworkopen.2023.25993

Bryant, N. S., Cimarolli, V. R., Falzarano, F., & Stone, R. (2023). Organizational factors associated with certified nursing assistants' job satisfaction during COVID-19. *Journal of Applied Gerontology*. Advance online publication. https://doi.org/10.1177/07334648231155017

Bunn, D., Brainard, J., Lane, K., Salter, C., & Lake, I. (2021). The lived experience of implementing infection control measures in care homes during two waves of the COVID-19 pandemic: A mixed-methods study. *MedRxiv*. https://doi.org/10.1101/2021.07.15.21260598

Castle, N. G., & Anderson, R. A. (2011). Caregiver staffing in nursing homes and their influence on quality of care: Using dynamic panel estimation methods. *Medical Care, 49*(6), 545–552.

Castle, N. G., & Engberg, J. (2007). The influence of staffing characteristics on quality of care in nursing homes. *Health Services Research, 42*(5), 1822–1847.

Castle, N. G., Engberg, J., & Men, A. (2007). Nursing home staff turnover: Impact on nursing home compare quality measures. *The Gerontologist, 47*(5), 650–661.

Chen, M. M., & Grabowski, D. C. (2015). Intended and unintended consequences of minimum staffing standards for nursing homes. *Health Economics, 24*(7), 822–839.

Cockshott, Z., Russell, S., Stocker, R., Knight, J., Mason, S., Hanratty, B., & Preston, N. (2024). 'In the shower crying…but we came back in the following day and did it all again': Distress and resilience in care home staff during the COVID-19 pandemic– A qualitative interview study. *BMC Geriatrics, 24*(1), 286–286. https://doi.org/10.1186/s12877-024-04804-w

CMS. (2019). Guide to improving nursing home employee satisfaction. https://www.cms.gov/files/document/cmprp-toolkit-3-guide-staff-satisfaction.pdf.

Danesh, B., Freeman, S., Jackson, P., Klassen-Ross, T., Freeman-Idemilih, A., & Banner, D. (2024). Staff resiliency in long-term care during the COVID-19 pandemic: A qualitative study. *COVID, 4*(6), 731–748.

de Perio, M. A., Srivastav, A., Razzaghi, H., Laney, A. S., & Black, C. L. (2023). Paid sick leave among US healthcare personnel, April 2022. *American Journal of Preventive Medicine, 65*(3), 521–527.

Dill, J., Frogner, B., & Travers, J. (2022). Taking the long view: Understanding the rate of second job holding among long-term care workers. *Medical Care Research and Review, 79*(6), 844–850. https://doi.org/10.1177/10775587221089414

Dohmen, M. D., van den Eijnde, C., Thielman, C. L., Lindenberg, J., Huijg, J. M., & Abma, T. A. (2022). A narrative approach to care home staff's.

Espinoza, R. (2020). *Competitive disadvantage: Direct care wages are lagging behind.* PHI. https://www.phinational.org/resource/competitive-disadvantage-direct-carewages-are-lagging-behind.

Estabrooks, C. A., Straus, S. E., Flood, C. M., Keefe, J., Armstrong, P., Donner, G. J., Boscart, V., Ducharme, F., Silvius, J. L., & Wolfson, M. C. (2020). Restoring trust: COVID-19 and the future of long-term care in Canada. *Facets, 5*(1), 651–691. https://doi.org/10.1139/facets-2020-0056

Gary, M., & Berlinger, N. (2020). Interdependent citizens: The ethics of care in pandemic recovery. *Hastings Center Report, 50*(3), 56–58.

Gasdaska, A., Segelman, M., Porter, K. A., Huber, B., Feng, Z., Barch, D., Squillace, M., Dey, J., & Oliveira, I. (2022, September 12). *Nursing home staffing disparities were exacerbated during the COVID-19 pandemic in 2020 (research brief).* Office of the Assistant Secretary for Planning and Evaluation, U.S. Department of Health and Human Services.

Geng, F., Stevenson, D. G., & Grabowski, D. C. (2019). Daily nursing home staffing levels highly variable, often below CMS expectations. *Health Aff (Millwood), 38*(7), 1095–1100. https://doi.org/10.1377/hlthaff.2018.05322

Giebel, C., Hanna, K., Marlow, P., Cannon, J., Tetlow, H., Shenton, J., Faulkner, T., Rajagopal, M., Mason, S., & Gabbay, M. (2022). Guilt, tears and burnout—impact of UK care home restrictions on the mental well-being of staff, families and residents. *Journal of Advanced Nursing, 78*(7), 2191–2202.

Gibson, D. M., & Greene, J. (2020). Risk for severe COVID-19 illness among health care workers who work directly with patients. *Journal of General Internal Medicine, 35*(9), 2804–2806.

Hackett, S. E., Peterson, L. J., Vogel, C. E., & Dobbs, D. (2023). "We did more damage": How COVID-19 collapsed the care convoys of residents living with dementia. *Journal of Applied Gerontology, 42*(7), 1565–1573.

Holmes, P., Santurri, L., Ewen, H. H., & Baggett, S. (2024). The experiences of skilled nursing staff in memory care units during the COVID-19 pandemic. *The Gerontologist, 64*(4), gnad108. https://doi.org/10.1093/geront/gnad108

Hutt, E., Radcliff, T. A., Liebrecht, D., Fish, R., McNulty, M., & Kramer, A. M. (2008). Associations among nurse and certified nursing assistant hours per resident per day and adherence to guidelines for treating nursing home-acquired pneumonia. *The Journals of Gerontology Series A: Biological Sciences and Medical Sciences, 63*(10), 1105–1111.

Hyer, K., Thomas, K. S., Branch, L. G., Harman, J. S., Johnson, C. E., & Weech-Maldonado, R. (2011). The influence of nurse staffing levels on quality of care in nursing homes. *The Gerontologist, 51*(5), 610–616.

Johnston, L., Malcolm, C., Rambabu, L., Hockley, J., & Shenkin, S. D. (2021). Practice based approaches to supporting the work related wellbeing of frontline care workers in care homes: A scoping review. *Journal of Long-Term Care, 2021*, 230–240.

Jutkowitz, E., Landsteiner, A., Ratner, E., Shippee, T., Madrigal, C., Ullman, K., et al. (2023). Effects of nurse staffing on resident outcomes in nursing homes: A systematic review. *Journal of the American Medical Directors Association, 24*(1), 75–81.

Kennedy, K. A., Abbott, K. M., & Bowblis, J. R. (2022). The one-two punch of high wages and empowerment on CNA retention. *Journal of Applied Gerontology, 41*(2), 312–321.

Kennedy, K. A., & Bowblis, J. R. (2023). Does higher worker retention buffer against consumer complaints? Evidence from Ohio nursing homes. *The Gerontologist, 63*(1), 96–107.

Kim, H., Kovner, C., Harrington, C., Greene, W., & Mezey, M. (2009). A panel data analysis of the relationships of nursing home staffing levels and standards to regulatory deficiencies. *Journals of Gerontology: Series B, 64*(2), 269–278.

Krein, S. L., Turnwald, M., Anderson, B., & Maust, D. T. (2022). “Sometimes it's not about the money… it's the way you treat people…”: A qualitative study of nursing home staff turnover. *Journal of the American Medical Directors Association, 23*(7), 1178–1184.

Konetzka, R. T., Stearns, S. C., & Park, J. (2008). The staffing–outcomes relationship in nursing homes. *Health Services Research, 43*(3), 1025–1042.

Kyler-Yano, J. Z., Tunalilar, O., Hasworth, S., Kohon, J., Winfree, J., Wilton, R., et al. (2022). “What keeps me awake at night”: Assisted living administrator responses to COVID-19. *The Gerontologist, 62*(2), 190–199.

Lai, J., Ma, S., Wang, Y., Cai, Z., Hu, J., Wei, N., Wu, J., Du, H., Chen, T., Li, R., Tan, H., Kang, L., Yao, L., Huang, M., Wang, H., Wang, G., Liu, Z., & Hu, S. (2020). Factors associated with mental health outcomes among health care workers exposed to coronavirus disease 2019. *JAMA Network Open, 3*(3), e203976. https://doi.org/10.1001/jamanetworkopen.2020.3976

Lakon, C. M., & Hipp, J. R. (2024). Socio-spatial health disparities in Covid-19 cases and deaths in United States skilled nursing facilities over 30 months. *American Journal of Infection Control, 52*(1), 3–14. https://doi.org/10.1016/j.ajic.2023.07.008

Lee, H. Y., Blegen, M. A., & Harrington, C. (2014). The effects of RN staffing hours on nursing home quality: A two-stage model. *International Journal of Nursing Studies, 51*(3), 409–417.

Leland, N. E., Prusynski, R. A., Shore, A. D., Cary, M. P., Jr., Falvey, J., Mroz, T., & Saliba, D. (2024). Skilled nursing facility staffing shortages: Sources, strategies, and impacts on staff who stayed. *Health Services Research*. https://doi.org/10.1111/1475-6773.14355

Lerner, N. B., Johantgen, M., Trinkoff, A. M., Storr, C. L., & Han, K. (2014). Are nursing home survey deficiencies higher in facilities with greater staff turnover. *Journal of the American Medical Directors Association, 15*(2), 102–107.

Lin, H. (2014). Revisiting the relationship between nurse staffing and quality of care in nursing homes: An instrumental variables approach. *Journal of Health Economics, 37*, 13–24.

Loomer, L., Grabowski, D. C., Yu, H., & Gandhi, A. (2022). Association between nursing home staff turnover and infection control citations. *Health Services Research, 57*(2), 322–332.

Martin, N., Frank, B., Farrell, D., Brady, C., Dixon-Hall, J., Mueller, J., & Rantz, M. (2023). Sharing lessons from successes: Long-term care facilities that weathered the storm of COVID-19 and staffing crises. *Journal of Nursing Care Quality, 38*(1), 19–25.

McGarry, B. E., Porter, L., & Grabowski, D. (2020, July 28). Nursing home workers now have the most dangerous jobs in America. They deserve better. 2020.[Opinion]. The Washington Post. https://www.washingtonpost.com/opinions/2020/07/28/nursing-home-workers-now-have-most-dangerous-jobs-america-they-deserve-better/.

McGilton, K. S., Escrig-Pinol, A., Gordon, A., Chu, C. H., Zúñiga, F., Sanchez, M. G., et al. (2020). Uncovering the devaluation of nursing home staff during COVID-19: Are we fueling the next health care crisis? *Journal of the American Medical Directors Association, 21*(7), 962–965.

Mileski, M., McIlwain, A. S., Scott Kruse, C., Lieneck, C., & Sokan, A. (2016). The effectiveness and need for facility based nurse aide training competency evaluation programs. *ABNF Journal, 27*(1).

Mukamel, D. B., Saliba, D., Ladd, H., & Konetzka, R. T. (2024). The relationship between nursing home staffing and health outcomes revisited. *Journal of the American Medical Directors Association, 105081*.

National Academies of Science, Engineering, and Medicine. (2022). *The national imperative to improve nursing home quality: Honoring our commitment to residents, families, and staff*. The National Academies Press. https://doi.org/10.17226/26526

Orth, J., Li, Y., Simning, A., Zimmerman, S., & Temkin-Greener, H. (2021). End-of-life care among nursing home residents with dementia varies by nursing home and market characteristics. *Journal of the American Medical Directors Association, 22*(2), 320–328.

PHI. (2021). Direct care workers in the United States: Key facts. https://phinational.org/resource/direct-care-workers-in-theunitedstates-key-facts-2/

Regan, T. "Average assisted living resident manages more than 14 chronic conditions." Senior Housing News, September 14, 2022.

Ramanan, H., Shensa, A., Guth, V., Rhoads, C., & Linkov, F. (2024). Attitudes and preferences about retention: A survey study of nursing home employees. *Geriatric Nursing (New York), 60*, 186–190. https://doi.org/10.1016/j.gerinurse.2024.08.044

Sarabia-Cobo, C., Pérez, V., de Lorena, P., Hermosilla-Grijalbo, C., Sáenz-Jalón, M., Fernández-Rodríguez, A., & Alconero-Camarero, A. R. (2021). Experiences of geriatric nurses in nursing home settings across four countries in the face of the COVID-19 pandemic. *Journal of Advanced Nursing, 77*(2), 869–878.

Shen, K., McGarry, B. E., Grabowski, D. C., Gruber, J., & Gandhi, A. D. (2022). Staffing patterns in US nursing homes during COVID-19 outbreaks. *JAMA Health Forum, 3*(7), e222151.

Shen, K., McGarry, B. E., & Gandhi, A. D. (2023). Health care staff turnover and quality of care at nursing homes. *JAMA Internal Medicine, 183*(11), 1247–1254.

Siskind, D., Dhansew, T., Burns, A., & Burns, E. (2024). Increasing illness severity of skilled nursing facility patients over time: Implications for readmission penalties. *Journal of the American Geriatrics Society, 72*(1), 160–169.

Snyder, R. L., Anderson, L. E., White, K. A., Tavitian, S., Fike, L. V., Jones, H. N., Jacobs-Slifka, K. M., Stone, N. D., & Sinkowitz-Cochran, R. L. (2021). A qualitative assessment of factors affecting nursing home caregiving staff experiences during the COVID-19 pandemic. *PLoS One, 16*(11), e0260055. https://doi.org/10.1371/journal.pone.0260055

Stepick, L., Hailer, L., Scales, K., & Wagner, L. M. (2024). *The increase in contract CNA staffing in U.S. nursing homes and associated care quality outcomes*. UCSF Health Workforce Research Center on Long-Term Care. https://healthworkforce.ucsf.edu/sites/healthworkforce.ucsf.edu/files/HWRC%20Report%20-%20Increase%20Contract%20CNA%20Staffing%20Jan2024.pdf.

Thomas, K. S., Mor, V., Tyler, D. A., & Hyer, K. (2013). The relationships among licensed nurse turnover, retention, and rehospitalization of nursing home residents. *The Gerontologist, 53*(2), 211–221.

Thomas, K. S., Zhang, W., Dosa, D. M., Carder, P., Sloane, P., & Zimmerman, S. (2021). Estimation of excess mortality rates among US assisted living residents during the COVID-19 pandemic. *JAMA Network Open, 4*(6), e2113411.

Travers, J.L., Choula, R., & Hado, E. (2024). Nursing home workforce issues and inequities. AARP Public Policy Institute. https://ltsschoices.aarp.org/resources-and-practices/nursing-home-workforce-issues-and-inequities.

Trinkoff, A. M., Han, K., Storr, C. L., Lerner, N., Johantgen, M., & Gartrell, K. (2013). Turnover, staffing, skill mix, and resident outcomes in a national sample of US nursing homes. *The Journal of Nursing Administration, 43*(12), 630–536.

U.S. Bureau of Labor Statistics. Nursing Assistants and Orderlies. Published August 2024. Accessed December 20, 2024. https://www.bls.gov/ooh/healthcare/nursing-assistants.htm.

U.S. House Committee on Oversight and Accountability. (2023, May 18). *Hearing wrap up: "Must-admit" COVID-19 nursing home mandates were deadly for elderly Americans, state officials responsible* [Press release]. https://oversight.house.gov/release/hearing-wrap-up-must-admit-covid-19-nursing-home-mandates-were-deadly-for-elderly-americans-state-officials-responsible%EF%BF%BC/

Vogel, C. E., Dobbs, D., Peterson, L., Meng, H., & Molinari, V. (2024). The impact of assisted living organizational structure and process characteristics on staff absence during COVID-19. *Journal of Aging & Social Policy*, 1–17.

Vogelsmeier, A., Popejoy, L. L., Johnson, A. H., Miller, S., Young, L., Thompson, R. A., et al. (2024). Nursing home leader response during COVID-19: A qualitative descriptive study about use of external resources during the pandemic. *BMC Health Services Research, 24*(1), 1–11.

White, E. M., Wetle, T. F., Reddy, A., & Baier, R. R. (2021). Front-line nursing home staff experiences during the COVID-19 pandemic. *Journal of the American Medical Directors Association, 22*(1), 199–203.

Yip, A., Yip, J., Tsui, Z., & Smith, G. D. (2024, August). Navigating uncertainty with compassion: Healthcare assistants' reflections on balancing COVID-19 and routine care through adversity. In *Healthcare* (Vol. 12, p. 1544). MDPI.

Zimmerman, S., Carder, P., Schwartz, L., Silbersack, J., Temkin-Greener, H., Thomas, K. S., et al. (2022). The imperative to reimagine assisted living. *Journal of the American Medical Directors Association, 23*(2), 225–234.

Chapter 8
Palliative Care in Long-Term Care

Frances M. Hawes and Lisa Quinn-Lee

Introduction

Palliative care originated from the hospice movement of the mid-twentieth century (Jakubów et al., 2023; MacDonald et al., 2022). As this movement evolved, it became clear that its core principles—such as pain management, symptom relief, and holistic support—were also valuable for patients with serious illnesses that were not necessarily terminal (Jakubów et al., 2023; Zehnder et al., 2022). This understanding led to the development of palliative care as a distinct specialty. In 1990, the World Health Organization recognized palliative care as a separate field, expanding its focus beyond end-of-life care to improve the quality of life for patients at any stage of a serious illness. In 2006, palliative care was officially recognized as a medical specialty in the United States by the American Board of Medical Specialties and the Accreditation Council for Graduate Medical Education (Morrison, 2013).

Palliative care programs encompass a range of services aimed at improving the quality of life for both the patient and their family. These services include minimizing pain and discomfort. Importantly, while palliative care focuses on enhancing comfort and quality of life, it is designed to complement rather than replace curative treatments. This means that palliative care can be provided alongside curative therapies, offering support throughout the treatment process and addressing symptoms that arise from both the illness and its treatments. The overall goal is to provide

F. M. Hawes (✉)
Health Care Administration Department, University of Wisconsin Eau Claire,
Eau Claire, WI, USA
e-mail: HAWESFM@uwec.edu

L. Quinn-Lee
Department of Social Work, University of Wisconsin Eau Claire, Eau Claire, WI, USA
e-mail: QUINNLLM@uwec.edu

K. K. Bhattacharyya (ed.), *Health Promotion in Long-Term Care Facilities*,
https://doi.org/10.1007/978-3-031-91038-8_8

holistic care that addresses the physical, emotional, and spiritual needs of individuals facing serious illness, ensuring that their experience is as comfortable and meaningful as possible. Despite its broader focus, significant confusion often surrounds the term *palliative care*, with many people mistakenly equating it with hospice care. While both services prioritize symptom management and the alleviation of suffering, they serve different purposes. Palliative care can be provided at any stage of a serious illness and does not require a terminal diagnosis. It offers benefits to patients of all ages. In contrast, hospice care is a specialized form of palliative care specifically designed for those nearing the end of life and requires a physician's certification of a terminal diagnosis with an expected lifespan of 6 months or less. Although hospice care falls under the broader umbrella of palliative care, not all palliative care is hospice care.

It is worth mentioning that individuals can transition between palliative care and hospice based on their evolving health needs. For example, if an individual's condition worsens, they may decide to move to hospice care for more intensive support. Conversely, if an individual's health improves or stabilizes, they might *graduate from hospice* (i.e., a patient's condition improves to the extent that they no longer qualify for hospice care) and be able to return to palliative care for ongoing symptom management and support. Both services emphasize flexibility and the patient's preferences, allowing families to navigate care options that best suit their circumstances.

Around 90 million Americans are currently living with serious illnesses, and this number is projected to more than double over the next 25 years as the baby boomer generation continues to age (Center to Advance Palliative Care, 2014). Yet, talking about death is frequently challenging and, combined with a general lack of understanding about palliative care, leads to insufficient use of these services. Globally, around 56.8 million people require palliative care each year, including 25.7 million who are in their final year of life. Despite this, only about 14% of those in need access palliative care (World Health Organization, 2022). In the United States, while approximately 12 million individuals could benefit from palliative care annually, only about 6 million actually receive it (Center to Advance Palliative Care, 2021).

The Role of Palliative Care in Health Promotion

During the later decades of the twentieth century, health promotion emerged as a response to the limitations of the biomedical model, which prioritized disease diagnosis, treatment, and cure while neglecting the complex interrelationships between physical, psychological, and social components of health (World Health Organization, 1995). This model's separation of disease from the person and the person from their social context led to calls for a more integrated approach to health.

The Ottawa Charter for Health Promotion, developed by the World Health Organization in 1986, marked a pivotal shift in this direction. It outlined five key action areas essential for improving health: building healthy public policy, creating supportive environments, strengthening community action, developing personal skills, and reorienting health services. The Charter emphasized that health promotion is a shared responsibility extending beyond the healthcare sector to include governments, social and economic sectors, industry, the media, and communities (World Health Organization, 1986).

Health-promoting palliative care (HPPC) began to take shape in the early 2000s, reflecting these principles by expanding the focus of traditional palliative care. HPPC integrates health promotion with palliative care, recognizing the need to address not only symptom management but also overall well-being and community engagement. Influenced by Allan Kellehear's (2013) "Compassionate Communities" model, HPPC advocates for embedding palliative care within community life, fostering a supportive environment that involves public participation in end-of-life care. To implement HPPC effectively, the comprehensive approach of the Ottawa Charter is applied to integrate palliative care into community life, addressing the full range of medical, social, emotional, and spiritual needs.

Benefits of Palliative Care

Holistic Approach to Care

A holistic approach to palliative care addresses patients' psychological, social, physical, and spiritual needs, aligning with health promotion goals even at the end of life. This approach acknowledges the multidimensional nature of health and well-being. The "National Consensus Project for Quality Palliative Care Guidelines" by the National Coalition for Hospice and Palliative Care (Ferrell et al.,, 2018) emphasizes enhancing patients' quality of life within this framework.

Psychological The psychological aspects of care emphasize the importance of addressing mental health processes, thoughts, feelings, and emotions. Addressing these needs is a critical component of palliative care, as patients with serious illnesses often experience a range of feelings, including anxiety, depression, fear, and uncertainty. Effective palliative care includes helping patients and families navigate and cope with the psychological challenges associated with illness and end of life. Support includes counseling and therapy, providing a safe space for open communication so patients feel heard and validated, and enhancing their emotional resilience and overall well-being. The goal is to not only alleviate psychological distress but also empower patients to express their feelings and concerns, fostering a sense of control and reducing the emotional burden on both patients and caregivers.

Social The social aspects of care may include factors like family dynamics, financial concerns, feeling cared for, having assistance available when needed, and being part of a social network. Cultural aspects stress the importance of culturally competent care that respects diverse backgrounds. Family support is also needed throughout the illness and into bereavement (Ferrel et al., 2018). Due to the patient- and family-centered nature of effective palliative care, there is greater satisfaction with the care (Cole et al., 2024; Unroe et al., 2023). Increased communication, extra support, and increased services are offered to both the patient and family (Cole et al., 2024), with one key aspect being bereavement services and other support to the family after the patient dies (Persson et al., 2022).

Physical Managing physical symptoms is a cornerstone of palliative care, aiming to improve the quality of life by managing pain and other distressing symptoms in order to improve comfort, function, and dignity. This can include the use of medications, physical therapy, and complementary therapies to control pain, ease nausea, reduce fatigue, manage breathlessness, and improve sleep, thereby improving the patient's overall physical well-being. This involves a tailored approach, including medications, physical therapy, and complementary and holistic therapies. By effectively managing these physical symptoms, patients can participate in daily activities and interact meaningfully with their loved ones.

Spiritual Spiritual and religious needs are acknowledged and respected in palliative care, recognizing that many patients find comfort and meaning through their spiritual beliefs and practices. Spiritual care involves providing support that respects patients' beliefs, values, and cultural practices and addressing existential concerns related to suffering, meaning, and death. By integrating spiritual care into the broader framework of palliative care, healthcare providers can help patients find peace and acceptance, enhancing their overall sense of well-being.

Advance Care Planning

Advance care planning (ACP) is part of palliative care and helps patients make informed decisions about their future medical care needs. Advance care planning is a process that involves discussions about a person's preferences and wishes for medical care in the event that they are unable to make decisions for themselves due to illness or incapacity. This process typically results in the documentation of these preferences in legal forms known as advance directives, which include living wills and healthcare proxies. In addition to outlining specific medical wishes, advance directives can also include the designation of a durable power of attorney for health care. This allows an individual to appoint a trusted person, known as a healthcare proxy or agent, to make medical decisions on their behalf if they are incapacitated. The healthcare proxy is responsible for ensuring that all aspects of the individual's advance directive are followed, thereby upholding the patient's end-of-life care preferences (National Institute on Aging, 2022). These documents guide healthcare providers and family members in making decisions that align with the individual's values, goals, and treatment preferences, particularly at the end of life (National Institute on Aging, 2022).

Advance care planning practices can vary significantly across different US states and internationally due to differences in legal frameworks, cultural norms, and healthcare policies. In the United States, for instance, each state has its own laws governing advance directives, including living wills, healthcare proxies, and medical power of attorney documents. These laws may dictate specific requirements regarding the format, witnessing, and validity of these documents.

Additional Benefits

Additional benefits of palliative care include cost savings (Cole et al., 2024; Miller et al., 2017; Naoum et al., 2024), lower rates of hospitalization (Lima & Miller, 2018; Liu et al., 2024; Miller et al., 2017; Unroe et al., 2023), reduced number of unnecessary medications (Lima & Miller, 2018) and medical interventions (Liu et al., 2024), and higher quality of life (Cole et al., 2024; Lima & Miller, 2018; Liu et al., 2024; Miller et al., 2017).

Quality/Practice Guidelines

Quality in palliative care is regulated and enforced by several standards and bodies. The Centers for Medicare & Medicaid Services play a major role by setting specific conditions of participation for palliative services and hospice care. The Joint Commission offers certification programs that require adherence to quality metrics, such as patient satisfaction, pain control, and care transitions. Additionally, palliative care programs must report data on outcomes like symptom burden, advance care planning, and readmission rates, which are evaluated during periodic reviews and audits. Organizations such as the National Quality Forum develop measures that ensure consistency in quality standards across different care settings.

Furthermore, compliance with the National Consensus Project Clinical Practice Guidelines is often evaluated during accreditation processes. These guidelines address eight key domains, including communication, spiritual care, and continuity, with measurable targets to assess the effectiveness of care. Failure to meet these regulatory requirements can lead to sanctions, loss of certification, or funding penalties, ensuring that quality standards are consistently enforced across the field (Ferrell et al., 2018).

Models of Palliative and Hospice Care Across Long-Term Care Settings

Palliative and hospice care are provided by an interdisciplinary team in various settings, including homes, communities, outpatient centers like pain and symptom management clinics, community living centers, and inpatient facilities. This broad availability ensures that palliative care can be tailored to meet the needs of patients at various stages and with different types of illnesses. However, the exact number of agencies delivering palliative care across all settings in the United States is not consistently tracked, as it can vary based on service models and regional availability (Center to Advance Palliative Care, 2022).

Home and Community-Based Care

Palliative care at home is usually provided by an interdisciplinary team that includes various professionals. Care can be delivered within the community or directly in a patient's home. Palliative home care can be offered to patients who encounter difficulties leaving home, without needing to be classified as homebound. The essential factor is that their medical condition makes traveling for care challenging. While not all members of the palliative care team may visit regularly, many offer home-based services. Palliative care physicians may conduct initial assessments and follow-up appointments at home and can also provide consultations via telehealth. Home health nurses typically visit to administer medications and monitor symptoms. Social workers often meet with patients and families at home to discuss resources and support, although some sessions may take place in the community or via phone or virtual meetings. Chaplains or spiritual care providers visit as needed to offer spiritual support, while home health and personal aides assist with personal care and daily activities regularly (e.g., instrumental activities of daily living and activities of daily living support). Occupational or physical therapists may conduct home visits based on patient needs, but they might also provide sessions at outpatient facilities. Meal delivery services can complement this care, and volunteers can also provide companionship and support in the home.

Hospice care can also be delivered at home, providing similar comprehensive support to patients with terminal illnesses and their families in a familiar environment. The hospice care team includes physicians, nurses, social workers, chaplains, and trained volunteers who work together to manage symptoms, provide emotional support, and assist with daily activities. They will visit the home regularly to ensure that the patient's needs are met and to help the family navigate the challenges of end-of-life care.

Overall, many services are provided at home, while others may be coordinated through clinics or virtual meetings, depending on the patient's circumstances and preferences.

Residential Care

In nursing homes, assisted living facilities, and continuing-care retirement communities, palliative care can be delivered through various approaches, including hospice partnerships, consultations with external clinical teams, and in-house teams or specialized palliative care units, each offering its own benefits (Kaasalainen et al., 2019; Tan, 2019).

Hospice In this model, the hospice organization takes the lead in providing end-of-life care through a multidisciplinary team that includes doctors, nurses, social workers, chaplains, and volunteers. Unlike other delivery models, the hospice agency assumes full responsibility for managing the patient's care, often reducing the involvement of the long-term care staff. The hospice team collaborates with the patient's primary care provider but takes the primary role in ensuring all aspects of care align with the hospice philosophy of comfort and dignity (Bull, 2016; Kelley & Meier, 2014). When nursing home residents enroll in hospice, the facility continues to provide room and board and ongoing clinical care and supportive services, while the hospice agency is responsible for overseeing the plan of care for the resident's terminal illness. The hospice agency supplements the resources available at the nursing home; additional services may include expert symptom assessment and management, personal care from the hospice agency's home health aides, spiritual counseling, social work services, and volunteer and bereavement services. The hospice agency also pays for medical supplies and medications but only for those related to the terminal condition.

External-Based Palliative Care The second model involves an external palliative care team working with the staff at a residential facility to provide care to a broader range of residents, including those with chronic conditions, without requiring them to forgo curative treatments. These external specialists bring expertise in managing complex symptoms, offering psychosocial support, and assisting with advance care planning. They collaborate with the facility's staff, who may lack specialized palliative care training, to ensure residents receive high-quality, personalized care. Unlike other models, this approach enhances care in complex cases but keeps overall responsibility with the facility's team. This model differs from hospice primarily in its focus and approach to care, as this external palliative care model is designed to support residents with serious or chronic illnesses, regardless of their stage in the disease process. In this model, residents can continue receiving curative treatments while also benefiting from palliative care. The focus is on managing symptoms and improving quality of life rather than exclusively on end-of-life care. Additionally, the overall responsibility for the resident's care remains with the nursing home staff, whereas in hospice care, the hospice team takes on primary responsibility (Bull, 2016; Kelley & Meier, 2014).

Facility-Based Palliative or Hospice Care The third model is facility-based palliative care, where nursing homes build their own palliative or hospice care capabilities internally, emphasizing staff training and creating a supportive culture. In this in-house end-of-life care model, the facility's staff—nurses, care aides, and on-site physicians—deliver end-of-life care, integrating palliative and hospice care into the daily routine. Hospice organizations may assist by providing training and resources (Bull, 2016; Kelley & Meier, 2014).

Who Pays for Palliative Care

Medicare

Medicare plans cover palliative care services, including inpatient care, outpatient care, and mental health counseling. Part A covers inpatient hospital stays, short-term skilled nursing facility care, limited home healthcare, and hospice care for those at the end of life. Part B includes doctor visits, durable medical equipment, outpatient rehabilitation therapy, and mental health counseling. Part C (Medicare Advantage) typically includes the same benefits as original Medicare, but it varies per plan. Part D covers prescription drugs, including those for symptom management in palliative care. However, individuals receiving palliative care but not enrolled in hospice may have out-of-pocket costs, such as premiums, deductibles, and co-payments.

To qualify for the Medicare Hospice Benefit, a patient must be certified as terminally ill with a life expectancy of 6 months or less and opt for comfort care over curative treatment. Hospice care is covered under Medicare Part A as a per diem rate and includes visits and services by an interprofessional team, medications and medical equipment related to the terminal diagnosis, volunteer services, and bereavement support for the family up to 13 months after the patient's death. Patients in nursing homes must pay for room and board separately. Medicare Part B, which generally covers outpatient medical services, plays a more limited role in hospice care. While Part A covers the core hospice services, Part B may still cover certain unrelated medical services that are not tied to the terminal illness (CMS, n.d.-a).

Medicaid

Medicaid is a state and federal assistance program that provides health coverage for individuals with very low incomes, regardless of age. Medicaid generally covers a range of palliative care services designed to enhance the quality of life for individuals with serious illnesses. These services typically include inpatient and outpatient care, home health services, and care coordination. However, coverage varies by state, and some palliative care team members, like chaplains, may not be covered.

Additionally, not all states clearly define palliative care services, leading to inconsistencies in coverage.

In contrast, Medicaid hospice care is a specialized program aimed specifically at providing care and comfort during the final months of a patient's life. The eligibility and services are similar to Medicare (CMS, n.d.-b).

Department of Veterans Health Administration (VHA)

The VHA covers a range of palliative care services for eligible veterans, including inpatient and outpatient care, and home-based services. The VHA also provides, purchases, or refers hospice care for more than 20,000 Veterans each year (U.S. Department of Veterans Affairs, n.d.). The eligibility is the same as it is under Medicare and Medicaid.

Insurance Policies

If a patient is not eligible for Medicare or Medicaid, private insurance may cover palliative care and/or hospice care. Coverage can vary widely based on the patient's plan. Patients may have co-payments or co-insurance, depending on their specific plan. For instance, there might be a co-payment for outpatient palliative care consultations or co-insurance for inpatient palliative care services (NIA, 2021).

Cross-Cultural Considerations in Palliative Care

Recognizing cultural rituals, beliefs, and values is essential throughout the care process, from diagnosis to the bereavement period after someone dies (Okan et al., 2019). The field of palliative care has recently recognized the importance of a cross-cultural approach to providing end-of-life care (Herbststomer & Stahl, 2021). However, due to having primarily White founders, palliative care as a specialty typically embodies beliefs, policies, and practices that encompass Western perspectives of death and dying. These approaches are not culturally accessible, safe, or appropriate for all groups. While global hospice use is rising, disparities persist among minority groups due to systemic racism, cultural differences around death and suffering, and language barriers (Bulle et al., 2023).

Some cultures may distrust hospice care because they have an inherent mistrust of physicians or Western medicine, whereas stigma or lack of awareness may also be factors for disparities (Herbststomer & Stahl, 2021). There may be differences in communication, family involvement, and pain management (Bulle et al., 2023; Herbststomer & Stahl, 2021). Also significant is how cultural norms around stoicism, how people express pain, and discrimination can all lead to inadequate pain assessment and management, alongside cultural values regarding opioid use, taboos around discussing death, place of death, and complementary medicine (Green et al., 2018).

Patients with limited English proficiency may face challenges in understanding their care, particularly as they tend to revert to their native language as they age. Relying on family interpreters can complicate accurate communication, while professional interpreters may present their own challenges. Cultural differences between collectivist and individualist cultures can impact decision-making, particularly respecting individual patient autonomy versus involving family members as a collective unit. This affects how information is shared and consent is obtained (Green et al., 2018). Family members often provide crucial support, but cultural leaders can also significantly impact care preferences (Herbststomer & Stahl, 2021).

Ethical and Legal Considerations

The World Health Organization defines *palliative care* as a practice that neither hastens nor postpones death. This is different from medical aid in dying and euthanasia, which hasten death. Medical aid in dying (MAID) is referred to by many different terms, including but not limited to assisted death, medically assisted death, physician-assisted death, physician-assisted suicide, assisted dying, aid in dying, compassionate dying, compassionate choices, death with dignity, compassionate death, and euthanasia. It is important to note that euthanasia and medical aid in dying are related concepts but differ in one important way. MAID involves a healthcare provider prescribing medication that a patient self-administers to end their life, whereas euthanasia involves a healthcare provider directly administering medication to the patient. Euthanasia is illegal in the United States, whereas as of 2024, medical aid in dying is legal in 10 US states and Washington, D.C. These states include California, Colorado, Hawaii, Maine, Montana, New Jersey, New Mexico, Oregon, Vermont, and Washington. In each jurisdiction, specific regulations govern the practice and provide oversight, typically requiring patients to have a terminal illness with a prognosis of 6 months or less to live. Each state has its own procedures and safeguards to ensure that the patients are eligible and their decisions are voluntary and informed.

Research indicates that 74%–88% of individuals opting for assisted dying also receive palliative or hospice care services (Gerson et al., 2020), underscoring the overlap between these two areas. The International Association for Hospice and Palliative Care opposes legalizing euthanasia and MAID without universal access to palliative care, including necessary medications (De Lima et al., 2017). Professional ethical standards sometimes conflict due to balancing a patient's right to autonomy versus the meaning of suffering and also what doing no harm means, which may vary based on values, religion, culture, and other factors. Practitioners need to remain unbiased and respect the wishes of patients, yet this may be difficult to do if their beliefs differ.

While some hospice and palliative care programs have policies that support patients pursuing medical aid in dying, others remain neutral or entirely opposed, creating dilemmas for healthcare staff. Studies show that nearly half of hospice programs permit moderate to full participation in medical aid in dying yet the policies may not provide clear guidance for practitioners, leaving confusion about legal and ethical boundaries. A range of views exists among hospice professionals. While many support patient choice and maintain a nonjudgmental stance, confusion persists about their roles under these laws. In Washington, for instance, many hospice institutions officially prohibit professionals from providing information about assisted dying or being present during the patient's self-administration of lethal medications, though some professionals still choose to be present in order to support the patient and family. Ultimately, the relationship between palliative care and medical aid in dying remains cooperative in some cases and conflicted in others, depending on individual values and institutional policies. Despite the legal framework, medical aid in dying is not fully integrated into palliative care practices, reflecting the ongoing dilemmas professionals face (Gerson et al., 2020).

The Future of Palliative Care in Long-Term Care

The future of palliative care in long-term care settings is influenced by demographic trends, staffing issues, and technological advancements. As chronic illnesses rise globally, the demand for palliative care support is expected to grow, requiring healthcare systems to adapt and allocate more resources for palliative and end-of-life care (Etkind et al., 2017).

Staffing challenges, such as high turnover and burnout, are prevalent in palliative care, just like they are in other healthcare professions. To ensure a stable workforce capable of delivering quality care, it is crucial to improve working conditions and support systems. Recent studies point to gaps in grief support and training for long-term care staff (Hawes, 2023; Hawes & Wang, 2024), highlighting the need for ongoing education in these activities to ensure they can effectively deliver this care.

Technological integration is another notable trend in enhancing care delivery. For example, telemedicine enables healthcare providers to remotely monitor patients, conduct virtual consultations, and implement timely interventions, thereby improving access to palliative care services, particularly for those in remote or underserved areas. While comprehensive studies on the use of telemedicine for delivering palliative care are lacking, existing research shows that home telemedicine can reduce hospitalizations and improve clinical outcomes for patients with chronic conditions like congestive heart failure (Bhatnager & Gupta, 2015). Additionally, advancements in wearable technology enable real-time monitoring of patients' vital signs and symptoms, allowing for proactive adjustments for pain management and other distressing symptoms (Sandic Spaho et al., 2023). Virtual reality also plays a vital role by providing immersive experiences that relieve pain and enhance emotional well-being, offering therapeutic environments that foster connection and relaxation (Moloney et al., 2023). These innovations not only improve the quality of care but also enhance the ability of patients to stay in their preferred environment, whether that be at home or in a long-term care facility.

Policy development is vital for integrating palliative care as standard practice. Changes are needed that support the integration of palliative care as a standard practice, including adequate funding, reimbursement, and resources for palliative care programs. The recent Hospice Care, Accountability, Reform, and Enforcement (CARE) Act of 2024 proposes significant reforms to the Medicare hospice benefit, including new payment mechanisms for high-acuity palliative care services, adjustments to daily hospice rates, and allowing nurse practitioners to certify patients for hospice. It also aims to combat fraud and improve quality data reporting, aimed at improving patient outcomes and care quality for vulnerable populations.

Acknowledgments The authors express their gratitude to Jeri Weiser for her contributions in editing this chapter.

References

Bhatnagar, S., & Gupta, M. (2015). Future of palliative medicine. *India Journal of Palliative Care, 21*(1), 95. https://doi.org/10.4103/0973-1075.150201

Bull J (2016) Palliative care in nursing homes: The role of the palliative care consultant. National Hospice and Palliative Care Organization. https://www.nhpco.org/wp-content/uploads/2019/04/PALLIATIVECARE_PC_NursingHome_0.pdf.

Bulle, S., Arya, A., & Dosani, N. (2023). From cultural safety to anti-racism: Reflections on addressing inequities in palliative care. *Current Oncology, 30*, 7920–7925. https://doi.org/10.3390/curroncol30090575

Center to Advance Palliative Care. (2014). Press kit: Palliative care facts and stats. https://media.capc.org/filer_public/68/bc/68bc93c7-14ad-4741-9830-86917296l8d0/capc_press-kit.pdf Accessed August 29, 2024.

Center to Advance Palliative Care. (2021). America's care of serious illness: 2021 state-by-state report card on access to palliative care in our nation's hospitals. https://www.capc.org/research-and-reports/state-by-state-report-card/. Accessed September 22, 2024.

Centers for Medicare & Medicaid Services. (n.d.-a). Hospice care. U.S. Department of Health and Human Services. https://www.medicare.gov/coverage/hospice-care.

Centers for Medicare & Medicaid Services. (n.d.-b) Medicare hospice benefits (Publication No. 02154). U.S. Department of Health and Human Services. https://www.medicare.gov/Pubs/pdf/02154-medicare-hospice-benefits.pdf.

Cole, C. S., Jackson, A. L., Fink, R. M., et al. (2024). Benefits and barriers of palliative care in nursing homes: A qualitative descriptive study. *Journal of Pain and Symptom Management, 67*(5), e710–e711. https://doi.org/10.1016/j.jpainsymman.2024.02.188

De Lima, L., Woodruff, R., Pettus, K., et al. (2017). International association for hospice and palliative care position statement: Euthanasia and physician-assisted suicide. *Journal of Palliative Medicine, 20*(1), 8–14. https://doi.org/10.1089/jpm.2016.0290

Etkind, S. N., Bone, A. E., Gomes, B., et al. (2017). How many people will need palliative care in 2040? Past trends, future projections and implications for services. *BMC Medicine, 15*, 1–10. https://doi.org/10.1186/s12916-017-0860-2

Ferrell, B. R., Twaddle, M. L., Melnick, A., et al. (2018). National consensus project clinical practice guidelines for quality palliative care guidelines. *Journal of Palliative Medicine, 21*(12), 1684–1689. https://doi.org/10.1089/jpm.2018.0431

Gerson, S. M., Koksvik, G. H., Richards, N., et al. (2020). The relationship of palliative care with assisted dying where assisted dying is lawful: A systematic scoping review of the literature. *Journal of Pain and Symptom Management, 59*(6), 1287–1303. https://doi.org/10.1016/j.jpainsymman.2019.12.361

Green, A., Jerzmanowska, N., Green, M., et al. (2018). Death is difficult in any language: A qualitative study of palliative care professionals' experiences when providing end-of-life care to patients from culturally and linguistically diverse backgrounds. *Palliative Medicine, 32*(8), 1419–1427. https://doi.org/10.1177/0269216318776850

Hawes, F. M. (2023). Leading through loss: Experiences of nursing home administrators-in-training during the COVID-19 pandemic. *OMEGA Journal of Death Dying*. https://doi.org/10.1177/00302228231189847

Hawes, F. M., & Wang, S. (2024). A comparative study of organizational grief support and burnout among nursing home staff. *Gerontologist, 64*(8). https://doi.org/10.1093/geront/gnae065

Herbstsomer, R. A., & Stahl, S. T. (2021). Cross-cultural experiences of hospice and palliative care services: A thematic analysis. *OMEGA Journal of Death Dying, 84*(2), 551–566. https://doi.org/10.1177/0030222820904205

Jakubów, P., Niedźwiecka, K., Kondracka, J., et al. (2023). Legal and medical aspects of the end of human life from the perspective of palliative medicine related to cardiac surgery. *Białostockie Studia Prawnicze, 28*(3), 53–70. https://doi.org/10.15290/bsp.2023.28.03.03

Kaasalainen, S., Sussman, T., McCleary, L., et al. (2019). Palliative care models in long-term care: A scoping review. *Nurse Leadersh, 32*(3), 8–26. https://doi.org/10.12927/cjnl.2019.25975

Kellehear, A. (2013). Compassionate communities: End-of-life care as everyone's responsibility. *QJM International Journal of Medicine, 106*(12), 1071–1075. https://doi.org/10.1093/qjmed/hct200

Kelley, A. S., & Meier, D. E. (2014). *Meeting the needs of older adults with serious illness*. Humana Press.

Lima, C., & Miller, S. C. (2018). Palliative care consults in U.S. nursing homes: Not just for the dying. *Journal of Palliative Medicine, 21*(2), 188–193. https://doi.org/10.1089/jpm.2017.0099

Liu, X., Chang, Y.-C., & Hu, W.-Y. (2024). The effectiveness of palliative care interventions in long-term care facilities: A systematic review. *Journal of Personalized Medicine, 14*, 700. https://doi.org/10.3390/jpm14070700

MacDonald, S., Herx, L., & Boyle, A. (Eds.). (2022). *Palliative medicine: A case-based manual* (4th ed.). Oxford Academic. https://doi.org/10.1093/oso/9780198837008.001.0001

Miller, S. C., Lima, J. C., Intrator, O., et al. (2017). Specialty palliative care consultations for nursing home residents with dementia. *Journal of Pain and Symptom Management, 54*(1), 9–16.e5. https://doi.org/10.1016/j.jpainsymman.2017.03.005

Moloney, M., Doody, O., O'Reilly, M., et al. (2023). Virtual reality use and patient outcomes in palliative care: A scoping review. *Digit Health, 9*. https://doi.org/10.1177/20552076231207574

Morrison, R. S. (2013). Models of palliative care delivery in the United States. *Current Opinion in Supportive and Palliative Care, 7*(2), 201–206. https://doi.org/10.1097/SPC.0b013e32836103e5

Naoum, P., Athanasakis, K., & Elpida Pavi, E. (2024). Is palliative care cost-effective? A systematic review of the literature. *Home Health Care Management and Practice, 36*(3), 205–216. https://doi.org/10.1177/10848223231209316

National Institute on Aging. (2022). Advance care planning: Advance directives for health care. U.S. Department of Health and Human Services. https://www.nia.nih.gov/health/advance-care-planning/advance-care-planning-advance-directives-health-care.

National Institute on Aging. (2021). What are palliative care and hospice care? U.S. Department of Health and Human Services. https://www.nia.nih.gov/health/hospice-and-palliative-care/what-are-palliative-care-and-hospice-care Accessed July 3, 2024.

Okan, I., Suren, M., Onder, Y., et al. (2019). An evaluation of the mourning tradition, the "First Feast," in the context of palliative care: The possibility of incorporating cultural rituals into palliative care. *Palliative & Supportive Care, 17*(4), 453–458. https://doi.org/10.1017/s1478951518000767

Persson, H. A., Ahlstrom, G., Arested, K., et al. (2022). Palliative care delivery at nursing homes before and after an educational intervention from professionals' perspectives: A pre-post design. *Scandinavian Journal of Caring Sciences, 37*, 229–242. https://doi.org/10.1111/scs.13084

Sandic Spaho, R., Uhrenfeldt, L., Fotis, T., et al. (2023). Wearable devices in palliative care for people 65 years and older: A scoping review. *Digit Health, 9*. https://doi.org/10.1177/20552076231181212

Tan, A. K., Jr. (2019). Models of palliative care in long-term care: An integrative review. *International Journal of Caring Sciences, 12*(2), 1–14.

Unroe, K. T., Ersek, M., Tu, W., et al. (2023). Using palliative leaders in facilities to transform care for people with Alzheimer's disease (UPLIFT-AD): Protocol of a palliative care clinical trial in nursing homes. *BMC Palliative Care, 22*. https://doi.org/10.1186/s12904-023-01226-0

U.S. Department of Veterans Affairs. (n.d.) Palliative and hospice care: VA's specialized programs for Veterans with serious and life-limiting illnesses. https://www.va.gov/geriatrics/docs/PHCFactSheet.pdf.

World Health Organization. (1986). Ottawa charter for health promotion, 1986 (No. WHO/EURO: 1986-4044-43803-61677). World Health Organization. Regional Office for Europe. https://iris.who.int/handle/10665/349652.

World Health Organization. (1995). Health promotion: Ottawa charter (No. WHO/HPR/HEP/95.1. Unpublished). World Health Organization. https://www.who.int/teams/health-promotion/enhanced-wellbeing/first-global-conference.

Zehnder, A. R., Pedrosa Carrasco, A. J., & Etkind, S. N. (2022). Factors associated with hospitalisations of patients with chronic heart failure approaching the end of life: A systematic review. *Palliative Medicine, 36*(10), 1452–1468. https://doi.org/10.1177/02692163221123422

Chapter 9
Cognitive and Mental Health Issues in Long-Term Care from a Health Disparities Perspective

Solange M. Marcel

Cognitive and mental health disparities in long-term care settings are increasingly recognized as critical issues that affect the quality of care and outcomes for older adults, particularly those with cognitive impairments. The interplay between cognitive health and care utilization is significant; cognitive impairment not only drives the need for healthcare services but also influences the trajectory of care utilization over time. Neurocognitive changes are vital indicators of future care needs, highlighting the importance of addressing cognitive health in long-term care planning and resource allocation (Atim et al., 2021).

The terms "neurocognitive disorder" and "dementia" are often used interchangeably in clinical settings; however, they represent different concepts within the field of mental health. Understanding the distinctions between these terms is essential for accurate diagnosis and treatment. According to the Diagnostic and Statistical Manual of Mental Disorders, Fifth Edition (DSM-5), neurocognitive disorders are characterized by a decline from a previously attained level of cognitive functioning, affecting memory, attention, language, and other cognitive domains (American Psychiatric Association, 2013). Dementia is a specific type of major neurocognitive disorder that is characterized by significant cognitive decline that interferes with daily life and independence. Neurocognitive disorder is often progressive and can result from various underlying conditions, such as Alzheimer's disease, vascular dementia, or frontotemporal degeneration (Livingston et al., 2017). DSM-5 has moved away from using the term "dementia" as a standalone diagnosis, instead classifying it under the domain of neurocognitive disorders; thus for the purposes of this chapter, we will do the same.

Neurocognitive disorders significantly impact activities of daily living (ADL) and require comprehensive care strategies in long-term care settings. As the

S. M. Marcel (✉)
NYU Grossman School of Medicine, NYU Langone, New York, NY, USA
e-mail: solange.marcel@nyulangone.org; sm10972@hunter.cuny.edu

K. K. Bhattacharyya (ed.), *Health Promotion in Long-Term Care Facilities*,
https://doi.org/10.1007/978-3-031-91038-8_9

population continues to age, the number of individuals living with neurocognitive disorder will increase, particularly in low- to middle-income countries (Livingston et al., 2017). The current global estimate of individuals living with dementia is approximately 55 million, according to the World Health Organization and various studies (Fujita et al., 2022; WHO, 2021; Wang et al., 2020). This figure reflects a significant increase from earlier estimates, highlighting the growing public health concern associated with neurocognitive disorder as populations age. The prevalence of neurocognitive disorders is projected to continue to rise, with estimates suggesting that the number of cases could reach 74.7 million by 2030 and 131.5 million by 2050 (Nakamura et al., 2020). As life expectancy increases, the incidence of neurocognitive disorders, which is significantly higher among older adults, is also expected to escalate. The prevalence among individuals aged 65 and older is estimated to be around 5–7%, with this figure increasing dramatically in those aged 85 and older, where it can exceed 30% (Gattas et al., 2020). Moreover, the global burden of dementia is not only measured in terms of prevalence but also in economic impact. The financial burden associated with dementia care is substantial, with estimates indicating that it exceeds 1 trillion USD annually (Lin et al., 2022). This economic strain is compounded by the fact that nearly 10 million new cases are diagnosed each year, emphasizing the urgent need for effective public health strategies to address this growing issue (Fujita et al., 2022; Wang et al., 2020). The prevalence of cognitive impairment in long-term care settings is compounded by the high incidence of delirium and other cognitive dysfunctions associated with critical illnesses. Research indicates that survivors of critical illness, including those who experienced delirium, often face long-term cognitive impairments that can persist for years, affecting their functional abilities and overall quality of life (Rengel et al., 2019). This underscores the need for comprehensive care strategies that not only address immediate health concerns but also consider the long-term cognitive health of patients. The World Health Organization (2021) has recognized that neurocognitive disorders are often accompanied by comorbid mental health issues, such as depression and anxiety, which further complicate the care of affected individuals (Livingston et al., 2017). For instance, late-onset depression has been shown to co-occur with neurocognitive impairment in up to 50% of cases, indicating a complex interplay between mood and cognitive disorders in older adults (Yasir et al., 2020). This dual burden highlights the necessity for integrated care approaches that address both cognitive and mental health needs.

Neurocognitive Disorders Related Health Disparities in Long-Term Care

Neurocognitive disorders represent a significant public health challenge in long-term care settings. The intersection of neurocognitive disorders and health equity is critical, as disparities in access to care, quality of treatment, and outcomes are evident across different demographic groups. Disparities in cognitive health outcomes are exacerbated by systemic issues within healthcare systems (Mansbach et al., 2015). A systematic review of older, minoritized populations demonstrates significant disparities in access to care and health outcomes in long-term care homes, which can be attributed to various factors including socioeconomic status, racial/ethnic backgrounds, and the quality of care provided (Scott, 2024). These disparities are not merely statistical; they translate into real differences in the quality of life and health outcomes for these populations, necessitating targeted interventions to address these inequities. Health equity is a crucial consideration in the management of neurocognitive disorders (Shepherd-Banigan et al., 2020). Research indicates that socio-demographic factors, including socioeconomic status, education, and geographic location, significantly influence the prevalence and management of neurocognitive disorders (Mansbach et al., 2015). This situation underscores the importance of training and education for healthcare workers to improve diagnostic practices and treatment options, particularly in underserved communities.

The stigma associated with neurocognitive disorders can hinder access to necessary care and support. In many cultures, cognitive decline is viewed as a normal part of aging, leading to underdiagnosis and delayed treatment (Kamoga et al., 2019). Addressing these misconceptions through public health campaigns and education can improve early detection and intervention, ultimately enhancing the quality of life for affected individuals and their families. Prioritizing health equity associated with neurocognitive disorders in long-term care settings requires a multifaceted approach. This includes improving access to care while supporting informal caregivers and combating stigma associated with cognitive decline. By focusing on these areas, a more equitable healthcare system that meets the needs of all individuals affected by neurocognitive disorders can be achieved.

Mental Illness-Related Disparities in Long-Term Care

Mental illness in LTC settings is a critical issue that intersects significantly with social determinants of health and health disparities. The deinstitutionalization movement of the 1960s and 1970s fundamentally reshaped the landscape of mental health care, transitioning from large psychiatric hospitals to community-based care models. This shift was driven by the recognition of inhumane conditions within institutions and the advent of psychotropic medications, which allowed many individuals with mental illnesses to live more independently (Chow & Priebe, 2013). Many individuals discharged from psychiatric hospitals were left to navigate a fragmented system that was ill-equipped to address their ongoing needs. This gap in care often led families to seek long-term care options, as they struggled to manage the demands of caregiving without sufficient resources or support (Muusse et al., 2020). Consequently, long-term care facilities became a refuge for those who could not thrive in community settings, leading to an increase in the population of mentally ill individuals in these environments (Mbadugha et al., 2023).

The prevalence of mental health disorders among older adults in long-term care facilities is notably high, often exacerbated by factors such as socioeconomic status, access to care, and systemic inequities. Understanding these relationships is essential for developing effective interventions aimed at improving mental health outcomes in this vulnerable population. Social determinants of health, including income, education, and social support, play a pivotal role in shaping mental health outcomes. Research has shown that individuals with lower socioeconomic status are at a higher risk for developing mental health disorders, contributing to worse health outcomes and increased mortality rates (Jayatilleke et al., 2017). This underscores the need for targeted interventions that address these disparities, particularly in long-term care settings where residents may have limited resources and support systems.

The stigma surrounding mental illness also plays a significant role in health disparities within long-term care. Negative attitudes toward mental health can deter individuals from seeking help and can lead to inadequate treatment (Carrara et al., 2020). Anti-stigma interventions through education and training are necessary to improve attitudes among healthcare providers and enhance the quality of care for individuals with mental health disorders (Carrara et al., 2020). Additionally, geographic disparities can influence access to mental health care in long-term care settings. Research indicates that individuals living in rural areas often face greater challenges in accessing mental health services compared to their urban counterparts (Cook et al., 2016; Pederson et al., 2013). This geographic divide can exacerbate existing health disparities, as residents in rural long-term care facilities may have limited access to specialized mental health care and fewer resources to address their needs (Cook et al., 2016). Racial and ethnic disparities also play a significant role in mental health outcomes within long-term care. Studies indicate that minority populations often experience higher rates of mental health disorders but have lower rates of treatment engagement (Jayatilleke et al., 2017). This can be attributed to a combination of stigma, cultural differences in the perception of mental health, and a lack of culturally sensitive services.

The COVID-19 pandemic has further highlighted the vulnerabilities of residents in long-term care regarding mental health. One of the most significant impacts of the pandemic within long-term care facilities has been the exacerbation of preexisting mental health conditions among residents (Eghtesadi, 2020; Murphy et al., 2021). Many individuals already had challenging depression and anxiety, which only intensified by the isolation and restrictions imposed during the pandemic (Eghtesadi, 2020; Zhong et al., 2022; Zaçe et al., 2021). The disruption of daily routines, limited social interactions, and the fear of infection have contributed to a deterioration in mental well-being among residents (Zhong et al., 2022; Reynolds et al., 2022). By fostering collaboration between mental health professionals and LTC providers, facilities can create a more holistic approach to care to address both physical and mental health needs. This integration is essential for ensuring that residents receive timely and appropriate mental health interventions, which can significantly enhance their quality of life.

Caregiver Disparities in Long-Term Care

Caregiving for individuals within LTC presents unique challenges and dynamics that differ significantly from those experienced by their community counterparts. Research indicates that cultural factors play a crucial role in shaping caregiving practices among ethnic minorities, often leading to distinct patterns of care that emphasize family involvement over formal services (Sagbakken et al., 2017; Nielsen et al., 2020). For many minority families, caregiving is not just a duty but a culturally ingrained responsibility (Sagbakken et al., 2017). The emotional and psychological burden of caregiving is particularly pronounced among family members of individuals with dementia. Studies have shown that caregivers often experience feelings of guilt, stress, and isolation, especially when they are unable to provide the level of care felt necessary (Midtbust et al., 2020). This burden is exacerbated in minority families, where caregivers may also face additional challenges such as language barriers and cultural misunderstandings within the healthcare system (Sagbakken et al., 2017; Toit et al., 2022). The dynamics of caregiving in minority families often involve a shared responsibility among several family members, which can lead to a more communal approach to care (Nielsen et al., 2020). This rotational care practice can alleviate some of the individual burden but may also introduce complexities in coordination and communication among caregivers (Nielsen et al., 2020; Toit et al., 2022). The need for culturally appropriate care is critical, as many minority families report dissatisfaction with the care provided in long-term care facilities, which often do not honor their cultural values and traditions (Toit et al., 2022). Support systems for caregivers are essential in mitigating the stress associated with dementia caregiving. Community-based programs that involve local ethnic organizations and volunteers have been shown to significantly enhance the support available to minority families (Moyle et al., 2014; Lee et al., 2017). Such initiatives not only provide practical assistance but also foster a sense of community and belonging, which is vital for the mental well-being of caregivers (Moyle et al., 2014; Lee et al., 2017).

Bridging Health Equity in Long-Term Care

Health equity ensures that all individuals, regardless of their socioeconomic status, race, or geographic location, have access to appropriate health services (Doykos et al., 2016). Advancing health equity is vital, especially for vulnerable populations within long-term care settings. Factors that make older adults at risk of inequitable care include frailty and physical and cognitive impairments, all of which make self-advocacy and self-determination more difficult requiring policy-driven and regulated care practices to meet these complex needs (Scott, 2024). Research indicates that individuals from marginalized communities often face barriers to accessing health care, including stigma, lack of culturally competent services, and financial constraints (Lama et al., 2018). Attaining equity in healthcare quality and cost for older adults remains unobtainable. Improving health equity for older adults requires identifying barriers, developing interventions designed to address the barriers, and implementing interventions (Huisingh-Scheetz et al., 2024). Health equity for older adults requires an approach that deliberately advances health equity along with research that applies an equity lens to quality and systems improvement that can inform tailored interventions (Huisingh-Scheetz et al., 2024). People who live in poverty are less healthy than those who are wealthier, regardless of physical or mental comorbidities (Institute for Research on Poverty, 2014). Roughly 26 percent of adults older than 65 in the United States live at or below 200 percent of the federal poverty level, and evidence demonstrates that Lesbian, Gay, Bisexual, and Transgender (LGBT) older adults are more economically disadvantaged than their heterosexual peers (Emlet, 2016). The interface between LGBT older adults and their social environment, particularly in long-term care, has the capacity to be supportive based on staff and community education efforts (Emlet, 2016).

Conclusion

Neurocognitive and mental health disorders in long-term care are deeply intertwined with health disparities and directly influenced by socioeconomic status, race, and systemic barriers. Addressing these disparities necessitates a multifaceted approach that includes integrating mental health services, supporting both lay and staff caregivers, and implementing culturally competent care practices. By focusing on these areas, we can work toward reducing inequities and improving the cognitive and mental health outcomes for all residents in long-term care facilities. Future research and policy efforts should focus on integrating cognitive health assessments into routine care practices well beyond the long-term care context in an effort to recognize early cognitive impairment. It is also paramount to develop targeted interventions that address the unique needs of this vulnerable population. It is essential to draw attention to the unique needs of minority caregivers through culturally sensitive support systems with anti-stigma education and training.

References

American Psychiatric Association. (2013). *Diagnostic and statistical manual of mental disorders* (5th ed.). https://doi-org.ezproxy.frederick.edu/10.1176/appi.books.9780890425596

Atim, L., Kaggwa, M., Mamun, M., Ashaba, S., & Maling, S. (2021). Prevalence of severe neurocognitive impairment and its association with socio-demographics and functionality among Ugandan older persons: a hospital-based study. *Clinical Interventions in Aging, 16*, 1415–1425. https://doi.org/10.2147/cia.s319891

Carrara, B., Fernandes, R., Bobbili, S., & Ventura, C. (2020). Health care providers and people with mental illness: An integrative review on anti-stigma interventions. *International Journal of Social Psychiatry, 67*(7), 840–853. https://doi.org/10.1177/0020764020985891

Chow, W. S., & Priebe, S. (2013). Understanding psychiatric institutionalization: A conceptual review. *BMC Psychiatry, 13*(1). https://doi.org/10.1186/1471-244x-13-169

Cook, B., Kim, G., Morgan, K., Chen, C., Nillni, A., & Alegría, M. (2016). Measuring geographic "hot spots" of racial/ethnic disparities: an application to mental health care. *Journal of Health Care for the Poor and Underserved, 27*(2), *663–684*. https://doi.org/10.1353/hpu.2016.0091

Doykos, P., Gray-Akpa, K., & Mitchell, F. (2016). New directions for foundations in health equity. *Health Affairs, 35*(8), 1536–1540. https://doi.org/10.1377/hlthaff.2016.0256

Eghtesadi, M. (2020). Breaking social isolation amidst covid-19: A viewpoint on improving access to technology in long-term care facilities. *Journal of the American Geriatrics Society, 68*(5), 949–950. https://doi.org/10.1111/jgs.16478

Emlet CA. (2016). Social, economic, and health disparities among LGBT older adults. *Generations. Summer, 40*(2):16–22. PMID: 28366981; PMCID: PMC5373809.

Fujita, K., Katsuki, M., Takasu, A., Kitajima, A., Shimazu, T., & Maruki, Y. (2022). Development of an artificial intelligence-based diagnostic model for Alzheimer's disease. *Aging Medicine, 5*(3), 167–173. https://doi.org/10.1002/agm2.12224

Gattas, B., Ibetoh, C. N., Stratulat, E., Liu, F., Wuni, G. Y., Bahuva, R., Shafiq, M. A., & Gordon, D. K. (2020). The impact of low hemoglobin levels on cognitive brain functions. *Cureus*. https://doi.org/10.7759/cureus.11378

Huisingh-Scheetz, M., Muramatsu, N., Konetzka, R. T., & Chin, M. H. (2024). Leveraging health services research to address aging health equity. *Generations: Journal of the American Society on Aging, 48*(2), 1–15. https://www.jstor.org/stable/48794767

Institute for Research on Poverty. (2014). *Health & Poverty*. www.irp.wisc.edu/research/health.htm

Jayatilleke, N., Hayes, R., Dutta, R., Shetty, H., Hotopf, M., Chang, C., & Stewart, R. (2017). Contributions of specific causes of death to lost life expectancy in severe mental illness. *European Psychiatry, 43*, 109–115. https://doi.org/10.1016/j.eurpsy.2017.02.487

Kamoga, R., Rukundo, G., Wakida, E., Nakidde, G., Obua, C., & Buss, S. (2019). Dementia assessment and diagnostic practices of healthcare workers in rural southwestern Uganda: A cross-sectional qualitative study. *BMC Health Services Research, 19*(1). https://doi.org/10.1186/s12913-019-4850-2

Lama, G., Alcala, E., & Capitman, J. (2018). Poor people are hospitalized three times more for mental health services than the non-poor in central valley. *California. Healthcare, 6*(1), 5. https://doi.org/10.3390/healthcare6010005

Lee, J., Nguyen, H., Park, J., Tran, L., Nguyen, T., & Huynh, Y. (2017). Usages of computers and smartphones to develop dementia care education program for Asian American family caregivers. *Healthcare Informatics Research, 23*(4), 338. https://doi.org/10.4258/hir.2017.23.4.338

Lin, Z., Ba, F., Allore, H., Liu, G. G., & Chen, X. (2022). Geographic variation in inpatient care utilization, outcomes and costs for dementia patients aged 65 years or older — China, 2017–2019. *China CDC Weekly, 4*(45), 997–1001. https://doi.org/10.46234/ccdcw2022.202

Livingston, G., Sommerlad, A., Orgeta, V., Costafreda, S., Huntley, J., Ames, D., Ballard, C., Banerjee, S., Burns, A., Cohen-Mansfield, J., Cooper, C., Fox, N., Gitlin, L., Howard, R., Kales, H., Larson, E. B., Ritchie, K., Rockwood, K., Sampson, E., & Mukadam, N. (2017). Dementia prevention, intervention, and care. *The Lancet, 390*(10113), 2673–2734. https://doi.org/10.1016/s0140-6736(17)31363-6

Mansbach, W., Mace, R., Clark, K., & Firth, I. (2015). A comparison of cognitive functioning in long-term care and short-stay nursing home residents. *Ageing and Society, 37*(1), 1–13. https://doi.org/10.1017/s0144686x15000926

Mbadugha, C. J., Ogbonnaya, N. P., Iheanacho, P., Omotola, N. J., Ogbonna, P. N., & Anetekhai, C. J. (2023). Exploring perceived impact of caregiving and coping strategies adopted by family caregivers of people with schizophrenia: A qualitative study in Enugu, south east Nigeria. *Qualitative Research Journal, 23*(3), 338–353. https://doi.org/10.1108/qrj-06-2022-0082

Midtbust, M. H., Alnes, R. E., Gjengedal, E., & Lykkeslet, E. (2020). Separation characterized by responsibility and guilt: Family caregivers' experiences with palliative care for a close family member with severe dementia in long-term care facilities. *Dementia, 20*(2), 518–533. https://doi.org/10.1177/1471301219898341

Moyle, W., Jones, C., Cooke, M., O'Dwyer, S., Sung, B., & Drummond, S. (2014). Connecting the person with dementia and family: A feasibility study of a telepresence robot. *BMC Geriatrics, 14*(1). https://doi.org/10.1186/1471-2318-14-7

Murphy, L., Markey, K., Donnell, C. O., Moloney, M., & Doody, O. (2021). The impact of the covid-19 pandemic and its related restrictions on people with pre-existent mental health conditions: A scoping review. *Archives of Psychiatric Nursing, 35*(4), 375–394. https://doi.org/10.1016/j.apnu.2021.05.002

Muusse, C., Kroon, H., Mulder, C. L., & Pols, J. (2020). Working on and with relationships: Relational work and spatial understandings of good care in community mental healthcare in trieste. *Culture, Medicine, and Psychiatry, 44*(4), 544–564. https://doi.org/10.1007/s11013-020-09672-8

Nakamura, T., Zou, K., Shibuya, Y., & Michikawa, M. (2020). Oral dysfunctions and cognitive impairment/dementia. *Journal of Neuroscience Research, 99*(2), 518–528. https://doi.org/10.1002/jnr.24745

Nielsen, R. T., Waldemar, G., & Nielsen, D. S. (2020). Rotational care practices in minority ethnic families managing dementia: A qualitative study. *Dementia, 20*(3), 884–898. https://doi.org/10.1177/1471301220914751

Pederson, K., Lutfiyya, M., Palombi, L., Simmons, D., Steenerson, D., Hohman, K., & Huot, K. (2013). Cross-sectional population-based study ascertaining the characteristics of us rural adults with mental health concerns who perceived a stigma regarding mental health issues. *Health, 05*(04), 695–702. https://doi.org/10.4236/health.2013.54092

Rengel, K., Hayhurst, C., Pandharipande, P., & Hughes, C. (2019). Long-term cognitive and functional impairments after critical illness. *Anesthesia & Analgesia, 128*(4), 772–780. https://doi.org/10.1213/ane.0000000000004066

Reynolds, K., Ceccarelli, L., Pankratz, L., Snider, T., Tindall, C., Omolola, D., Feniuk, C., & Turenne-Maynard, J. (2022). Covid-19 and the experiences and needs of staff and management working at the front lines of long-term care in central Canada. *Canadian Journal on Aging, 41*(4), 614–619. https://doi.org/10.1017/s0714980821000696

Sagbakken, M., Spilker, R. S., & Ingebretsen, R. (2017). Dementia and migration: Family care patterns merging with public care services. *Qualitative Health Research, 28*(1), 16–29. https://doi.org/10.1177/1049732317730818

Scott, M. (2024). Building evidence to advance health equity: A systematic review on care-related outcomes for older, minoritized populations in long-term care homes. *Age and Ageing, 53*(4). https://doi.org/10.1093/ageing/afae059

Shepherd-Banigan, M., James, H., Smith, V., Plassman, B., Jutkowitz, E., Bélanger, E., & Houtven, C. (2020). Drivers of long-term care considerations by persons with cognitive impairment. *Journal of Applied Gerontology, 40*(6), 648–660. https://doi.org/10.1177/0733464820903908

Toit, S. H. J.d., Bagul, D., Jessup, G. M., & McGrath, M. (2022). Providing culturally appropriate residential dementia care for older adults with an Indian heritage: Perspectives from Sydney-based stakeholders. *Australian Occupational Therapy Journal, 70*(2), 159–174. https://doi.org/10.1111/1440-1630.12840

Wang, H., Li, T., Barbarino, P., Gauthier, S., Brodaty, H., Molinuevo, J. L., Xie, H., Sun, Y., Yu, E., Tang, Y., Weidner, W., & Yu, X. (2020). Dementia care during covid-19. *The Lancet, 395*(10231), 1190–1191. https://doi.org/10.1016/s0140-6736(20)30755-8

World Health Organization (2021). World failing to address dementia challenge. https://www.who.int/news/item/02-09-2021-world-failing-to-address-dementia-challenge

Yasir, S., Yasir, S., Haider, N., Fatima, S., Mazhar, M., Chaudhry, S., & Tamizuddin-Nizami, A. (2020). Magnitude of neurocognitive impairment and severity of depression in geriatric population. *Biomedica, 36*(4), 400–404. https://doi.org/10.51441/biomedica/5-87

Zaçe, D., Hoxhaj, I., Orfino, A., Viteritti, A. M., Janiri, L., & Pietro, M. L. D. (2021). Interventions to address mental health issues in healthcare workers during infectious disease outbreaks: A systematic review. *Journal of Psychiatric Research, 136*, 319–333. https://doi.org/10.1016/j.jpsychires.2021.02.019

Zhong, S., Huisingh-Scheetz, M., & Huang, E. S. (2022). Delayed medical care and its perceived health impact among us older adults during the covid-19 pandemic. *Journal of the American Geriatrics Society, 70*(6), 1620–1628. https://doi.org/10.1111/jgs.17805

Chapter 10
Cultural Perspectives for Promoting Residents' Quality of Life in Long-Term Care

David Hage

The Relationship Between Aging, Culture, and Quality of Life in Long-Term Care

Culture involves determined customs, traditions, beliefs, and values shared by people located in a particular place and time (Basirico et al., 2021; Spencer & Lu, 2022). The way in which customs, traditions, beliefs, and values are perceived and experienced varies according to societal types and sociocultural evolution. Age became a more prominent point of focus as rapid changes impacted older adults. Burgess (1960) first highlighted an archetype of a "roleless role" for older adults after retirement, whereby migration from rural to urban environments took place as industrialization rapidly emerged (p. 20). Since then, a postindustrial societal structure advanced in many countries that are increasingly now technology-based economically, with an organizational approach similar to industrial societies that largely use machinery to produce goods (Macionis & Bhatia, 2019). Long-term care approaches must progress to account for important variables in cultural perspectives that promote improvement in residents' quality of life. This approach would be consistent with Havighurst's (1961) notion of "successful aging," which introduced an orientation toward the importance of defining what successful aging entails, how it could be measured, and what outcomes would be consistent with the achievement of aging success (Williams et al., 2017). An emerging body of literature that continues to center around successful aging promotes three categories of focus, including the dimensions and principles of successful aging and appreciating factors that influence a successful aging experience (Estebsari et al., 2020).

D. Hage (✉)
Department of Social Work & Affiliate Faculty at Shady Rest Institute on Positive Aging, Florida Gulf Coast University, Fort Myers, FL, USA
e-mail: dhage@fgcu.edu

K. K. Bhattacharyya (ed.), *Health Promotion in Long-Term Care Facilities*,
https://doi.org/10.1007/978-3-031-91038-8_10

The way in which individual agency is approached in the activity theory of aging serves to inform continued efforts to keep older adults active concordantly with their preferences and varied abilities, consistent with the concept of successful aging (Bengtson et al., 2016). This is in contrast to the decreased acceptance of disengagement theory, which posited that successful aging required voluntarily disengaging from social roles and activities for the benefit of societies (Cumming & Henry, 1961; Rose, 1964; Hochschild, 1975; Marshalla & Clarke, 2007). Neugarten's (1996) work on the meaning of aging clarified chronological aging categorization by defining what is "young old" (55–75 years) vs. "old old" (75+ years); addressed aging norms, constraints, and stereotypes; and determined the level of satisfaction older adults self-assessed in their own lives. Where negative appraisals of aging emerged, the concept of the social disease of "ageism" was coined by Robert Butler (1990), who encouraged a much-needed shift away from pathological aging. He further asserted that the medical industry also perpetuated "medical ageism" and called for medical schools to educate students in the study of gerontology and geriatrics (Butler, 1990). This focus on a broader context of positively impacting aging is consistent with life-course and life-span perspectives on aging, which promote evaluating the impact of macro-level forces on individuals who exist in institutional settings like long-term care facilities (Bengtson et al., 2016).

Global Variance Across Long-term Care Types

Among a network of 30 global member countries, an alliance developed in pursuit of economic collaboration called the Organisation for Economic Co-Operation and Development (OCED) (Baker et al., 2010). These OCED member countries were compared and analyzed to compare how long-term care is embedded in the welfare state and how it relates to other welfare state institutions (Ariaans, et al., 2021). Six typological constructs of long-term care solutions were identified, including a type of public supply (Sweden), a type of private supply (Germany), a residual public type (Poland), an emerging public supply type (Korea), a need-based supply type (Switzerland), and an emerging need-based type (United States) (Ariaans et al., 2021). Within these varied global constructions of long-term care, there are varied fiscal models, care types, services, and supports that emerge (Applebaum et al., 2016).

In an effort to ensure a more globally integrated continuum of long-term care, the World Health Organization (WHO) identified three essential approaches to long-term care that exist or are being developed in many global long-term care settings. These include (1) long-term care as part of a universal coverage initiative, (2) developing and sustaining an adequately trained long-term care workforce, and (3) ensuring long-term care quality (WHO, n.d.a). In individualistic and independence-driven societies, family care is less utilized in long-term care contexts when compared to more group and family-centric societies (Fang & Yang, 2023). One way to view variations in these individualistic vs. collectivistic long-term care approaches might be as "cultural expressions" that all necessarily require a person-centered approach to care provision in different ways relative to the dominant culture and diverse needs of residents and families receiving care at long-term facilities internationally (Ågotnes & Øye, 2017, p. 480).

Cultural Competence and Cultural Humility in Long-Term Care

Cultural competence requires a commitment to learning new cultural information and integrating that information into practice (Sue et al., 2016). Failing to do so, despite even positive intentions, can create a misalignment between care providers and long-term care residents, thus negatively impacting health and quality-of-life experience (Spencer & Lu, 2022). When care providers demonstrate insufficient knowledge of long-term care residents' customs, traditions, beliefs, and values, this can contribute to resident disengagement, perceived lack of respect, or even prejudice and harm. In addition to individuals within long-term care facilities pursuing cultural competence themselves, long-term care facilities need to more broadly pursue organizational behaviors, strategies, policies, and procedures that serve the diverse, multiethnic, and linguistic needs of long-term care facilities and communities (White & Griffith, 2019).

Roles and contexts of family culture aid in further understanding of social meaning related to aging in long-term care environments. Family structure and relationships are known to influence these social forces (Burgess, 1960), and this can, in turn, provide older adults with fulfillment and personal satisfaction (Thompson et al., 1960) and promote familial satisfaction as well (Song & Jang, 2020). When familial ethics, levels of contact and interdependence, and caregiving meaning and practice are explored, differences in individualistic and collectivistic family systems become more apparent (Pyke & Bengtson, 1996). Individualistic families typically offer less caregiving support and employ formal support more often, whereas collectivist families utilize caregiving to develop family connectedness (Pyke & Bengtson, 1996). Individualistic vs. collectivistic approaches to long-term care approaches occur in relation to localized preferences, leadership, and broader regulatory and legislative forces (Ågotnes & Øye, 2017). During the final stage of caregiving, many family caregivers can no longer provide long-term care services at home, even with formal in-home caregiver support, and need to relinquish primary care responsibility to a long-term care facility (Bengtson et al., 2016), such as an assisted living facility or skilled nursing facility. Families who utilize long-term care services also benefit when facilities account for factors contributing to their resilience, such as identifying stressors, family beliefs, coping approaches, external supports, and adaptive potential (Kuang et al., 2022).

Therefore, long-term care providers, staff, and facilities have a duty to enhance their cultural competence for the benefit of residents, their family members, and social support resources (Spencer & Lu, 2022). Augmenting cultural competence in combination with cultural humility, or a sustained commitment to self-reflection and acceptance of cultural feedback, with a known mechanism for addressing errors and imbalances in perspectives and actions, can promote a healthier and more productive long-term living environment (Tervalon & Murray-García, 1998). Combining cultural competence and cultural humility has been described as producing five desirable results: (1) increasing cultural awareness, (2) improving cultural knowledge, (3) promoting cultural skills, (4) enhancing cultural desire, and (5) creating opportunities for more cultural encounters (Hook et al. 2016).

Integrating these cultural competence results involves awareness of beliefs, values, and biases, perspectives of diverse stakeholders themselves, intervening as appropriate, and recognizing the role of organizational and institutional forces (Sue et al., 2016). Identifying and care planning for cultural factors relevant to long-term care residents' cultural identities is essential to enhancing residents' quality of life. According to the WHO (n.d.b), quality of life involves a person's view of their life position relative to the culture and value systems where they reside and relative to their intentions, principles, and concerns. Individualizing person-centered care can potentially enhance long-term care residents' quality of life by accounting for preferences, increasing the ability to self-determinate, and revealing how diverse factors relate to perceived life satisfaction and engagement (Andrew & Meeks, 2016). However, persistent staffing shortages (Abbasi, 2020) and regulatory compliance challenges like documentation burden (Wang et al., 2024) frequently serve as barriers to having sufficient time and resources to achieve culturally competent care in long-term care settings.

The recent COVID-19 pandemic further stressed preexisting long-term care staffing shortages (Abbasi, 2020). The International Centre for Nurse Migration alarmingly reports that if only an additional 4% of the global nursing workforce leaves healthcare, the global nursing shortfall will increase to a seven million nurse shortage across the world (Buchan et al., 2022). Documentation burden remains a significant challenge in long-term care environments, and regulatory documentation burden makes evidence-based, culturally informed assessment and care provision a more complex task to achieve. In a comprehensive literature review including data from 2010 through 2023, the Agency for Healthcare Research and Quality (AHRQ) identified that clinical documentation burdens often center on time spent writing medical orders, billing and insurance-related tasks, workforce fragmentation, and electronic medical record (EMR) issues that are significant challenges to time availability for other important aims (Wang, et al., 2024). Despite these barriers, long-term care facilities must find ways forward to provide culturally competent care for an increasingly diverse societal population. The proceeding section of this chapter will describe practical resources that can be applied and modified as needed in long-term care facilities in support of cultural competence and humility as a mechanism to positively influence the quality-of-life experience of residents and families.

Resources for Cultural Assessment and Intervention in Long-term Care

Person-centered and culturally competent care necessitates understanding variable unique factors experienced and valued by each long-term care recipient. While each discipline involved in care provision at long-term care facilities across the world engages in various focused assessments per their training and scope of practice, driven by regulatory requirements and facility policies and procedures, obtaining additional data about resident perceptions of care provider's cultural competence within a facility could be a valuable starting point toward developing a culturally competent long-term care organization. Pacquiao et al. (2021) developed the 23-item Client Perceptions of Care Providers Cultural Competence tool (Cronbach's alpha of .89) that evaluates cultural competence as evaluated by residents who detail the behavior of care providers, with an emphasis on nurses in healthcare environments. Long-term care healthcare staff can self-assess cultural competence via tools like the Cultural Competence of Healthcare Providers (HCPs) (Cronbach's alpha ranging from .54 -.84), which is concurrently an initial framework to guide reducing healthcare disparities (Bernhard, et al., 2015). From an organizational lens, the American Nurse Credentialing Center (ANCC) has created a valuable self-assessment guide for appraising long-term care organizational culture that can help long-term care facilities evaluate elements of performance, their achievement of a desired organizational state, gaps in performance, and an action plan for improvement (ANCC, 2017). These and other related cultural competence assessment tools can be a foundational resource for gathering resident, family, and healthcare staff self-appraisal and organization critiques of cultural competence attainment.

Once sufficient cultural competence data are collected, Spencer and Lu (2022) indicate that the roles of culture, cultural understanding, and competence in long-term care should be the points of focus in moving toward improved resident quality of life. Practical domains for making incremental changes that contribute to cultural improvement often include communication and language choices, socialization and activity engagement, quality-of-life needs related to religion, ethnicity, race, values, and beliefs, and organizational focus (Spencer & Lu, 2022). Long-term care staff can also increasingly acknowledge family involvement when desired to increase participation with residents, which can strengthen familial, family-facility, and staff relationships (Lao et al., 2019). This can include involvement in care planning meetings, social visitation, external activities, participation in surveys, and engagement with cultural opportunities in activity programming, especially on important cultural and religious calendar dates.

Another important policy-level intervention opportunity that could be modified in a positive direction might include reducing prescriptive requirements of facilities concerning the role of resident councils to voice resident preferences by allowing for more interpretive guidance that can enhance resident quality of life in accordance with their own preferences over regulatory mandates (Hande et al., 2021). This collaborative alignment of collecting facility-wide and individual resident cultural data, improving cultural performance, and engagement with all members of the long-term care community is essential to becoming a culturally competent long-term care facility.

Care Preferences

Race, gender, ethnicity, spiritual/religious beliefs, and other cultural considerations commonly impact long-term care residents' care preferences and choices. For example, racial and ethnic minorities are less likely to develop advanced directives, Black residents might use hospice supports less frequently, and Hispanic residents are more likely to experience hospitalization at end-of-life compared to White residents (Estrada et al., 2021). Universal and gender-specific needs should be considered concerning preferences for personal care and bathing (Heusinger & Dummert, 2016). Since Hindus are religiously required to attend to cleanliness before religious, cultural, or social events (Bista, 2023), they may not engage in daily activities, care, or meals until hygiene and bathing activities are completed, and therefore, they may require early and more frequent bathing than other residents. Informed older adult consumers of healthcare services are more frequently expecting compassionate care that is regularly evaluated for quality in support of the goal of providing desired care (Moustafa Ibrahim et al., 2021).

Greater recognition of the role of sexuality in later adulthood in general, combined with scientific advances for sexual dysfunction, makes a strong case for long-term care staff having discussions with residents about the role of sexuality in their lives and associated health needs (Agronin, 2022). The literature further reflects that long-term care environments are not often welcoming of sexual and gender minorities (Skeldon & Jenkins, 2022). Increased need for staff training on sexual and gender minority health issues and attitudes of care providers remain areas to assess and improve (Caceres et al., 2019). Spirituality and religion are known to frequently be protective to many long-term care residents, and therefore, individual beliefs and preferences should be evaluated on admission and re-evaluated periodically. Faith can be a positive health predictor and could involve ritual activity, possibly including visitation from an interfaith chaplain (Zhang et al., 2019), or might involve in-facility religious services or spiritual activities, visits from faith practitioners, or leaving the facility for these supports, when appropriate.

Assessing health beliefs is critical as these ways of perceiving one's medical conditions can range greatly from Western biomedical approaches to blended, holistic, and folk or spiritual beliefs (Levkoff et al., 2000). Another important factor to consider is residents' social determinants of health (SDoH), which are based on biological/physiological status, psychological stressors, health behaviors, social issues, and disparate access to healthcare. Some diverse health considerations might include African American distrust of the health system related to past unethical treatment in the Tuskegee Experiment (Ford et al., 2024), Jehovah's Witnesses (JWs) generally refusing to accept blood products (Scharman et al., 2017), or

Buddhists choosing to reject pain medications to maintain mindfulness (Stonington 2022). When Minimum Data Set (MDS) and other assessments are conducted, culturally related health information can be clarified at these contact points, such as if interpreter services are needed or preferred, determining past experiences with healthcare systems and providers, desired healthcare support or interventions consistent with preferences, and the role of culture in diet, among other health topics.

Dietary Culture

Dietary preferences vary greatly across time and culture. A contemporary framework to conceptualize traditional and modern approaches to eating is the TEP 10 framework of traditional and modern eating (Sproesser et al., 2019). What is eaten includes ingredients, processing, preparation, temporal origins, spatial origins, and variety (Sproesser et al., 2019). How food is eaten involves temporal aspects, spatial aspects, social aspects, meals, appreciation, and concerns (Sproesser et al., 2019). When applying this to considering what and how food is approached through the cultural lens of residents, enhancing cultural food strategies becomes more readily accessible to long-term care facility staff. There are commonly shared cultural experiences of eating and individual and group preferences to consider.

Dining environments often vary due to physical environment, social factors, political will and constraint, and related to cost factors (Wierda et al., 2024). In Canada, resident dining usually occurs in large communal areas due to most long-term care facilities having been built between the 1950s and 1990s (Estabrooks et al., 2020). Dutch long-term care facilities vary between having meals in household-like settings, in restaurants, and in centralized facility locations (Wierda et al., 2024). A European model of comprehensive non-medicalized dementia care is the Dementia Village (DV) model, which creates a community-like setting for all services, including dining in restaurant-like settings to avoid medical connotations, where staff modify their approach to care as opposed to traditional models requiring residents to adapt to institutional environments (Roberts, 2023).

In addition to intentional consideration of dining spaces, other notable themes that can modulate dining experiences include communicating clearly about dining, supply chain accountability, and clarifying staff abilities and related goals (Hoefnagels et al., 2023). A recent integrative review of the Five Aspects Meal Model (FAMM) highlights the importance of resident input into mealtime, food that is eaten, and how food is consumed as a way to positively impact meal intake and socialization (Heikkilä et al., 2022). In populations with cognitive impairment, staff training, consistent staffing ratios, considering way finding approaches, safety, comfort, and sensory issues remain important dining considerations as well (Seetharaman et al., 2020). The Japan Gerontological Evaluation Study (JAGES) was recently analyzed and found trends of higher happiness associated with eating with others, and interestingly, the association was even stronger in people who lived alone, alluding to some potential benefits of eating as a beneficial socialization opportunity within communal long-term care settings (Wang et al., 2023). The CHOICE+ Program is an emerging relationship-focused mealtime training strategy to improve dining in long-term care that stands for Connecting, Honoring Dignity, Offering Support, Supporting Identity, Creating Opportunities, and Enjoyment that shifts focus from the tasks of eating to enhancing the resident quality of life through relational eating (Keller et al., 2021). This approach demonstrates promising increases in physical and social environments, relationship-centered eating practices, and perceived quality at mealtime (Keller et al., 2021).

While sensory experiences of human beings vary, a recent international study found that only 6% of the variance was observed cross-culturally when ranking single individual molecules that produce smell (Arshamian, et al., 2022). This may explain why skilled nursing facilities often bake bread to feed and engage residents in social activity, as "breaking bread" daily has long been culturally practiced, harkening to Christian religious concepts, like in Luke 11:3, which orients adherents to seek daily sustenance provided by God and to consider how they treat others (English Standard Version Bible, 2001), as can be experienced in communal eating. Baking bread also involves basic known and enjoyed ingredients, such as wheat and oil, and simple processing and preparation that families are often familiar with. Bread types will vary greatly across time and culture, and considerations should be made for residents with celiac disease and non-celiac wheat sensitivity (Tovoli et al., 2019). Bread is also often enjoyed with others in abundant quantity and is cost-effective to make.

Health factors such as adequate protein consumption for well-being and healing are often focused on in long-term care, but cultural variations in preferred protein sources vary. For example, sources of protein in Mexican cuisine can frequently include seafood, meat, and poultry with spiced sauces, while Chinese cuisine includes a yin/yang balance between cold and hot foods with proteins like beef, tofu, and chicken, which are often stewed. In contrast, Middle Eastern protein sources more typically include fermented dairy, chickpeas, and other nuts and seeds (Nemec, 2020). Offering different cultural food options, particularly on important holidays and religious occasions, could address this culturally mediated variation in protein and other dietary preferences. Residents could be provided with additional cultural education information on menus and activity calendars in combination with meal variations. Substitute options from regional ethnic restaurants or caterers could be an occasional resource of benefit for facilities, or where there are individual cultural dietary needs but not sufficient justification for altering menus for a whole facility.

An emerging consideration in long-term menu planning is plant-based, vegan, or vegetarian (plants + dairy) dietary options that feature certain health benefits such as lower saturated fat and increased fiber, but that may also present nutritional risks like vitamin B12 and D deficiencies, particularly among vegans, and require dietary planning and monitoring (Key et al., 2022). While some long-term care residents may pursue plant-based diets for health reasons and/or general preferences, others eat this way for religious reasons. Hindus practice ahimsa (non-violence), especially by avoiding beef consumption (Arslan & Aydın, 2024), and Buddhist diets are often plant-based, related to practicing moderation and mindfulness (Donovan, 2018). Other religious traditions also prescribe specific dietary guidance, like Kosher eating laws in Judaism and Halal eating laws in Islam, both of which prohibit the consumption of pork (Arslan & Aydın, 2024).

Activities and Programming

Long-term care residents commonly demonstrate low social engagement; however, racial and ethnic minority groups can be less engaged in social activities than white residents (Li & Cai, 2014; Shippee et al., 2020). This gap in social engagement is detrimental to quality-of-life experience and must be accounted for in activities and other programming approaches, especially because racial and ethnic minority adults are increasing in numbers across the United States (Campbell et al., 2016). The role of individual personality also remains an important domain of inquiry, as specific personality traits may correlate to tendencies to participate in activities (Newton et al., 2016). Ensuring that activities offered are personally meaningful to long-term residents is correlated to improved mood and positive life satisfaction (Hooker et al., 2019).

Practical opportunities in long-term care settings might optimally include the creation of a cultural activity committee with resident, family, and staff involvement. One such example observed by the author in an assisted living memory care facility was a weekly geographic knowledge activity, where residents were invited to learn about the cultures of people from varied countries across the map. Other facilities may include multicultural fairs, music, and other rich cultural celebrations and gatherings. Religious holidays in the spring season could include the Christian Easter holiday, the Hindu Festival of Colors, the Jewish Passover, or the Muslim holy month of Ramadan (Sheikh, 2023).

Clinical arts and non-clinical arts programs support holistic health engagement, mental health well-being, and general health (Jensen & Bonde, 2018) and can be encouraged in the general population, with less verbal residents, and those with various levels of physical ability and social engagement. As cultural institutions are finding ways to virtually connect with broader audiences, museums, music venues, and other cultural events are becoming more digitally accessible to global long-term care environments (Alnasser & Yi, 2023). Upon searching the Metropolitan Museum of Art's (n.d.) website online, full collections are virtually accessible, including African art, ancient American art, ancient Near Eastern art, Egyptian art, European art, Islamic art, and Medieval art, among others. Resources like this can be readily used on a large presentation screen in groups or for individual residents with computers, tablets, or phones with Internet access.

Organizational Culture

An example of an organizational response that impacted social engagement within long-term care can be found in the development of COVID-19 policies and procedures. While many of the related social distancing policies were beneficial in protecting resident safety, some may have contributed to increased social isolation and/or other adverse consequences, like in the case of reducing access of families to dying family members (Strang et al., 2020). Large numbers of older adults in long-term care also experienced threats to mental well-being, including higher incidences of anxiety and depression (Grolli et al., 2021). Adaptive strategies to promote social well-being, even during public health crises, are possible and ought to be implemented. Some possible strategies might include policies and resources that support Internet-driven groups and religious services, simulated presence therapies, or encouraging family engagement through windows and safety barriers (Simard & Volicer, 2020), or online meeting applications like Facetime or Zoom during periods of social isolation.

Another looming societal challenge that will continue to impact long-term care culture significantly is the complex care needs of 78 million people who are expected to have dementia by 2030, which is predicted to climb to just under 140 million by 2050 (WHO, 2021). The Chinese government has attempted a three-tier system to approach this problem, preferring home care primarily, adding supportive community care, and lastly, relying on institutional support (Wang et al., 2018). Minority ethnic groups in Norway note barriers to dementia care services and a lack of culturally different care at times that illustrate the need for more patient-centered dementia care approaches, especially for ethnic minority groups in long-term care settings (Czapka & Sagbakken, 2020). When global organizations tackle these issues within governmental and long-term organizational contexts, cultural dementia beliefs, roles of family and caregivers, and integrating increasing numbers of migrant health workers will continue to be significant areas of focus for long-term care organizations (Brooke et al., 2017).

The role of cultural differences within long-term care organizations includes appreciating contexts between staff, staff and residents, and among personal and organizational stakeholders (Kilaberia, 2021). Some of the cultural themes within long-term care organizations impacting diverse staff include shared norms and needs for challenges to what is normative, flexibility, the context of language, understanding of roles, and prejudice and harassment (Debesay et al., 2022). Tools like the interRAI Self-Reported Quality of Life Survey for Long-Term Care Facilities (SQOL-LTCF) can help long-term care facilities better understand the quality-of-life and service-related data (Morris et al., 2018). This tool was developed and tested internationally by researchers in over 35 countries and has been adopted in Canada, Europe, South Africa, and New Zealand (Morris et al., 2018).

Conclusion

In summary, as society focuses on health promotion in long-term care for various reasons, current context and future considerations should be points of strategic focus. This involves appreciating the relationship between a rapidly aging society and culture as related to global perspectives on long-term care. Different countries have determined varied economic and structural approaches to long-term care provision, and ensuring basic quality of care is an essential public health aim. Variations in individualistic and collectivist cultures will naturally vary in the way long-term care organizations respond to institutional older adult care needs in varied geographic locations. Successfully navigating these cultural long-term care differences involves a commitment to enhancing cultural knowledge in combination with cultural competence and openness to needed changes as a product of cultural humility. When combined with emerging strategies and tools for cultural assessment and practical resources for responsive intervention in long-term care settings, allied health professionals can better attend to the present scenario and future demands of culturally appropriate health promotion in long-term care environments.

References

Abbasi, J. (2020). "Abandoned" nursing homes continue to face critical supply and staff shortages as covid-19 toll has mounted. *JAMA, 324*(2), 123. https://doi.org/10.1001/jama.2020.10419

Ågotnes, G., & Øye, C. (2017). Facilitating resident community in nursing homes: A slippery slope? an analysis on collectivistic and individualistic approaches. *Health: An Interdisciplinary Journal for the Social Study of Health, Illness and Medicine, 22*(5), 469–482. https://doi.org/10.1177/1363459317708825

Agronin, M. (2022). Sexuality and aging. *The American Psychiatric Association Publishing Textbook of Geriatric Psychiatry*, 399.

Alnasser, N. S., & Yi, L. J. (2023). Strategies applied by different arts and cultural organizations for their audience development: A comparative review. *Heliyon, 9*(5). https://doi.org/10.1016/j.heliyon.2023.e15835

American Nurse Credentialing Center. (2017). *Self-Assessment of Organizational Culture* (for Long Term … https://www.nursingworld.org/globalassets/organizational-programs/self-assessment-of-organizational-culture-for-long-term-care.pdf

Andrew, N., & Meeks, S. (2016). Fulfilled preferences, perceived control, life satisfaction, and loneliness in elderly long-term care residents. *Aging and Mental Health, 22*(2), 183–189. https://doi.org/10.1080/13607863.2016.1244804

Applebaum, R., Robins, E., & Bardo, A. (2016). Long-term services & supports. In *Global aging* (pp. 183–185). Chapter, Springer.

Ariaans, M., Linden, P., & Wendt, C. (2021). Worlds of long-term care: A typology of OECD countries. *Health Policy, 125*(5), 609–617. https://doi.org/10.1016/j.healthpol.2021.02.009

Arshamian, A., Gerkin, R. C., Kruspe, N., Wnuk, E., Floyd, S., O'Meara, C., Garrido Rodriguez, G., Lundström, J. N., Mainland, J. D., & Majid, A. (2022). The perception of odor pleasantness is shared across cultures. *Current Biology, 32*(9). https://doi.org/10.1016/j.cub.2022.02.062

Arslan, S., & Aydın, A. (2024). Religious dietary practices: Health outcomes and psychological insights from various countries. *Journal of Religion and Health, 63*(5), 3256–3273. https://doi.org/10.1007/s10943-024-02110-8

Baker, E., McGaw, B., & Peterson, P. (2010). *International Encyclopedia of Education. vol. 3 eds.-in-chief Penelope Peterson; Eva Baker; Barry McGaw*. Elsevier Academic.

Basirico, L. A., Cashion, B. G., & Eshleman, J. R. (2021). *Introduction to sociology*. BVT Publishing.

Bengtson, V. L., Settersten, R. A., Kennedy, B. K., Morrow-Howell, N., & Smith, J. (2016). *Handbook of theories of aging*. Springer Publishing Company, LLC.

Bernhard, G., Knibbe, R. A., von Wolff, A., Dingoyan, D., Schulz, H., & Mösko, M. (2015). Development and psychometric evaluation of an instrument to assess cross-cultural competence of healthcare professionals (CCCHP). *PLOS ONE, 10*(12). https://doi.org/10.1371/journal.pone.0144049

Bista, C. B. (2023). Socio-cultural practice: A case study on personal hygienic behavior in the Hindu society. *Patan Pragya, 12*(01), 1–12. https://doi.org/10.3126/pragya.v12i01.61466

Brooke, J., Cronin, C., Stiell, M., & Ojo, O. (2017). The intersection of culture in the provision of dementia care: A systematic review. *Journal of Clinical Nursing, 27*(17–18), 3241–3253. https://doi.org/10.1111/jocn.13999

Buchan, J., Catton, H., & Shaffer, F. (2022). *(Tech.). Sustain and retain in 2022 and beyond*. International Centre on Nurse Migration.

Burgess, E. W. (1960). Aging in Western Culture. In E. W. Burgess (Ed.), *Aging in Western societies*. University of Chicago Press.

Butler, R. N. (1990). A disease called ageism. *Journal of the American Geriatrics Society., 38*(2), 178–180. https://doi.org/10.1111/j.1532-5415.1990.tb03483.x

Caceres, B. A., Travers, J., Primiano, J. E., Luscombe, R. E., & Dorsen, C. (2019). Provider and LGBT individuals' perspectives on LGBT issues in long-term care: A systematic review. *The Gerontologist, 60*(3). https://doi.org/10.1093/geront/gnz012

Campbell, L. J., Cai, X., Gao, S., & Li, Y. (2016). Racial/ethnic disparities in nursing home quality of life deficiencies, 2001 to 2011. *Gerontology and Geriatric Medicine, 2*, 233372141665356.

Cumming, E., & Henry, W. E. (1961). *Growing old: The process of disengagement*. Basic Books.

Czapka, E. A., & Sagbakken, M. (2020). "It is always me against the Norwegian system." barriers and facilitators in accessing and using dementia care by minority ethnic groups in Norway: A qualitative study. *BMC Health Services Research, 20*(1). https://doi.org/10.1186/s12913-020-05801-6

Debesay, J., Arora, S., & Fougner, M. (2022). Organisational culture and ethnic diversity in nursing homes: A qualitative study of healthcare workers' and ward nurses' experiences. *BMC Health Services Research, 22*(1), 843. https://doi.org/10.1186/s12913-022-08184-y

Donovan, M. M. (2018). Mindful eating: A guide to rediscovering a healthy and joyful relationship with food. *Journal of Nutrition Education and Behavior, 50*(7), 752. https://doi.org/10.1016/j.jneb.2018.02.010

English Standard Version Bible. (2001). *ESV Online*. https://esv.literalword.com/

Estabrooks, C. A., Straus, S. E., Flood, C. M., Keefe, J., Armstrong, P., Donner, G. J., Boscart, V., Ducharme, F., Silvius, J. L., & Wolfson, M. C. (2020). Restoring trust: Covid-19 and the future of long-term care in Canada. *FACETS, 5*(1), 651–691. https://doi.org/10.1139/facets-2020-0056

Estebsari, F., Dastoorpoor, M., Khalifehkandi, Z. R., Nouri, A., Mostafaei, D., Hosseini, M., Esmaeili, R., & Aghababaeian, H. (2020). The concept of Successful aging: A review article. *Current Aging Science, 13*(1), 4–10. https://doi.org/10.2174/1874609812666191023130117

Estrada, L. V., Agarwal, M., & Stone, P. W. (2021). Racial/ethnic disparities in nursing home end-of-life care: A systematic review. *Journal of the American Medical Directors Association, 22*(2). https://doi.org/10.1016/j.jamda.2020.12.005

Fang, F., & Yang, X. (2023). Socioeconomic status, cultural values, and elderly care: An examination of elderly care preference in OECD countries. *Aging and Health Research, 3*(3), 100153. https://doi.org/10.1016/j.ahr.2023.100153

Ford, M., Grandpre, A., Harmon, N., Mwenechanya, T., & Wang, N. (2024). Ethical advancements from the Tuskegee Experiment. *2024 Systems and Information Engineering Design Symposium (SIEDS)*, pp 189–194. https://doi.org/10.1109/sieds61124.2024.10534655

Global status report on the public health response to dementia. Geneva: World Health Organization; 2021. License: CC BY-NC-SA 3.0 IGO.

Grolli, R. E., Mingoti, M. E., Bertollo, A. G., Luzardo, A. R., Quevedo, J., Réus, G. Z., & Ignácio, Z. M. (2021). Impact of covid-19 in the mental health in elderly: Psychological and biological updates. *Molecular Neurobiology, 58*(5), 1905–1916. https://doi.org/10.1007/s12035-020-02249-x

Hande, M. J., Keefe, J., & Taylor, D. (2021). Long-term residential care policy guidance for staff to support resident quality of life. *The Gerontologist, 61*(4), 540–551. https://doi.org/10.1093/geront/gnaa176

Havinghurst, R. J. (1961). Successful aging. *The Gerontologist, 1*, 4–7.

Heikkilä, K., Andersson, S., Lagerbielke, E., Persson, C., Sandgren, A., & Harstäde, C. W. (2022). Mealtime interventions and their outcomes in care homes for older people considering the five aspects meal model: An integrative review. *Geriatric Nursing, 47*, 171–182. https://doi.org/10.1016/j.gerinurse.2022.07.011

Heusinger, J., & Dummert, S. (2016). "Genderspezifische Bedürfnisse von Pflegeheimbewohner_innen": Fokus Körperpflege ["Gender-specific needs of nursing home residents" : Focus on personal hygiene]. *Zeitschrift fur Gerontologie und Geriatrie, 49*(8), 685–691. https://doi.org/10.1007/s00391-016-1146-6

Hochschild, A. R. (1975). Disengagement theory: A critique and proposal. *American Sociological Review*, 553–569.

Hoefnagels, F. A., Patijn, O. N., Meeusen, M. J., & Battjes-Fries, M. C. (2023). The perceptions of food service staff in a nursing home on an upcoming transition towards a healthy and sustainable food environment: A qualitative study. *BMC Geriatrics, 23*(1). https://doi.org/10.1186/s12877-023-04493-x

Hook, J. N., Watkins, C. E., Jr., Davis, D. E., Owen, J., Van Tongeren, D. R., & Ramos, M. J. (2016). Cultural humility in psychotherapy supervision. *American Journal of Psychotherapy, 70*(2), 149–166. https://doi.org/10.1176/appi.psychotherapy.2016.70.2.149

Hooker, S. A., Masters, K. S., Vagnini, K. M., & Rush, C. L. (2019). Engaging in personally meaningful activities is associated with meaning salience and psychological well-being. *The Journal of Positive Psychology, 15*(6), 821–831. https://doi.org/10.1080/17439760.2019.1651895

Jensen, A., & Bonde, L. (2018). The use of arts interventions for mental health and well-being in Health Settings. *Perspectives in Public Health, 138*(4), 209–214. https://doi.org/10.1177/1757913918772602

Keller, H. H., Wu, S. A., Iraniparast, M., Trinca, V., Morrison-Koechl, J., & Awwad, S. (2021). Relationship-centered mealtime training program demonstrates efficacy to improve the dining environment in long-term care. *Journal of the American Medical Directors Association, 22*(9). https://doi.org/10.1016/j.jamda.2020.11.008

Key, T. J., Papier, K., & Tong, T. Y. N. (2022). Plant-based diets and long-term health: findings from the EPIC-Oxford study. *The Proceedings of the Nutrition Society, 81*(2), 190–198. https://doi.org/10.1017/S0029665121003748

Kilaberia, T. R. (2021). Negotiating Social Diversity in Residential Care for Older Persons. *Journal of Contemporary Ethnography, 50*(4), 466–496. https://doi.org/10.1177/0891241621991638

Kuang, Y., Wang, M., Yu, N. X., Jia, S., Guan, T., Zhang, X., Zhang, Y., Lu, J., & Wang, A. (2022). Family resilience of patients requiring long-term care: A meta-synthesis of qualitative studies. *Journal of Clinical Nursing, 32*(13–14), 4159–4175. https://doi.org/10.1111/jocn.16500

Lao, S. S. W., Low, L. P. L., & Wong, K. K. Y. (2019). Older residents' perceptions of family involvement in residential care. *International Journal of Qualitative Studies on Health and Well-Being, 14*(1). https://doi.org/10.1080/17482631.2019.1611298

Levkoff, S., Chee, Y. K., Reynoloso-Vallejo, H., & Mendez, J. (2000). Culturally appropriate geriatric care: fund of knowledge. In G. Yeo (Ed.), *Core curriculum in Ethnogeriatrics* (2nd ed.). Stanford Geriatric Education Center.

Li, Y., & Cai, X. (2014). Racial and ethnic disparities in social engagement among US nursing home residents. *Medical Care, 52*(4), 314–321. https://doi.org/10.1097/MLR.0000000000000088

Macionis, J. J., & Bhatia, R. (2019). *Sociology*. Pearson India Education Services Pvt. Ltd.

Marshalla, V., & Clarke, P. J. (2007). Theories of aging: Social. In J. E. Birren (Ed.), *Encyclopedia of gerontology* (2nd ed., pp. 621–630). Academic Press.

Morris, J. N., Declercq, A., Hirdes, J. P., Finne-Soveri, H., Fries, B. E., James, M. L., Geffen, L., Kehyayan, V., Saks, K., Szczerbińska, K., & Topinkova, E. (2018). Hearing the voice of the resident in long-term care facilities—an internationally based approach to assessing quality of life. *Journal of the American Medical Directors Association, 19*(3), 207–215. https://doi.org/10.1016/j.jamda.2017.08.010

Moustafa Ibrahim, E., Mahmod, A., Elmaghwry, A., & Elzeblawy Hassan, H. (2021). Compassionate care delivery: Elderlies' perception. *Research in Psychology and Behavioral Sciences, 9*(1), 24–32. https://doi.org/10.12691/rpbs-9-1-4

Nemec, K. (2020). Cultural awareness of eating patterns in the health care setting. *Clinical Liver Disease, 16*(5), 204–207. https://doi.org/10.1002/cld.1019

Neugarten, B. L. (1996). *The meanings of age: Selected papers of Bernice L. Neugarten*. Chicago University Press.

Newton, N. J., Pladevall-Guyer, J., Gonzalez, R., & Smith, J. (2016). Activity engagement and activity-related experiences: The role of personality. *The Journals of Gerontology Series B: Psychological Sciences and Social Sciences*. https://doi.org/10.1093/geronb/gbw098

Pacquiao, D. F., Katz, J. R., Sattler, V., Zha, P., & Daub, K. F. (2021). Development of the clients' perceptions of providers' cultural competency instrument. *Journal of Transcultural Nursing: Official Journal of the Transcultural Nursing Society, 32*(5), 539–550. https://doi.org/10.1177/1043659620962559

Pyke, K. D., & Bengtson, V. L. (1996). Caring more or less: Individualistic and collectivist systems of family eldercare. *Journal of Marriage and the Family, 58*(2), 379. https://doi.org/10.2307/353503

Roberts, E. (2023). A conversation about the ethics of past and future memory care models: Perspectives from the first two European dementia villages. *INQUIRY: The Journal of Health Care Organization, Provision, and Financing, 60*. https://doi.org/10.1177/00469580221150565

Rose, A. M. (1964). A current theoretical issue in social gerontology. *The Gerontologist, 4*(1), 46–50.

Scharman, C. D., Burger, D., Shatzel, J. J., Kim, E., & DeLoughery, T. G. (2017). Treatment of individuals who cannot receive blood products for religious or other reasons. *American Journal of Hematology, 92*(12), 1370–1381. https://doi.org/10.1002/ajh.24889

Seetharaman, K., Chaudhury, H., Kary, M., Stewart, J., Lindsay, B., & Hudson, M. (2020). Best practices in dementia care: A review of the grey literature on guidelines for staffing and physical environment in long-term care. *Canadian Journal on Aging / La Revue Canadienne Du Vieillissement, 41*(1), 55–70. https://doi.org/10.1017/s0714980820000392

Sheikh, F. (2023). Celebrating cultural diversity and spirituality in long-term care facilities. *Caring for the Ages, 24*(4), 14–15. https://doi.org/10.1016/j.carage.2023.04.007

Shippee, T. P., Ng, W., & Bowblis, J. R. (2020). Does living in a higher proportion minority facility improve quality of life for racial/ethnic minority residents in nursing homes? *Innovation in Aging, 4*(3). https://doi.org/10.1093/geroni/igaa014

Simard, J., & Volicer, L. (2020). Loneliness and isolation in long-term care and the COVID-19 pandemic. *Journal of the American Medical Directors Association, 21*(7), 966–967. https://doi.org/10.1016/j.jamda.2020.05.006

Skeldon, L., & Jenkins, S. (2022). Experiences and attitudes of the LGBTQ+ community on care/nursing homes. *Journal of Homosexuality, 70*(13), 3075–3107. https://doi.org/10.1080/00918369.2022.2086751

Song, E. O., & Jang, H. Y. (2020). Predictors of satisfaction with care services among family members of older adult residents of long-term care facilities. *International Journal of Environmental Research and Public Health, 17*(9), 3298. https://doi.org/10.3390/ijerph17093298

Spencer, L., & Lu, K. (2022). Infusing culture into the long-term care environment to improve public health and quality-of-life experience. *European Journal of Environment and Public Health, 6*(1), em0091. https://doi.org/10.21601/ejeph/11336

Sproesser, G., Ruby, M. B., Arbit, N., Akotia, C. S., dos Alvarenga, M., Bhangaokar, R., Furumitsu, I., Hu, X., Imada, S., Kaptan, G., Kaufer-Horwitz, M., Menon, U., Fischler, C., Rozin, P., Schupp, H. T., & Renner, B. (2019). Understanding traditional and modern eating: The TEP10 framework. *BMC Public Health, 19*(1). https://doi.org/10.1186/s12889-019-7844-4

Stonington, S. (2022). Ontological collateral: The entanglement of "Cancer pain" and "chronic non-cancer pain" in Thailand. *Cultural Anthropology, 37*(1) https://doi.org/10.14506/ca37.1.09

Strang, P., Bergström, J., Martinsson, L., & Lundström, S. (2020). Dying from covid-19: Loneliness, end-of-life discussions, and support for patients and their families in nursing homes and hospitals. A National Register Study. *Journal of Pain and Symptom Management, 60*(4). https://doi.org/10.1016/j.jpainsymman.2020.07.020

Sue, D. W., Rasheed, M. N., & Rasheed, J. M. (2016). *Multicultural social work practice: A competency-based approach to diversity and social justice*. Jossey-Bass.

Tervalon, M., & Murray-García, J. (1998). Cultural humility versus cultural competence: A critical distinction in defining physician training outcomes in multicultural education. *Journal of Health Care for the Poor and Underserved, 9*(2), 117–125. https://doi.org/10.1353/hpu.2010.0233

The met collection. Metropolitan Museum of Art. (n.d.). https://www.metmuseum.org/art/collection

Thompson, W. E., Streib, G. F., & Kosa, J. (1960). The effect of retirement on personal adjustment: A panel analysis. *Journal of Gerontology, 15*, 165–169.

Tovoli, F., Granito, A., Negrini, G., Guidetti, E., Faggiano, C., & Bolondi, L. (2019). Long term effects of gluten-free diet in non-celiac wheat sensitivity. *Clinical Nutrition, 38*(1), 357–363. https://doi.org/10.1016/j.clnu.2017.12.017

Wang, H., Tsuji, T., Ide, K., Nakagomi, A., Ling, L., & Kondo, K. (2023). Does eating with others promote happiness among older adults living alone? A 3-year longitudinal study of the japan gerontological evaluation study. *International Journal of Geriatric Psychiatry, 38*(12). https://doi.org/10.1002/gps.6033

Wang, S., Cheung, D. S., & Leung, A. Y. (2018). Overview of dementia care under the three-tier long-term care system of china. *Public Health Nursing, 36*(2), 199–206. https://doi.org/10.1111/phn.12573

Wang, Z., West, C. P., Vaa Stelling, B. E., Hasan, B., Simha, S., Saadi, S., Firwana, M., Nayfeh, T., Viola, K. E., Prokop, L. J., Murad, M. H. (2024) *Measuring documentation burden in iii healthcare*. Technical Brief No. 47. (Prepared by the Mayo Clinic Evidence-based Practice Center under Contract No. 75Q80120D00005.) AHRQ Publication No. 24-EHC023. Rockville, MD: Agency for Healthcare Research and Quality; May 2024. https://doi.org/10.23970/AHRQEPCTB47. Posted final reports are located on the Effective Health Care Program search page.

White, K. R., & Griffith, J. R. (2019). *The well-managed healthcare organization*. Health Administration Press; Association of University Programs in Health Administration.

Wierda, J. J., de Vet, E., Troost, E., & Poelman, M. P. (2024). Characterizing food environments of hospitals and long-term care facilities in the Netherlands: A mixed methods approach. *BMC Health Services Research, 24*(1), 31. https://doi.org/10.1186/s12913-023-10399-6

Williams, R. H., Tibbitts, C., & Donahue, W. T. (2017). *Process of aging: Social and psychological perspectives*. Routledge.

World Health Organization. (n.d.-a). *Integrated continuum of long-term care*. World Health Organization. https://www.who.int/teams/maternal-newborn-child-adolescent-health-and-ageing/ageing-and-health/integrated-continuum-of-long-term-care

World Health Organization. (n.d.-b). *WHOQOL - measuring quality of life| The World Health Organization*. World Health Organization. https://www.who.int/tools/whoqol

Zhang, Q., Shenkel, J., Paasche-Orlow, S., Cadge, W., Howard, E., Bryan, M., & Morris, J. N. (2019). Effect of chaplaincy visits in an elder care setting: A pilot analysis of existing data. *Journal of Health Care Chaplaincy, 26*(3), 103–116. https://doi.org/10.1080/08854726.2019.1599257

Chapter 11
How Social Determinants of Health Influence Health Promotion in Long-Term Care

Romil Rakesh Parikh

Introduction

A key aim of health promotion in long-term care (LTC) settings is to ensure that residents live with dignity, independence, and a good quality of life (Doty et al., 1985). Services provided across the LTC continuum, including in nursing homes, residential care (such as assisted living), and home- and community-based settings, are designed to support individuals who have chronic illnesses, disabilities, or other needs that require assistance with daily activities (Rowles & Teaster, 2015). LTC settings serve a vulnerable population, often elderly individuals who may experience a range of physical, mental, and emotional health challenges. However, the health outcomes of older adults utilizing LTC are not solely determined by the care they receive (Broyles et al., 2016; Holt, 2017). Social determinants of health (SDOH)—the conditions in the environments where people are born, live, learn, work, play, and age—play a crucial role in shaping their health and well-being (World Health Organization, n.d.). These determinants include factors such as socioeconomic status, education, physical environment, employment, social support, and access to healthcare (Andermann, 2016). The SDOH may have profound implications for how health promotion is implemented and how effective these interventions for health promotion are in LTC settings (Rowles & Teaster, 2015). Although the SDOH have been studied in-depth for hospital-based care, their impact on health, specifically in different LTC settings, remains a relatively understudied, unorganized, and emerging area of research.

This chapter explores how the SDOH influence health promotion in LTC. By examining these factors in depth, we aim to understand how they affect the overall

R. R. Parikh (✉)
Division of Health Policy and Management, School of Public Health, University of Minnesota, Minneapolis, MN, USA
e-mail: parik075@umn.edu

K. K. Bhattacharyya (ed.), *Health Promotion in Long-Term Care Facilities*,
https://doi.org/10.1007/978-3-031-91038-8_11

quality of care and health outcomes and offer strategies for addressing these determinants within LTC environments.

SDOH Vary Across the LTC Continuum

The World Health Organization (n.d.) defines SDOH as the conditions in which people are born, grow, live, work, and age, as well as the wider set of forces and systems shaping the conditions of daily life. These determinants are key drivers of health inequities and include several dimensions such as economic stability, education, social connectedness, community engagement, healthcare access and quality, neighborhood and built environment, and cultural and societal factors (Andermann, 2016; Office of Disease Prevention and Health Promotion, 2020; World Health Organization, n.d.). Examples of factors within these dimensions are displayed in Fig. 11.1. The SDOH may influence older adults in every setting across the LTC continuum (Rowles & Teaster, 2015; Broyles et al., 2016; Holt, 2017). Nursing homes, assisted living, memory care units, home care, and adult day care each present distinct challenges and advantages in terms of healthcare access, social engagement, economic stability, and cultural and environmental factors (Rowles & Teaster, 2015). Furthermore, the interplay of these factors can impact residents differently based on age, sex, gender, race, ethnicity, physical and mental disabilities, the intersectionality of identities, and experiences of related discrimination, creating additional barriers for marginalized groups (Broyles et al., 2016; Scott et al., 2024). Understanding these differences in SDOH across the LTC continuum is essential for improving care delivery and developing interventions that address the unique needs

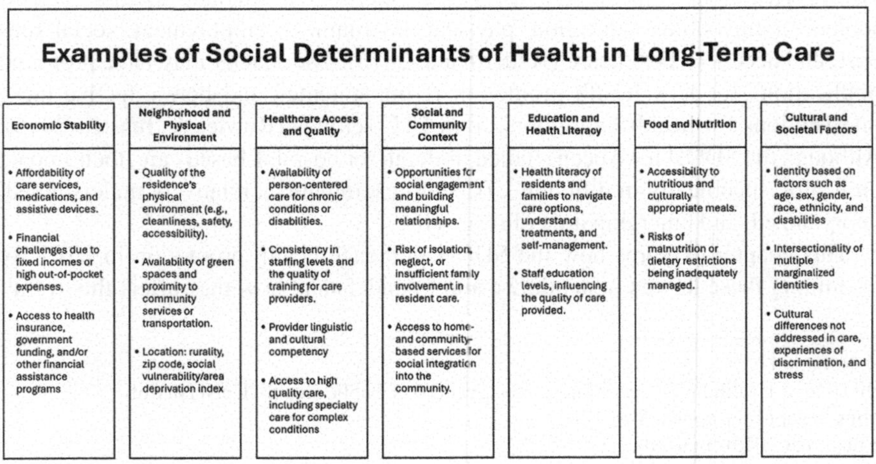

Fig. 11.1 Examples of social determinants of health in long-term care

of older adults in various LTC environments (Rowles & Teaster, 2015; Broyles et al., 2016; Holt, 2017; Barreira et al., 2023).

Nursing Homes

In nursing homes, which are designed for individuals with significant medical needs, such as chronic conditions or cognitive impairments, the SDOH are largely shaped by the level of healthcare access provided (Hedinger et al., 2015; Rowles & Teaster, 2015; Barreira et al., 2023). Nursing homes offer 24/7 medical care, including physical, occupational, and speech therapies, which can improve the management of complex health conditions. However, disparities in the quality of care, staff-to-resident ratios, and access to specialized treatments can affect health outcomes (National Academies of Sciences, Engineering, and Medicine, 2022). Economic stability in nursing homes is often linked to residents relying on governmental funding programs, for example, Medicaid in the United States, which can limit access to certain services or higher-quality care (Mor et al., 2004; Broyles et al., 2016; National Academies of Sciences, Engineering, and Medicine, 2022). The social environment in nursing homes can be challenging, as residents may experience higher levels of social isolation compared to other settings. This isolation is compounded by the institutionalized nature of many facilities, which may lack meaningful community integration. The physical environment, such as room layouts and facility design, can limit mobility and accessibility, leading to higher risks of falls or injury (National Academies of Sciences, Engineering, and Medicine, 2022). Age is an essential SDOH, as older adults typically have more complex health needs and are more vulnerable on account of being easier targets for discrimination, and these issues can be further compounded by physical disabilities. Sexual and gender identity can also influence the care provided; for example, women, who represent a larger proportion of nursing home residents, may experience different health challenges, including higher rates of chronic diseases and frailty. Race and ethnicity are crucial factors, as older adults from minority backgrounds often face healthcare disparities, including lower access to quality care, discrimination from staff, and cultural insensitivity in treatment (Shippee et al., 2022). For instance, Black and Hispanic older adults may encounter biases in pain management or less access to specialized care. Additionally, nursing home residents with mental disabilities, such as dementia or depression, may face stigma and less personalized care (National Academies of Sciences, Engineering, and Medicine, 2022). Intersectionality, where factors such as race, gender, and age interact, can amplify the challenges individuals face (Shippee et al., 2022). For example, an older Black woman with dementia may experience compounded discrimination, receiving lower-quality care due to both racial and cognitive biases. Furthermore, for older individuals with physical disabilities, the institutional ambiance, as well as physical barriers in the environment, can exacerbate social isolation by preventing meaningful engagement with others. These physical barriers, combined with mental disabilities, can lead to reduced participation in social activities, further exacerbating the risk of depression and poor health outcomes (National Academies of Sciences, Engineering, and Medicine, 2022).

Assisted Living

Assisted living facilities, designed for individuals who need assistance with activities of daily living but do not require intensive medical care, offer a different set of SDOH (Zimmerman et al., 2022; Shippee et al., 2024). The cost of assisted living is often higher and typically requires private payment, which can limit access to additional services or higher-quality care. Residents in assisted living facilities usually experience a higher degree of autonomy and social engagement compared to those in nursing homes, but their quality of life is still influenced by their ability to access healthcare and social services (Zimmerman et al., 2022; Shippee et al., 2024). Many assisted living facilities provide communal dining, social events, and outings that promote socialization, though the quality and frequency of these activities can vary. Healthcare access in assisted living is generally less intensive, with fewer on-site medical services available (Zimmerman et al., 2022; Shippee et al., 2024). This can create gaps in health management, particularly for residents with complex needs. The neighborhood and built environment in assisted living facilities are often more residential and community-oriented, providing easier access to local services such as grocery stores, public transportation, and recreational opportunities, which can improve mobility and social participation for residents (Shippee et al., 2024). Age-related physical decline is a common issue in this setting, with many residents experiencing chronic conditions such as arthritis, hypertension, or diabetes. Gender can also influence the experience of care, as older women in assisted living may experience higher rates of conditions such as osteoporosis or dementia. Ethnic and racial differences are particularly significant in this setting, as minority groups may experience poorer health outcomes due to systemic discrimination, less access to healthcare, or a lack of culturally competent care (Shippee et al., 2022). Older adults with minoritized identities, for example, in the United States, Black, Hispanic, and Indigenous identifying older adults in assisted living facilities with a majority white population, may face barriers to receiving care that addresses their cultural needs and may struggle with mistrust toward LTC systems due to historical discrimination (Shippee et al., 2022). Mental and physical disabilities also play a role, as individuals with conditions like mobility impairments or mental health disorders such as depression may find it more difficult to navigate an assisted living facility (Zimmerman et al., 2022). Intersectionality is relevant here as well, as an elderly Asian woman with limited English proficiency may face multiple barriers to accessing the resources and services she needs, including discrimination based on both race and language, in addition to age-related health issues. Social engagement is also crucial in assisted living, but residents with disabilities, particularly those with mental health disorders, may find it more challenging to participate in communal activities, leading to increased feelings of isolation and loneliness (Zimmerman et al., 2022).

Memory Care Units

Memory care units cater to individuals with Alzheimer's disease or other dementias, and their SDOH are influenced by specialized care environments (Orth et al., 2023). Socialization in memory care units can be more structured due to cognitive impairments, and residents often engage in therapeutic activities tailored to their condition. However, communication barriers and cognitive decline may heighten the risk of social isolation (Orth et al., 2023). Memory care units also provide specialized care for dementia-related conditions; however, gaps may exist in managing co-existing health conditions, as these settings tend to focus primarily on memory-related care (Orth et al., 2023). The physical environment in memory care units is designed with safety in mind, featuring secure spaces to prevent wandering and to reduce the risk of falls. However, these environments can sometimes lack stimulation or cognitive engagement unless designed with therapeutic activities in mind (Orth et al., 2023). Additionally, societal attitudes and stigma surrounding dementia can affect residents' emotional well-being, influencing their quality of life. Age is, of course, a central factor, as dementia typically affects older adults, with a higher prevalence among those aged 85 and above. Gender influences the experience of care, as women are more likely to develop dementia than men, leading to higher demand for memory care services among women. Therefore, ageism and sexism are a risk factor among a considerable portion of the older adult population in this LTC setting. Additionally, race and ethnicity can play a role in the prevalence and progression of dementia, with some studies indicating that in the United States, Blacks and Hispanics have higher rates of dementia compared to white populations but are often less likely to receive early diagnosis or access to specialized care (Hinton et al., 2024). Serious mental illness and mental health, including neuropsychiatric symptoms of dementia such as agitation, anxiety, and depression, are a key focus of memory care units; however, these conditions are often compounded by physical disabilities, making the management of care more complex (Orth et al., 2023). Moreover, individuals with mental disabilities may experience stigma, which can affect their quality of care. Discrimination related to cognitive disabilities is common, as staff may have lower expectations or provide less engaging care for individuals with dementia, viewing them as less capable of participating in activities (Shippee et al., 2022). Intersectionality is evident in memory care as well; for example, an elderly Black man with dementia may face challenges not only related to his cognitive impairment but also the biases and discrimination tied to his racial identity. This can impact his access to care, the quality of interactions with staff, and the overall care environment. In some cases, residents from marginalized backgrounds may not receive care that acknowledges their cultural preferences, leading to a sense of alienation and poorer outcomes.

Home- and Community-Based Settings

Home care allows individuals to remain in their own homes while receiving assistance with medical or personal care (Rowles & Teaster, 2015). The types of services provided in-home care are not limited to healthcare. Instead, they include non-medical personal care, assistance with activities of daily living, home modifications to support aging in place, and many other types of assistance. They include a wide range of services such as assistive technology and devices, attendant care /personal care, care/case management, caregiver training, chore services, community transition services, prevocational training services and employment seeking and retaining supports, companion services, durable and home medical equipment, environmental accessibility adaptations (home modifications), financial management services, home-delivered meals, home healthcare, homemaker services, non-medical transportation, nursing services, personal emergency response systems, caregiver support/respite care, and transportation (Fabius et al., 2024). These services can vary greatly in availability, eligibility, administration, policies, and funding sources, even within a country; for example, these services vary greatly between states within the United States. Home care presents its own unique SDOH challenges (Bucy et al., 2023). This LTC setting offers personalized care plans and flexibility, allowing caregivers to adjust services based on individual needs. However, home care may limit access to immediate medical interventions or specialized care available in institutional settings. Economic factors also play a significant role, as home care can be expensive and may require out-of-pocket payments, leading to financial strain for many families (Bucy et al., 2023). Family caregivers often bear the responsibility of care, which can contribute to stress, caregiver burnout, and social isolation. The lack of formal support systems can exacerbate these issues, especially when family members are juggling multiple roles and financial pressures (Bucy et al., 2023). The neighborhood and environment in home care settings are highly variable, depending on whether the home is equipped with accessibility features and how integrated it is within the broader community (Bucy et al., 2023). Homes with accessibility modifications are better suited to aging in place, while those without may present challenges to mobility and safety. Ethnic and racial disparities also affect home care, with minority groups facing barriers such as limited access to quality services, lower-income levels, and language barriers. For example, in the United States, Asian older adults may experience difficulties in finding culturally competent caregivers, leading to inadequate care that does not consider their cultural values or communication needs. Intersectionality is particularly relevant here, as an older disabled Black woman may face multiple challenges, including racial discrimination, gendered expectations about caregiving, and accessibility issues in her home environment.

Adult day care programs provide daytime supervision and care for older adults, often those with chronic illnesses or dementia. These programs are designed to offer structured activities, socialization, and therapeutic interventions, fostering social connections and mental stimulation (Ellen et al., 2017). Adult day care can help alleviate social isolation, but the level of healthcare services provided is generally less comprehensive than in nursing homes or assisted living facilities (Ellen et al., 2017). Financially, adult day care is usually a more affordable option compared to full-time institutional or residential care, though it can still present challenges for low-income families. The neighborhood and environment of adult day care programs tend to be more accessible, with many programs located in community settings that allow residents to engage with their broader neighborhoods. However, the physical resources available within each facility can vary, influencing the quality of care and the types of activities offered (Ellen et al., 2017). The experiences of older adults receiving care in adult day programs are also shaped by factors such as age, gender, and race (Ellen et al., 2017; Shippee et al., 2022). Gender influences care needs, as women are more likely to experience conditions like dementia, leading to a higher representation of women in adult day care programs. Age-related health conditions, such as arthritis or diabetes, are common in these settings as well. Race and ethnicity are crucial factors in adult day care, as older adults from minority backgrounds may face challenges in accessing care that is culturally sensitive and responsive to their needs. Additionally, individuals with mental disabilities, particularly dementia or depression, may face stigma or less engaging care in these programs. Discrimination based on mental health conditions can further marginalize these individuals, leading to a diminished quality of care and socialization opportunities (Ellen et al., 2017). Intersectionality also plays a role, as an older Latino man with depression may face compounded stigma based on both his mental health and ethnic background, leading to less supportive care and reduced participation in activities.

Thus, the SDOH framework for older adults underscores the importance of a multidimensional approach to aging. It suggests that regardless of the type of LTC setting, health and well-being are not solely the result of individual behaviors or biological processes but are improving economic security, enhancing social support, improving healthcare access, or implementing culturally tailored person-centered care—are essential to improving the quality of life and promoting health equity in older adult populations in LTC. Apart from differences in how SDOH vary across LTC settings, targeting SDOH requires consideration of differences in services provided, target populations, needs, policies, and administrative factors (such as how services are delivered, evaluated, and reimbursed) for each unique LTC setting. Understanding and addressing the setting-specific SDOH is critical for developing effective policies and programs that support healthy aging and reduce health disparities by assuring equitable and culturally competent care for older adults across the LTC continuum.

SDOH Impact Health Outcomes in LTC

Different SDOH, such as economic stability, education and literacy, social connectedness, built environment, healthcare access and quality, neighborhood and built environment, social identities, and cultural factors, have a profound impact on health outcomes, healthcare utilization outcomes, quality of care outcomes, and quality of life outcomes for older adults in each LTC setting. Given the variations in SDOH across the LTC continuum, we will discuss their impact on different health-related and healthcare-related outcomes in different types of LTC settings, including residential care settings such as nursing homes and assisted living, home care, and community-based care settings such as the adult day programs.

Economic Factors and Access to Quality Healthcare

Economic stability is a critically important SDOH, perhaps one of the most important factors, because the effects of several other SDOH often converge downstream onto this factor, and this factor has direct implications on healthcare access and quality (Mor et al., 2004; Broyles et al., 2016; National Academies of Sciences, Engineering, and Medicine, 2022). Older adults requiring LTC often face financial limitations that affect their access to care and overall health outcomes. Many residents in nursing homes, assisted living facilities, and memory care units rely on pensions, social security, or family support; however, these financial resources may not always be sufficient to cover the high costs of care. In contrast, residents with greater wealth/economic resources—who often have better access to private healthcare and higher-quality nursing homes—are more likely to receive timely care, better management of chronic conditions, and regular medical assessments. These differences in access and quality are linked to disparities in health outcomes, with residents in lower socioeconomic settings having worse physical and mental health outcomes than their wealthier counterparts (National Academies of Sciences, Engineering, and Medicine, 2022).

In nursing homes, older adults with limited financial resources may struggle to access critical medications, specialized treatments, and advanced healthcare services (Perez et al., 2022). These challenges can lead to poor management of chronic conditions, increased hospital admissions, and preventable health complications. For example, a resident with chronic conditions such as diabetes may have difficulty affording insulin or other diabetic medications, leading to fluctuating blood sugar levels, which can result in preventable hospitalizations for conditions like diabetic ketoacidosis or stroke. When financial limitations restrict access to health services, residents may also fail to receive necessary follow-up care after hospitalizations, increasing the risk of readmission (National Academies of Sciences, Engineering, and Medicine, 2022). Nursing homes with limited resources may also experience challenges in staffing, which can directly impact the quality of care. If a facility cannot afford to hire enough staff members, there may be delays in responding to residents' needs, leading to an increased risk of complications such as pressure ulcers or infections. Moreover, limited financial resources can lead to substandard living conditions, which in turn may affect residents' physical and mental well-being (Broyles et al., 2016; National Academies of Sciences, Engineering, and Medicine, 2022).

Systemic economic factors such as insurance and reimbursement mechanisms can also have a significant influence on the health of nursing home residents (Artiga & Hinton, 2018). For example, in the United States, nursing home residents who rely on public insurance programs like Medicaid are often at a disadvantage compared to those who can afford private insurance or pay out-of-pocket for more expensive care options. Research has shown that Medicaid residents frequently face lower-quality care, including reduced access to healthcare providers, fewer medical interventions, and a higher likelihood of being treated in understaffed facilities (Mor et al., 2004). This disparity can potentially result in poorer health outcomes, such as a greater risk of preventable conditions like pressure ulcers, infections, and malnutrition, as well as higher rates of utilizing emergency services and hospitalization (Mor et al., 2004; National Academies of Sciences, Engineering, and Medicine, 2022).

Similarly, in other LTC settings, economic challenges can manifest as difficulty accessing specialized health services or timely interventions, leading to unnecessary emergency department (ED) visits or potentially preventable hospitalizations (Zimmerman et al., 2022; Shippee et al., 2024). For instance, in assisted living, a resident with congestive heart failure who cannot afford regular check-ups with a cardiologist may experience a sudden exacerbation, requiring an ED visit. Additionally, the cost of assisted living services can vary greatly, and many residents may not be able to afford higher-end facilities that provide comprehensive care. Those in lower-income settings may experience reduced care quality, contributing to poorer health outcomes, such as malnutrition, dehydration, or untreated infections. Memory care units, if underfunded, may struggle to provide specialized dementia care, leading to increased agitation, confusion, and behavioral issues among residents (Orth et al., 2023). This struggle may escalate into preventable hospitalizations due to falls or medical complications related to untreated conditions. Regular medical appointments are crucial for managing comorbid conditions that often accompany dementia, such as diabetes, hypertension, or cardiovascular disease. When these conditions are not managed effectively due to financial limitations, residents may face increased hospitalizations and adverse health outcomes.

Home care provides support with daily tasks, such as bathing, dressing, and eating, and can be a cost-effective alternative to institutional care. However, those with limited financial resources may not be able to afford the level of care they need. For example, a senior with limited income might only be able to afford a few hours of home care per week, resulting in gaps in essential support. This could lead to falls, untreated medical conditions, or preventable hospitalizations due to a lack of adequate caregiving. In some cases, economic instability in home care settings can also result in a caregiver shortage (Bucy et al., 2023). Families may need to provide unpaid care, which can lead to caregiver burnout. If family caregivers do not have the resources or training to manage their loved one's health needs effectively, it can result in a failure to detect early signs of health problems, leading to ED visits and hospitalizations that could have been avoided with proper care. Similarly, restricted access to adult day programs due to financial constraints may prevent older adults from benefiting from social interaction and medical oversight. This lack of access can lead to greater isolation and poorer health outcomes, including depression and physical decline, which increase the risk of adverse outcomes (Ellen et al., 2017). In adult day programs that serve low-income populations, staff may face challenges in providing comprehensive care due to resource constraints (Ellen et al., 2017). Without sufficient funding, these programs may not be able to offer the range of services required to preserve health, such as nutrition support, cognitive engagement, and exercise programs.

Education and Health Literacy

Education access and quality, pertaining to past education, continued education efforts, and health literacy initiatives, are powerful SDOH that influence clinical outcomes, health outcomes, and the overall experience of care (Berkman et al., 2011). Education pertaining to both older adults and their care providers can impact outcomes in LTC (National Academies of Sciences, Engineering, and Medicine, 2022; Bucy et al., 2023). The impact of education on older adults in LTC settings is often seen through health literacy, which affects residents' ability to understand their medical conditions, follow treatment plans, and engage with healthcare providers. For example, in a residential LTC setting like a nursing home or assisted living, an older resident with heart disease who has not received sufficient education about the condition may miss the importance of taking prescribed medications, leading to a worsening of their symptoms and possibly resulting in hospitalization. On the other hand, continued education is important for LTC providers who may have varying levels of training and education pertaining to caring for medically complex older adults. Nursing home staff with higher levels of education are often better equipped to provide quality care and deliver health education to residents (National Academies of Sciences, Engineering, and Medicine, 2022). Educating residents on how to manage their conditions or recognize early warning signs of deterioration can reduce hospitalizations and improve overall health outcomes. For instance, a well-educated nursing home staff can help residents with diabetes monitor their blood sugar levels, preventing complications like diabetic neuropathy or ulcers that would otherwise lead to hospital stays. Residents who receive education about their health conditions and are actively engaged in managing their own care are more likely to experience improved health outcomes. For instance, assisting residents with understanding dietary restrictions or helping them organize their medications can help prevent complications from conditions such as chronic kidney disease or heart failure. In memory care units, the importance of education and health literacy is compounded due to the greater prevalence of cognitive impairments among residents (Orth et al., 2023). Trained staff members are aware of the unique issues faced by these residents and can create individualized, person-centered, dementia-friendly care plans grounded in the SDOH framework. They can also educate families on how to optimally support their loved ones in managing their health and well-being. Additionally, cognitive therapies and activities designed to promote memory retention may potentially help slow the progression of dementia and reduce the risk of hospitalization (Orth et al., 2023).

Education and health literacy are crucial in home- and community-based settings because the responsibility for managing one's health often falls on the individual and their caregivers (Berkman et al., 2011). Older adults with limited education may struggle to understand medical instructions, such as how to manage chronic conditions like diabetes or high blood pressure. This lack of understanding can lead to poor self-management, medication errors, and ultimately, unnecessary hospitalizations (Bucy et al., 2023). For example, a resident with high blood pressure may fail to recognize the importance of regular medication adjustments or diet modifications, leading to a hypertensive crisis that results in a preventable ED visit. Training home care staff to recognize signs of health literacy challenges is essential (Berkman et al., 2011; Bucy et al., 2023). When caregivers are equipped with the knowledge to educate patients and their families, they can help prevent ED visits and hospitalizations by ensuring that medical instructions are clearly communicated and followed. Furthermore, involving family members in the care process can help reinforce important health education, improving residents' health outcomes. Adult day programs often provide educational sessions on topics like chronic disease management, fall prevention, and nutrition. When older adults participate in educational activities that improve their health literacy, they may become better equipped to manage their conditions and make informed decisions about their care (Berkman et al., 2011; Perez et al., 2022). For example, an adult day program that teaches participants about the importance of exercise in managing arthritis may help reduce the number of hospitalizations caused by falls or complications of mistreated arthritis. Similarly, staff in these settings can be trained to provide regular health screenings, which might help identify early signs of medical issues. Early detection of conditions like hypertension or diabetes can prevent adverse health outcomes.

Social and Community Context

Social and community context plays a major role in the health and well-being of older adults across the LTC continuum (Perez et al., 2022). Strong social networks and community involvement can improve both clinical outcomes and quality of life by reducing isolation, encouraging healthy behaviors, and providing emotional support. Conversely, social isolation and lack of community engagement can contribute to poor mental and physical health outcomes. In nursing homes, social connectedness through group activities, friendships, and family support reduces the risks of social isolation, leading to better mental health outcomes such as lower risk of depression and cognitive decline (National Academies of Sciences, Engineering, and Medicine, 2022). For example, nursing home residents with family support are more likely to seek help early for medical issues, preventing avoidable hospitalizations. Similarly, in assisted living facilities, residents who participate in social activities and maintain connections tend to have better physical and mental health, with fewer hospitalizations and falls (Zimmerman et al., 2022; Shippee et al., 2024). In memory care units or other LTC settings providing dementia care, meaningful social interactions can alleviate agitation and improve cognitive function in residents with dementia. Family and caregiver involvement can help reduce confusion and improve communication, leading to fewer hospitalizations. Activities such as group therapy, music, or art therapy stimulate cognitive function and provide opportunities for relationship-building, improving overall quality of life (Perez et al., 2022; Orth et al., 2023). In contrast, social isolation can lead to depression and rapid cognitive decline, increasing the risk of preventable hospitalizations (National Academies of Sciences, Engineering, and Medicine, 2022). In home care, social isolation is a significant concern. Homebound seniors often face challenges in accessing transportation, limiting their social engagement and healthcare appointments. Home care workers, such as personal care aides and other paid caregivers, can provide companionship, facilitate social connections, and help coordinate community services like meal delivery or transportation, which might confer favorable health outcomes (Artiga & Hinton, 2018). Adult day programs also offer valuable social engagement, reducing isolation and improving both mental and physical health. These programs also support family caregivers by reducing burnout, leading to better care for older adults, which may translate to favorable health outcomes. In sum, social engagement across various LTC settings can potentially play a critical role in improving health outcomes (Perez et al., 2022).

Physical Environment and Neighborhood

The physical environment and neighborhood surrounding any LTC setting can have a significant influence on health outcomes (Perez et al., 2022). Older adults who reside in areas with poor infrastructure or unsafe conditions are at greater risk for falls, accidents, and preventable hospitalizations, such as those caused by fractures or injuries. For residential care, the design of an LTC facility itself—such as having adequate space for mobility, accessible features, and safe outdoor areas—can reduce the risk of falls and improve overall clinical outcomes. Inadequate access to outdoor spaces, for instance, could lead to sedentary behavior, which contributes to conditions like obesity or cardiovascular disease that may result in ED visits or hospitalizations (National Academies of Sciences, Engineering, and Medicine, 2022). Conversely, well-maintained facilities that promote physical activity and social engagement can enhance health and well-being (Perez et al., 2022). Similarly, for home- and community-based settings, the built environment can either promote mobility, independence, and social connectedness or hinder these based on funding availability, infrastructure, and geographic location. Adverse health outcomes of depriving these economic and social connectedness-related SDOH have been discussed in detail above for each LTC setting, including residential care as well as home- and community-based settings.

Cultural Factors

Cultural factors based on sociodemographic identities also influence both the quality of care and clinical outcomes for older adults across the LTC continuum (Shippee et al., 2022; Scott et al., 2024). Cultural sensitivity in care ensures that residents' beliefs, values, and preferences are respected, leading to better communication and higher adherence to care plans. Without this, misunderstandings between older adults and their care providers (including professional, skilled, and non-skilled staff)—such as cultural differences in pain expression or dietary restrictions—can result in preventable complications and hospitalizations. For instance, a resident may refuse to take a prescribed medication due to cultural beliefs, which can result in worsened health and unnecessary ED visits. A culturally competent care environment improves trust and satisfaction, which ultimately supports better quality of care and quality of life in every LTC setting (Shippee et al., 2022).

Food Insecurity and Nutrition

Food insecurity and nutrition are essential factors in maintaining good health for older adults in LTC. Poor nutrition can lead to malnutrition, dehydration, and other related complications that result in hospitalizations. For example, a nursing home resident who does not receive adequate nutrition may develop pressure ulcers, which increase the risk of infections and necessitate hospitalization. Ensuring that older adults in residential LTC settings receive nutritious meals tailored to their needs helps prevent these complications, reducing the risk of hospitalizations and improving overall health. Moreover, culturally minoritized residents might face a greater risk of poor nutrition because of cultural differences in meal preferences, which may not be honored due to factors such as lack of awareness of staff or financial/resource constraints. Due to these factors, culturally minoritized groups (e.g., Black and Asian residents in predominately white population serving facilities) might face a greater risk of malnutrition and related adverse health outcomes (Shippee et al., 2022). Similarly, in home- and community-based settings, lack of access to nutritious fresh food (e.g., among older adults living in areas recognized as a food desert) can confer a greater risk of malnutrition and its adverse health consequences and greater healthcare utilization (Fabius et al., 2024). In home care, there are specific services provided to address food insecurity such as home-delivered meal programs (e.g., Meals-on-Wheels), transportation (to grocery stores), and homemaker assistance (to aid grocery shopping). However, these services are not provided uniformly in every place (e.g., a limited number of states in the United States provide coverage or reimbursement for home-delivered meal programs), and in some instances, despite the existence of services, there aren't sufficient service providers or staff to provide these services to all older adults requiring these services (Artiga & Hinton, 2018). Proper nutrition is critically important to the health and well-being of older adults as it contributes to energy levels, mood, and physical functionality, enhancing the quality of life in LTC.

In conclusion, SDOH have a wide-ranging impact on the clinical outcomes, health outcomes, quality of care, and quality of life for older adults in long-term care settings (Perez et al., 2022). These factors influence hospitalization rates, including preventable hospitalizations, and affect how well residents manage chronic conditions and engage with healthcare services. There exists a complex interplay between several SDOH, which is unique to individual LTC settings. Addressing these determinants through holistic, person-centered care models can lead to better health outcomes, reduced hospitalizations, and an enhanced quality of life for older adults in LTC (National Academies of Sciences, Engineering, and Medicine, 2022).

Integration of SDOH with Health Promotion in LTC

The integration of SDOH into health promotion efforts in LTC settings offers a proactive, culturally grounded, equitable, and person-centered strategy to enhance overall well-being, improve health outcomes, and mitigate the negative impact of aging (McGilton et al., 2018; Perez et al., 2022). The first step in this integration involves conducting thorough assessments that go beyond just clinical health metrics. In settings such as assisted living communities, where residents may have varying degrees of independence, personalized care plans should be developed based on a comprehensive understanding of each resident's economic, social, and environmental context (Zimmerman et al., 2022). This approach allows healthcare providers to identify specific SDOH barriers affecting an individual and create tailored interventions that address those needs. For example, in a nursing home, a resident's financial status and access to social services can be assessed to ensure they receive the necessary support while also evaluating their social network to reduce feelings of loneliness. These personalized care plans can include strategies to improve access to resources, enhance social engagement, and foster a more supportive living environment that promotes physical activity, social interaction, and mental well-being (Perez et al., 2022). Additionally, LTC providers may adopt collaborative care models that involve interdisciplinary teams working together to address the physical, mental, and social needs of residents. This approach ensures that all aspects of residents' health are addressed and integrated into health promotion efforts (McGilton et al., 2018).

Incorporating community engagement is also vital for addressing social isolation, a key SDOH in LTC. Long-term care settings, including nursing homes and home care, can benefit from building strong partnerships with local community organizations, social service agencies, and volunteer networks (National Academies of Sciences, Engineering, and Medicine, 2022; Zimmerman et al., 2022). These collaborations can provide additional resources such as companionship programs, educational workshops, and recreational activities. In some assisted living facilities, peer-led initiatives or resident-led social groups have proven effective in fostering a sense of belonging and improving mental health. Peer mentorship programs, where residents support each other through shared experiences, can also reduce isolation and create stronger bonds among residents. For residents in home care, technology can offer a means to stay connected with family, friends, and healthcare providers, ensuring that they do not become disconnected from their support networks (Artiga & Hinton, 2018). Virtual platforms for social interaction, health consultations, or even fitness programs can be invaluable in preventing isolation for those who may have difficulty leaving their homes.

Health promotion efforts in LTC settings must also focus on policy and environmental changes that address SDOH (Artiga & Hinton, 2018). For instance, ensuring food security is a critical aspect of long-term care. In nursing homes, where dietary needs are essential for maintaining health, improving meal options and providing nutrition education can make a significant difference in residents' health outcomes. Residential LTC facilities can also create supportive physical environments by implementing design modifications that enhance accessibility and safety (National Academies of Sciences, Engineering, and Medicine, 2022). These may include installing ramps, wider doorways, or non-slip flooring, which can prevent falls and promote mobility. Creating spaces that encourage physical activity—whether it is an in-house gym, safe walking paths, or outdoor areas for gardening—can also significantly improve residents' physical health, reduce frailty, and prevent the onset of chronic conditions such as heart disease or diabetes (Andermann, 2016). In home care, providing residents with adaptive equipment and ensuring their homes are free from hazards can empower them to maintain independence and engage in physical activity. Advocacy and policy interventions can establish frameworks that prioritize SDOH in LTC (Hinton & Diana, 2021). For instance, legislation promoting equitable funding for facilities in underserved areas can address disparities in access to quality care. Similarly, policies mandating culturally competent training for LTC staff ensure services are tailored to the diverse social and cultural needs of residents (Shippee et al., 2022; Shippee et al., 2024).

Training and capacity building for care providers is another crucial aspect of integrating SDOH with health promotion (National Academies of Sciences, Engineering, and Medicine, 2022). Whether in nursing homes or assisted living facilities, long-term care staff play an essential role in identifying and addressing the broader social factors that influence residents' health. Regular training on cultural competence, understanding diverse backgrounds, and person-centered care can help staff recognize the unique needs of residents and offer more individualized, compassionate care (Shippee et al., 2022). In home care settings, where caregivers often work in isolation with little oversight, training programs that focus on identifying and addressing SDOH in the home environment can be especially beneficial. Additionally, interdisciplinary collaboration among healthcare providers, social workers, dietitians, and therapists ensures that all aspects of a resident's well-being are considered and that health promotion efforts are comprehensive and effective (Hinton & Diana, 2021; National Academies of Sciences, Engineering, and Medicine, 2022).

Conclusion

The SDOH have a profound impact on the health promotion efforts across the LTC continuum. By addressing these determinants, LTC providers can improve the health and quality of life for their residents. Economic stability, education, social and community context, access to healthcare, and the built environment are all factors that must be considered in health promotion initiatives in LTC. Only by taking a holistic approach to care that considers the broader social determinants can we hope to provide the highest standard of care in every LTC setting, ranging from nursing homes and assisted living to home- and community-based settings. Incorporating these factors into daily practice is essential for improving health outcomes and ensuring that older adults relying on LTC live with dignity, autonomy, optimal physical, mental, and emotional health, and a sense of overall well-being. Health promotion activities in LTC can be effectively grounded in SDOH through a combination of policy changes, community engagement, staff education, and personalized care plans, with the goal of equitably addressing the complex needs of the vulnerable aging population requiring LTC.

References

Andermann, A., & CLEAR Collaboration. (2016). Taking action on the social determinants of health in clinical practice: A framework for health professionals. *CMAJ: Canadian Medical Association Journal = journal de l'Association medicale canadienne, 188*(17-18), E474–E483. https://doi.org/10.1503/cmaj.160177

Artiga, S., & Hinton, E. (2018). *Beyond health care: The role of social determinants in promoting health and health equity - issue brief.* Kaiser Family Foundation. Retrieved December 4, 2024, from https://www.kff.org/report-section/beyond-health-care-the-role-of-social-determinants-in-promoting-health-and-health-equity-issue-brief/#endnote_link_412056-1

Barreira, L. F., Paiva, A., Araújo, B., & Campos, M. J. (2023). Challenges to systems of long-term care: Mapping of the central concepts from an umbrella review. *International Journal of Environmental Research and Public Health, 20*(3), 1698. https://doi.org/10.3390/ijerph20031698

Berkman, N. D., Sheridan, S. L., Donahue, K. E., Halpern, D. J., & Crotty, K. (2011). Low health literacy and health outcomes: An updated systematic review. *Annals of Internal Medicine, 155*(2), 97–107. https://doi.org/10.7326/0003-4819-155-2-201107190-00005

Broyles, I. H., Sperber, N. R., Voils, C. I., Konetzka, R. T., Coe, N. B., & Van Houtven, C. H. (2016). Understanding the context for long-term care planning. *Medical Care Research and Review: MCRR, 73*(3), 349–368. https://doi.org/10.1177/1077558715614480

Bucy, T. I., Mulcahy, J. F., Shippee, T. P., Fashaw-Walters, S., Dahal, R., Duan, Y., & Jutkowitz, E. (2023). Examining satisfaction and quality in home- and community-based service programs in the United States: A scoping review. *The Gerontologist, 63*(9), 1437–1455. https://doi.org/10.1093/geront/gnad003

Doty, P., Liu, K., & Wiener, J. (1985). An overview of long-term care. *Health Care Financing Review, 6*(3), 69–78.

Ellen, M. E., Demaio, P., Lange, A., & Wilson, M. G. (2017). Adult day center programs and their associated outcomes on clients, caregivers, and the health system: A scoping review. *The Gerontologist, 57*(6), e85–e94. https://doi.org/10.1093/geront/gnw165

Fabius, C. D., Parikh, R., Wolf, J. M., Giordano, S., Fashaw-Walters, S., Jutkowitz, E., & Shippee, T. (2024). Racial and ethnic differences in unmet needs among older adults receiving publicly-funded home and community-based services. *Journal of the American Geriatrics Society, 72*(11), 3520–3529. https://doi.org/10.1111/jgs.19153

Hedinger, D., Hämmig, O., Bopp, M., & Swiss National Cohort Study Group. (2015). Social determinants of duration of last nursing home stay at the end of life in Switzerland: A retrospective cohort study. *BMC Geriatrics, 15*, 114. https://doi.org/10.1186/s12877-015-0111-3

Hinton, E., & Diana, A. (2021). *Medicaid authorities and options to address social determinants of health (SDOH)*. Kaiser Family Foundation. Retrieved December 4, 2024, from https://www.kff.org/medicaid/issue-brief/medicaid-authorities-and-options-to-address-social-determinants-of-health-sdoh/

Hinton, L., Tran, D., Peak, K., Meyer, O. L., & Quiñones, A. R. (2024). Mapping racial and ethnic healthcare disparities for persons living with dementia: A scoping review. *Alzheimer's & Dementia, 20*(4), 3000–3020. https://doi.org/10.1002/alz.13612

Holt, J. D. (2017). Navigating long-term care. *Gerontology & Geriatric Medicine, 3*, 2333721417700368. https://doi.org/10.1177/2333721417700368

McGilton, K. S., Vellani, S., Yeung, L., Chishtie, J., Commisso, E., Ploeg, J., Andrew, M. K., Ayala, A. P., Gray, M., Morgan, D., Chow, A. F., Parrott, E., Stephens, D., Hale, L., Keatings, M., Walker, J., Wodchis, W. P., Dubé, V., McElhaney, J., & Puts, M. (2018). Identifying and understanding the health and social care needs of older adults with multiple chronic conditions and their caregivers: A scoping review. *BMC Geriatrics, 18*(1), 231. https://doi.org/10.1186/s12877-018-0925-x

Mor, V., Zinn, J., Angelelli, J., Teno, J. M., & Miller, S. C. (2004). Driven to tiers: Socioeconomic and racial disparities in the quality of nursing home care. *The Milbank Quarterly, 82*(2), 227–256. https://doi.org/10.1111/j.0887-378X.2004.00309.x

National Academies of Sciences, Engineering, and Medicine. (2022 April 6). *Health and Medicine Division; Board on Health Care Services; Committee on the Quality of Care in Nursing Homes. The National Imperative to Improve Nursing Home Quality: Honoring Our Commitment to Residents, Families, and Staff*. National Academies Press (US)

Office of Disease Prevention and Health Promotion. (2020). *Social determinants of health*. Healthypeople.gov; Office of Disease Prevention and Health Promotion. https://www.healthypeople.gov/2020/topics-objectives/topic/social-determinants-of-health

Orth, J., Flowers, D., Betz, G., & Cagle, J. G. (2023). A systematic review of specialty dementia care units in long-term care settings. *International Journal of Geriatric Psychiatry, 38*(4), e5907. https://doi.org/10.1002/gps.5907

Perez, F. P., Perez, C. A., & Chumbiauca, M. N. (2022). Insights into the social determinants of health in older adults. *Journal of Biomedical Science and Engineering, 15*(11), 261–268. https://doi.org/10.4236/jbise.2022.1511023

Rowles, G. D., & Teaster, P. B. (Eds.). (2015). *Long-term care in an aging society: Theory and practice*. Springer Publishing Company.

Scott, M. M., Ménard, A., Sun, A. H., Murmann, M., Ramzy, A., Rasaputra, P., Fleming, M., Orosz, Z., Huynh, C., Welch, V., Cooper-Reed, A., & Hsu, A. T. (2024). Building evidence to advance health equity: A systematic review on care-related outcomes for older, minoritised populations in long-term care homes. *Age and Ageing, 53*(4), afae059. https://doi.org/10.1093/ageing/afae059

Shippee, T. P., Akosionu-DeSouza, O., Beebe, T. J., Parikh, R. R., & Brasure, M. (2024). Measurement of quality in assisted living in the United States of America: A scoping review. *Journal of American Medical Directors Association, 26*(1), 105355. https://doi.org/10.1016/j.jamda.2024.105355

Shippee, T. P., Fabius, C. D., Fashaw-Walters, S., Bowblis, J. R., Nkimbeng, M., Bucy, T. I., Duan, Y., Ng, W., Akosionu, O., & Travers, J. L. (2022). Evidence for action: Addressing systemic racism across long-term services and supports. *Journal of American Medical Directors Association, 23*(2), 214–219. https://doi.org/10.1016/j.jamda.2021.12.018

World Health Organization. (n.d.). *Social Determinants of Health*. World Health Organization. Retrieved November 26, 2024, from https://www.who.int/health-topics/social-determinants-of-health#tab=tab_1

Zimmerman, S., Sloane, P. D., Wretman, C. J., Cao, K., Silbersack, J., Carder, P., Thomas, K. S., Allen, J., Butrum, K., Chicotel, T., Giorgio, P., Hernandez, M., Kales, H., Katz, P., Klinger, J. H., Kunze, M., Laxton, C., McNealley, V., Meeks, S., O'Neil, K., et al. (2022). Recommendations for medical and mental health care in assisted living based on an expert Delphi Consensus Panel: A consensus statement. *JAMA Network Open, 5*(9), e2233872. https://doi.org/10.1001/jamanetworkopen.2022.33872

Chapter 12
Aging in Place *or* Long-term Care? Changing the Narrative to Promote Aging in Place *in* Long-Term Care

Elizabeth Braungart Fauth, Gavin Green, and Josey Batura

Aging in Place refers to the movement focused on enabling older adults to live safely, independently, and comfortably in their own homes or communities, regardless of age, income, or functional ability (Vasunilashorn et al., 2012). The concept of *Place* is broader than just the "home"; it includes both a territory, that is, a geographic area of dwelling, and relational aspects like connections and networks that form and may change over time (Yarker et al., 2024). It is a preference for many older adults to remain in place (and specifically in their home) as they age (Ratnayake et al., 2022) or to be key decision makers in transitioning to a different home or community (Egan et al., 2022). It is also economically advantageous for individuals, families, and housing/medical assistance programs for individuals to stay in their home residence and not transition to more expensive residential long-term care (Crowley et al., 2022; Ratnayake et al., 2022).

As such, research on Aging in Place has often involved ways to enable older individuals to remain at home if they wish. Studies examine environmental design and housing modifications to facilitate aging at home (Hwang et al., 2011; Hjelle et al., 2016), as well as community support, healthcare services, and technology (Van Dijk et al., 2016; Jeste et al., 2016; Ollevier et al., 2020). Additionally, Aging in Place incorporates psychological components, like feeling there is a "fit" with one's home environment, quality of life in one's personal space, and maintaining a sense of mastery (Golant, 2011) and autonomy (Wiles et al., 2011). This chapter reviews these key components of the Aging in Place construct, as well as how individuals can be supported at home if they desire. While it may seem that Aging in Place and transitioning to residential long-term care (LTC) are incompatible with one another, this chapter describes that when long-term care environments become necessary, Aging in Place concepts can still be fostered within residential care.

E. B. Fauth (✉) · G. Green · J. Batura
Alzheimer's Disease and Dementia Research Center, Utah State University, Logan, UT, USA
e-mail: beth.fauth@usu.edu; gavin.green@usu.edu; j.batura@usu.edu

K. K. Bhattacharyya (ed.), *Health Promotion in Long-Term Care Facilities*,
https://doi.org/10.1007/978-3-031-91038-8_12

Aging in Place: Environment Aspects

At the environmental micro-level, the territory of *Place* is the physical dwelling or home. Home ownership is common in older adults in the USA, with the most common dwelling for this age group being a single-family detached house (Engelhardt et al., 2013). Many older adults have lived in the same home for a long time, and this age group relocates less often than other age groups (Joint Center for Housing Studies of Harvard University, 2019). It should be noted, however, that homes purchased in one phase of adulthood may not meet the needs of homeowners as they age. Aging in Place research has reviewed the safety implications of houses that were not designed to support functional impairment and provided recommendations for home modification (see, for example, Lau et al., 2007). Features of the home are important in Aging in Place decisions; when moving by choice, relocations in late life are more driven by dislikes about the current dwelling than by dislikes about the neighborhood or community (Hillcoat-Nallétamby & Ogg, 2014). Home maintenance needs can also inhibit Aging in Place (Fausset et al., 2011).

At the environmental macro-level, the territory of *Place* encompasses aspects of the neighborhood and community that support Aging in Place. These include neighborhood safety, transportation, opportunities for social or civic engagement, opportunities for leisure, affordability, and more. Some individuals want to stay within their long-lived communities; however, population and economic shifts in neighborhoods and communities over time can present challenges for Aging in Place and may be reasons why older people want to move to a new community (Lewis & Buffel, 2020). There is an extensive crossover between Aging in Place research and the "Age-Friendly Communities" movement, which posits that aspects of the built community and community health and service provisions support individuals to remain in place as they age (Kim et al., 2024; van Hoof & Marston, 2021).

In sum, extensive global research (with scoping reviews and meta-analyses) shows that micro-level and macro-level aspects of the built environment impact the physical health, functional impairment, and mental health of older adults (Garin et al., 2014). The built environment can support independent living, keep older people at home longer, and improve quality of life, *or* a poorer/incompatible built environment can increase disablement, increase risks of falls, or otherwise decrease quality of life.

Aging in Place: Psychosocial Aspects

Aging in Place research has encompassed psychological experiences related to *Place*, such as attachment to home and community, mental health outcomes related to physical space, preferences about housing, and quality of life. Imrie (2004) and Rowles et al. (2004) review the positive psychological aspects of "home," including privacy, safety, being able to navigate with ease (mental map of where things are), and having a place for peace and rest. They report that the home reflects people's identity; people design and use their space to reflect their personal expression and values. Their memories are tied to artifacts, décor, and comfort items in the home. Attachment to the community is similarly documented: people find comfort in knowing how to navigate their neighborhood, town, or city. They have memories attached to buildings and the natural environment. They feel "rooted in" their community and glean identity from their broader environment (Erickson et al., 2012).

The social attachments and relationships within the home, the neighborhoods, and larger communities are immensely important to the well-being of older people. The home itself may have been a shared dwelling, either prior in life or currently; thus, the home reflects social relationships with humans or pets, not just individual identity. The home may be a physical location to bring in friends or host family events. A scoping review covers the vast ways in which neighborhood and community social engagement promote well-being for older people in rural areas (Carver et al., 2018). Older people have (prior or currently) supported their neighbors, volunteered, or otherwise engaged in social organizations that evoke feelings of pride, pleasure, and a sense of self. The community can be developed to support such meaningful engagement, quality of life, and well-being fostered by age-friendly homes and communities with social engagement in mind (Sharifi et al., 2024).

In sum, psychological attachment to space is well-documented across the lifespan and may be even more salient for older people who have had more time to develop attachment to their home and to the people that occupy their home and community. Recent reviews have highlighted this more complex multifaceted nature of Aging in Place, showing a shift toward more integrated approaches that consider psychological well-being, social networks, place attachment, and community interventions (Ahn et al., 2017; Greenfield, 2015; Graham et al., 2015; Campbell, 2015). These studies emphasize that successful Aging in Place is not only about adapting to the physical environment but also ensuring access to resources that support the social and emotional world of the older person (Seo & Lee, 2023).

Aging in Place *or* Long-term Care

Older adults are at risk for chronic health conditions, physical or cognitive impairment, falls, and more, which strain their ability to stay in their home and/or community. Scoping and systematic reviews of in-home monitoring technologies (Kim et al., 2022) and in-home care (Boland et al., 2017; Dostalova et al., 2021) support that Aging in Place (in the home) can be realized for many older people with increased care needs. Reviewing at-home care coordination, best practices in community-based care, or outcomes for older individuals receiving at-home care is outside the scope of this chapter; however, it is a recognized and valued care option that supports Aging in Place. That being said, and moving toward the purpose of this chapter, there are times when transitioning to long-term care (LTC) is necessary. Making this decision is a deeply emotional and complex process and often involves people other than the older adult, such as family caregivers. *Here we review common personal and contextual factors that precipitate the transition to LTC.*

Safety risks in the home are often a driving factor in transitioning to LTC. Falls are caused by a combination of functional and environmental factors (Ambrose et al., 2013). While home modification can mitigate some risks, certain features at the home may not be amenable to support a person at risk for falls. Living alone may increase the health impact of a fall when it occurs, and in many scenarios, living alone cannot be modified without the older person relocating. Mobility and accessibility features impact the quality of life and well-being (Costa-Font et al., 2009), and when mobility and accessibility are compromised, individuals may feel vulnerable in their homes. Imrie (2004) notes that people with impairment may not feel like their home is a sanctuary at all; instead, it enforces parameters around their mobility, accessibility, social opportunities, and independence. Older adults with dementia incur additional safety risks (Yin et al., 2023). They may wander from home and leave doors unlocked or stoves/heaters on. They may become targets of financial fraud or lose their ability to perform self-care and hygiene. In sum, when the built environment of the home or the safety of the neighborhood cannot be modified, or when extensive supervision or monitoring is required, a transition to LTC may ensure a safer living situation.

Much of the care of older people at home is provided by family members. While family members willingly support their older loved ones, caring for an older person can result in physical and emotional strain and burden (Liu et al., 2020). Conditions like dementia may yield behavioral symptoms like aggression or serious agitation, as well as grief over the loss of the reciprocal relationship with their family members. Caregivers' own well-being may be compromised; for example, they may feel clinically significant levels of depression based on the behavioral and emotional symptoms of the person they care for (Fauth & Gibbons, 2014). Caregiving for an older person may continue for years, resulting in exhaustion, burnout, or poorer health for caregivers over the long-term.

A "tipping point" in at-home family-based care can be defined as a significant and decisive event that breaks down the (often fragile) stability of the caregiving arrangement (McGrath et al., 2021). It may be caused by a medical event that exacerbates care needs, or a shift in the mental or physical health of the caregiver. Multimorbidity and cognitive impairment add significant complexity to geriatric home care (Murtaugh et al., 2009). Even when a family caregiver is supported by at-home medical care, the reality is that some conditions require more skilled nursing care, more advanced medical equipment, or medical interventions that exceed what is feasible to be delivered at home.

Aging in Place *in* Long-Term Care

As described, Aging in Place is not an end goal of never leaving one's home, despite health or care circumstances. Aging in Place is a dynamic and evolving process of evaluating the "fit" of the micro- and macro-environments within the changing contexts of health, functional abilities, psychosocial needs, and caregiver well-being. A shift into LTC should not be perceived as an Aging in Place failure; rather is a new environment to foster Aging in Place principles. We also should not presume that all moves into LTC are contrary to the wishes of the older individual or naturally result in poorer well-being (Hillcoat-Nallétamby & Ogg, 2014). A new living environment, including into LTC may bring about improvements in the quality of the lived space, freedom from having to maintain a home, a safer space designed to improve mobility and accessibility, opportunities for socialization, relief for family caregivers, and more immediate response to daily needs and health challenges with more advanced interventions.

A key concept proposed by Golant (2011) is to understand *residential normalcy* for older adults as defined as such. *Residential comfort* is found when people feel that their residence brings them pleasure, is free of (or low on) hassles, and builds positive memorable experiences. *Residential mastery* is found when people feel control of, and competent in their lived environment. Residential normalcy occurs when both comfort and mastery are present, however these states are perceived and thereby individualized, and dynamic. For example, a feature that may make an individual feel safe may not make them feel autonomous. Or something that initially brought pleasure may later lose its appeal. When discordant experiences emerge, older adults either accommodate or assimilate to cope with the complexity (Golant, 2011). Moreover, while not all older people will reach or sustain residential normalcy in their own homes or residential care settings, the concept helps guide LTC facilities to prioritize building residential comfort and opportunities for residential mastery for the individuals who live there.

Living in residential care congruently with Aging in Place principles includes both design features and psychosocial approaches to care and daily life. Above, we listed features of "home" that are important for people and can be integrated into LTC. Personal and shared spaces can be modified to reflect person- and community-level identity. Including artifacts, décor, and comfort items are important for all residents, and easily recognizable landmarks have been shown to improve orientation and reduce agitation among residents with dementia (Marquardt et al., 2014; Day et al., 2000). People like to have competence (e.g., a mental map) to easily navigate their space. Design that is purposeful in enhancing functionality and reducing potential confusion has been shown to be particularly helpful for the well-being of residents with dementia (Fleming & Purandare, 2010; Marquardt et al., 2014). These include clear signage, contrasting colors, and access to secure outdoor spaces to assist individuals in navigating their environments safely while fostering opportunities for social interaction and physical activity (Fleming et al., 2014; Waller & Masterson, 2015). People want privacy and a place for peace and rest. Closing doors and knocking before entering may not be design features, per se, but are staff behaviors that promote both dignity and the sense of relaxation associated with home. The integration of smart home technologies and other monitoring technologies is promising in supporting safety, independence, and privacy in LTC (Ma et al., 2021; Calkins, 2009).

Aging in Place involves the interplay between environmental and psychosocial factors. Aging in Place principles in LTC, therefore, also require attention to residents' autonomy and supporting decision-making. Residents can help plan and choose activities, music, food choices, and social opportunities, as well as what they wear or how/when they want their care provided. Additionally, involving residents in daily activities, such as meal preparation, setting tables, folding towels, etc., enhances their sense of purpose and engagement and promotes control and mastery (Van Hoof & Kort, 2009; Marquardt & Schmieg, 2009). As stated earlier, *Place* is not just territory; it also involves relational components. A significant amount of research in residential care (and Age-Friendly Communities) emphasizes fostering opportunities to build relationships among residents and relationships between residents, staff, and their families; facilitating connection to family or friends can be in-person or virtual (Chapman et al., 2024). A scoping review identified the protective effects of social engagement on physical health and mortality in LTC, but the mechanisms by which social connectedness impacts health and mortality in LTC were less studied. It was posited that mechanisms may involve improved mental health, improved physical activity, or improved nutritional intake fostered by social engagement (Lem et al., 2021).

While no single model exists as a "gold standard" for integrating Aging in Place in LTC, the integration of these concepts is not merely theoretical. Small-house models, like The Green House Project, are examples of *how* Aging in Place principles can be integrated into residential care settings (Chapin & Dobbs-Kepper, 2001). These models prioritize smaller, self-contained living spaces that mimic the comfort and familiarity of a traditional home while emphasizing communal areas for socialization and participation in daily routines (Fleming et al., 2014; Zeisel et al., 2003). Empirical studies have shown that residents in such settings experience higher satisfaction levels and improved quality of life compared to traditional nursing homes (Chapin & Dobbs-Kepper, 2001; Mitchell & Burton, 2010).

Conclusion

While early discourse on Aging in Place emphasized living at home and resisting leaving, even with increased impairment, the construct has evolved to understand that this may not be desired by or be possible for all older people. Staying put may increase distress for some older people as they navigate home maintenance or neighborhood changes. Some features of the home or the consequences of being home alone may impair mobility or independence and be unsafe. Instead of seeing Aging in Place and transitioning to LTC as an Aging in Place failure or incompatible with the construct, residential long-term care facilities have the capacity to design environmental spaces and support the psychosocial aspects of Aging in Place that people value. Health promotion activities can include training architects and interior designers of LTC facilities, LTC administrators, and direct care providers on elements that foster Aging in Place within LTC. By creating environments, communities, care practices, and meaningful leisure activities, LTC can foster social engagement, attachment to place, residential comfort, and residential mastery, and thus align with important features of Aging in Place, concurrent with the residential transition.

References

Ahn, M., Kwon, H. J., & Kang, J. (2017). Supporting aging-in-place well: Findings from a cluster analysis of the reasons for aging-in-place and perceptions of well-being. *Journal of Applied Gerontology, 39*(1), 3–15. https://doi.org/10.1177/0733464817748779

Ambrose, A. F., Paul, G., & Hausdorff, J. M. (2013). Risk factors for falls among older adults: A review of the literature. *Maturitas, 75*(1), 51–61. https://doi.org/10.1016/j.maturitas.2013.02.009

Boland, L., Légaré, F., Perez, M. M. B., Menear, M., Garvelink, M. M., McIsaac, D. I., et al. (2017). Impact of home care versus alternative locations of care on elder health outcomes: An overview of systematic reviews. *BMC Geriatrics, 17*, 1–15. https://doi.org/10.1186/s12877-017-0471-1

Calkins, M. P. (2009). Evidence-based long-term care design. *Neurorehabilitation, 25*(3), 145–154. https://doi.org/10.3233/NRE-2009-0513

Campbell, N. (2015). Designing for social needs to support aging in place within continuing care retirement communities. *Journal of Housing and the Built Environment, 30*, 645–665. https://doi.org/10.1007/s10901-015-9437-6

Carver, L. F., Beamish, R., Phillips, S. P., & Villeneuve, M. (2018). A scoping review: Social participation as a cornerstone of successful aging in place among rural older adults. *Geriatrics, 3*(4), 75. https://doi.org/10.3390/geriatrics3040075

Chapin, R., & Dobbs-Kepper, D. (2001). Aging in place in assisted living: Philosophy versus policy. *The Gerontologist, 41*(1), 43–50. https://doi.org/10.1093/geront/41.1.43

Chapman, H., Bethell, J., Dewan, N., Liougas, M. P., Livingston, G., McGilton, K. S., & Sommerlad, A. (2024). Social connection in long-term care homes: A qualitative study of barriers and facilitators. *BMC Geriatrics, 24*(1), 857. https://doi.org/10.1186/s12877-024-04177-9

Costa-Font, J., Elvira, D., & Mascarilla-Miró, O. (2009). 'Ageing in place'? Exploring elderly people's housing preferences in Spain. *Urban Studies, 46*(2), 295–316. https://doi.org/10.1177/0042098008099356

Crowley, R., Atiq, O., Hilden, D., Beachy, M. W., Brislen, H. C., Curry, W. A., Engel, L. S., Hollon, M., Mathew, S. M., Southworth, M., Tan, M. J., Mellacheruvu, P., Shoushtari, C. S., Sagar, A., Beachy, M. W., Brislen, H. C., Curry, W. A., Engel, L. S., Hollon, M., & Hilden, D. (2022). Long-term services and supports for older adults: A position paper from the American College of Physicians. *Annals of Internal Medicine, 175*(8), 1172–1174. https://doi.org/10.7326/m22-0864

Day, K., Carreon, D., & Stump, C. (2000). The therapeutic design of environments for people with dementia: A review of the empirical research. *Gerontologist, 40*(4), 397–416. https://doi.org/10.1093/geront/40.4.397

Dostalova, V., Bártová, A., Blahova, H., & Holmerova, I. (2021). The needs of older people receiving home care: A scoping review. *Aging Clinical and Experimental Research, 33*, 495–504. https://doi.org/10.1007/s40520-020-01564-4

Egan, C., Naughton, C., Caples, M., & Mulcahy, H. (2022). Shared decision-making with adults transitioning to long-term care: A scoping review. *International Journal of Older People Nursing, 18*(1). https://doi.org/10.1111/opn.12518

Engelhardt, G. V., Eriksen, M. D., & Greenhalgh-Stanley, N. (2013). *A Profile of Housing and Health Among Older Americans* (SSRN Scholarly Paper 2359676). Social Science Research Network. https://papers.ssrn.com/abstract=2359676Erickson et al 2012

Erickson, L. D., Call, V. R., & Brown, R. B. (2012). SOS—satisfied or stuck, why older rural residents stay put: Aging in place or stuck in place in rural Utah. *Rural Sociology, 77*(3), 408–434. https://doi.org/10.1111/j.1549-0831.2012.00084.x

Fausset, C. B., Kelly, A. J., Rogers, W. A., & Fisk, A. D. (2011). Challenges to aging in place: Understanding home maintenance difficulties. *Journal of Housing for the Elderly, 25*(2), 125–141. https://doi.org/10.1080/02763893.2011.571105

Fauth, E. B., & Gibbons, A. (2014). Which behavioral and psychological symptoms of dementia are the most problematic? Variability by prevalence, intensity, distress ratings, and associations with caregiver depressive symptoms. *International Journal of Geriatric Psychiatry, 29*(3), 263–271. https://doi.org/10.1002/gps.4002

Fleming, R., Goodenough, B., Low, L. F., Chenoweth, L., & Brodaty, H. (2014). The relationship between the quality of the built environment and the quality of life of people with dementia in residential care. *Dementia, 15*(4), 663–680. https://doi.org/10.1177/1471301214532460

Fleming, R., & Purandare, N. (2010). Long-term care for people with dementia: Environmental design guidelines. *International Psychogeriatrics, 22*(7), 1084–1096. https://doi.org/10.1017/S1041610210000438

Garin, N., Olaya, B., Miret, M., Ayuso-Mateos, J. L., Power, M., Bucciarelli, P., & Haro, J. M. (2014). Built environment and elderly population health: A comprehensive literature review. *Clinical Practice and Epidemiology in Mental Health, 10*, 103–115. https://doi.org/10.2174/1745017901410010103

Golant, S. M. (2011). The quest for residential normalcy by older adults: Relocation but one pathway. *Journal of Aging Studies, 25*(3), 193–205. https://doi.org/10.1016/j.jaging.2011.03.003

Graham, L. T., Gosling, S. D., & Travis, C. K. (2015). The psychology of home environments. *Perspectives on Psychological Science, 10*(3), 346–356. https://doi.org/10.1177/1745691615576761

Greenfield, E. A. (2015). Healthy aging and age-friendly community initiatives. *Public Policy and Aging Report, 25*(2), 43–46. https://doi.org/10.1093/ppar/prv002

Hillcoat-Nallétamby, S., & Ogg, J. (2014). Moving beyond 'ageing in place': Older people's dislikes about their home and neighbourhood environments as a motive for wishing to move. *Ageing and Society, 34*(10), 1771–1796. https://doi.org/10.1017/S0144686X13000482

Hjelle, K. M., Tuntland, H., Førland, O., & Alvsvåg, H. (2016). Driving forces for home-based reablement; A qualitative study of older adults' experiences. *Health & Social Care in the Community, 25*(5), 1581–1589. https://doi.org/10.1111/hsc.12324

Hwang, E., Cummings, L., Sixsmith, A., & Sixsmith, J. (2011). Impacts of home modifications on aging-in-place. *Journal of Housing for the Elderly, 25*(3), 246–257. https://doi.org/10.1080/02763893.2011.595611

Imrie, R. (2004). Disability, embodiment and the meaning of the home. *Housing Studies, 19*(5), 745–763. https://doi.org/10.1080/0267303042000249189

Jeste, D. V., Blazer, D. G., Buckwalter, K. C., Cassidy, K.-L. K., Fishman, L., Gwyther, L. P., Levin, S. M., Phillipson, C., Rao, R. R., Schmeding, E., Vega, W. A., Avanzino, J. A., Glorioso, D. K., & Feather, J. (2016). Age-friendly communities initiative: Public health approach to promoting successful aging. *The American Journal of Geriatric Psychiatry, 24*(12), 1158–1170. https://doi.org/10.1016/j.jagp.2016.07.021

Joint Center for Housing Studies of Harvard University. (2019). *Housing America's older adults 2019*. Author.

Kim, D., Bian, H., Chang, C. K., Dong, L., & Margrett, J. (2022). In-home monitoring technology for aging in place: A scoping review. *Interactive Journal of Medical Research, 11*(2), e39005. https://doi.org/10.2196/39005

Kim, S., Kim, J., Kim, K., & Buckley, T. (2024). Age-friendly environment and aging in place: Findings from latent profile analysis. *International Journal of Aging & Human Development, 98*(4), 499–514. https://doi.org/10.1177/00914150231194236

Lau, D. T., Scandrett, K. G., Jarzebowski, M., Holman, K., & Emanuel, L. (2007). Health-related safety: A framework to address barriers to aging in place. *Gerontologist, 47*(6), 830–837. https://doi.org/10.1093/geront/47.6.830

Lem, K., McGilton, K. S., Aelick, K., et al. (2021). Social connection and physical health outcomes among long-term care home residents: A scoping review. *BMC Geriatrics, 21*, 722. https://doi.org/10.1186/s12877-021-02638-4

Lewis, C., & Buffel, T. (2020). Aging in place and the places of aging: A longitudinal study. *Journal of Aging Studies, 54*, 100870. https://doi.org/10.1016/j.jaging.2020.100870

Liu, Z., Heffernan, C., & Tan, J. (2020). Caregiver burden: A concept analysis. *International Journal of Nursing Sciences, 7*(4), 438–445. https://doi.org/10.1016/j.ijnss.2020.07.012

Ma, C., Guerra-Santin, O., & Mohammadi, M. (2021). Smart home modification design strategies for ageing in place: A systematic review. *Journal of Housing and the Built Environment, 37*(2), 625–651. https://doi.org/10.1007/s10901-021-09888-z

Marquardt, G., Bueter, K., & Motzek, T. (2014). Impact of the design of the built environment on people with dementia: An evidence-based review. *Health Environments Research & Design Journal, 8*(1), 127–157. https://doi.org/10.1177/193758671400800111

Marquardt, G., & Schmieg, P. (2009). Dementia-friendly architecture: Environments that facilitate wayfinding in nursing homes. *American Journal of Alzheimer's Disease & Other Dementias, 24*(4), 333–340. https://doi.org/10.1177/1533317509334959

McGrath, T., Blundell, B., & Morrisby, C. (2021). The 'tipping point': Exploring the factors associated with entry into residential care for people with dementia in Western Australia. *Dementia, 20*(7), 2494–2508. https://doi.org/10.1177/14713012211001265

Mitchell, L., & Burton, E. (2010). Designing dementia-friendly neighborhoods: Helping people with dementia to get out and about. *Journal of Integrated Care, 18*(6), 11–18. https://doi.org/10.5042/jic.2010.0647

Murtaugh, C., Peng, T., Totten, A., Costello, B., Moore, S., & Aykan, H. (2009). Complexity in geriatric home healthcare. *Journal for Healthcare Quality, 31*(2), 34–43. https://doi.org/10.1111/j.1945-1474.2009.00017.x

Ollevier, A., Aguiar, G., Palomino, M., & Simpelaere, I. S. (2020). How can technology support ageing in place in healthy older adults? A systematic review. *Public Health Reviews, 41*(1). https://doi.org/10.1186/s40985-020-00143-4

Ratnayake, M., Lukas, S., Brathwaite, S., Neave, J., & Henry, H. (2022). Aging in place. *Delaware Journal of Public Health, 8*(3), 28–31. https://doi.org/10.32481/djph.2022.08.007

Rowles, G. D., Oswald, F., & Hunter, E. G. (2004). Interior living environments in old age. In H.-W. Wahl, R. Scheidt, & P. G. Windley (Eds.), *Aging in context: Socio-physical environments (Annual Review of Gerontology and Geriatrics, 2003)* (pp. 167–193). Springer.

Seo, E., & Lee, S. (2023). Implications of aging in place in the context of the residential environment: Bibliometric Analysis and literature review. *International Journal of Environmental Research and Public Health, 20*(20), 6905. https://doi.org/10.3390/ijerph20206905

Sharifi, S., Mosafer, H., Rahmati, M., Babaei Khorzoughi, K., & Parandeh, A. (2024). Dwelling characteristics and mental well-being in older adults: A systematic review. *Heliyon, 10*(18), e37676. https://doi.org/10.1016/j.heliyon.2024.e37676

Van Dijk, H. M., Cramm, J. M., & Nieboer, A. P. (2016). How to build an integrated neighborhood approach to support community-dwelling older people? *International Journal of Integrated Care, 16*(2), 4. https://doi.org/10.5334/ijic.1596

Van Hoof, J., & Kort, H. S. M. (2009). Supportive living environments: A first concept of a dwelling designed for older adults with dementia. *Dementia, 8*(2), 293–316. https://doi.org/10.1177/1471301209103276

van Hoof, J., & Marston, H. R. (2021). Age-friendly cities and communities: State of the art and future perspectives. *International Journal of Environmental Research and Public Health, 18*(4), 1644. https://doi.org/10.3390/ijerph18041644

Vasunilashorn, S., Steinman, B. A., Liebig, P. S., & Pynoos, J. (2012). Aging in place: Evolution of a research topic whose time has come. *Journal of Aging Research, 120952*. https://doi.org/10.1155/2012/120952

Waller, S., & Masterson, A. (2015). Designing dementia-friendly hospital environments. *Future Hospital Journal, 2*(1), 63–68. https://doi.org/10.7861/futurehosp.15.017

Wiles, J. L., Leibing, A., Guberman, N., Reeve, J., & Allen, R. E. (2011). The meaning of "aging in place" to older people. *Gerontologist, 52*(3), 357–366. https://doi.org/10.1093/geront/gnr098

Yarker, S., Doran, P., & Buffel, T. (2024). Theorizing "place" in aging in place: The need for territorial and relational perspectives. *Gerontologist, 64*(2), gnad002. https://doi.org/10.1093/geront/gnad002

Yin, G., Lin, S., & Chen, L. (2023). Risk factors associated with home care safety for older people with dementia: Family caregivers' perspectives. *BMC Geriatrics, 23*(1). https://doi.org/10.1186/s12877-023-03893-3

Zeisel, J., Silverstein, N. M., Hyde, J., Levkoff, S., Lawton, M. P., & Holmes, W. (2003). Environmental correlates to behavioral health outcomes in Alzheimer's special care units. *Gerontologist, 43*(5), 697–711. https://doi.org/10.1093/geront/43.5.697

Chapter 13
Person-Centered Care and the Culture Change Movement in Long-Term Care

Michelle Goonasekera, Kristina M. Kokorelias, Erica Dove, and Maurita T. Harris

Introduction

Person-centered care is a transformative approach that places the preferences, values, and needs of long-term care (LTC) residents and their families at the heart of care. In LTC settings, this approach promotes holistic care by fostering meaningful relationships, supporting resident autonomy, and actively involving families in care decisions. The COVID-19 pandemic brought to light the significant challenges within LTC facilities, particularly around isolation, staff shortages, and inadequate emotional and social support for residents. These issues have driven the need to rethink and reform care practices to prioritize the well-being of residents.

A key element in this transformation is the culture change movement, which aims to create more flexible, compassionate, and person-centered environments in LTC. This chapter will delve into the foundations of person-centered care, examine the goals of the culture change movement, and address how person-centered care

M. Goonasekera
Dalla Lana School of Public Health, University of Toronto, Toronto, ON, Canada
e-mail: michelle.goonasekera@mail.utoronto.ca

K. M. Kokorelias
Division of Geriatric Medicine, Department of Medicine, Sinai Health, University Health Network, Toronto, ON, Canada
e-mail: kristina.kokorelias@sinaihealth.ca

E. Dove
University of Toronto, Toronto, ON, Canada
e-mail: erica.dove@mail.utoronto.ca

M. T. Harris (✉)
Faculty of Liberal Arts, User Experience Design, Wilfrid Laurier University, Brantford, ON, Canada
e-mail: mauharris@wlu.ca

K. K. Bhattacharyya (ed.), *Health Promotion in Long-Term Care Facilities*,
https://doi.org/10.1007/978-3-031-91038-8_13

can be tailored to meet the unique needs of people living with dementia. It will also provide an analysis of the barriers that hinder and facilitators that support the successful implementation of person-centered care in LTC settings.

Understanding Person-Centered Care

Defining Person-Centered Care and Its Core Elements

While **person-centered care** may seem like a universally accepted approach in healthcare, it is not consistently practiced across all settings, especially in (LTC) (Evans, 2017). To explore why this inconsistency exists, it is first essential to establish a clear understanding of what person-centered care is and its evolution over the years.

Person-centered care originated from the concept of patient-centered care, first introduced by psychologist Carl Rogers in the 1950s and further refined by psychiatrist George Engle in the 1970s as a challenge to the conventional paternalistic medical model of care (Latimer et al., 2017). In recent years, the shift in philosophy from patient to person-centered care marks a deeper recognition of the individual's humanity beyond their illness, acknowledging that healthcare is only one part of a person's complex, multifaceted life (Evans, 2017; Håkansson Eklund et al., 2019). Person-centered care as a concept is consistently evolving, making it difficult to define; however, most definitions share common elements related to care delivery, the people involved, and communication. NEJM Catalyst (2017) outlined seven elements of person-centered care: (1) the healthcare system's mission and values are aligned with the patient's goals; (2) care is collaborative, coordinated, and accessible; (3) care focuses on physical comfort and emotional well-being; (4) patient and family viewpoints are respected and valued; (5) patient and family are included in decisions at the patient and system level; (6) family members are welcomed and encouraged to participate in the care setting; and lastly (7) full transparency and fast delivery of information to patients and families.

Based on these elements of person-centered care, core ideas emerge. Firstly, care is regarded as person-specific—that is, each person requires holistic, coordinated, and personalized care that works for *them*; there is no one-size-fits-all solution (The Health Foundation, 2016). Secondly, there is a shift in control from the clinician or institution to the person, giving the individual a say in their care as equal partners (Evans, 2017). Thirdly, those who matter most to the individual—such as unpaid caregivers (care provided by family and friends) and paid caregivers (care provided by an institution or individual)—are recognized as care partners. They are welcomed and actively involved in care decisions alongside the person receiving care. Lastly, philosophies of treating the individual with respect, dignity, and compassion are evident throughout the approach (The Health Foundation, 2016). However, a consensus definition that clarifies approaches to operationalize person-centered care in care settings is still needed (Kogan et al., 2015).

The Importance of Person-Centered Care in LTC Settings

The global population is aging rapidly, and with increasing longevity, the demand for LTC among older adults is projected to rise significantly (PAHO, 2019). Person-centered care is particularly crucial in LTC settings due to the unique challenges and needs of individuals receiving care over long periods of time and, for some, over a lifetime (Kane et al., 1998). Unlike acute care, where interventions are focused on treating immediate medical concerns, LTC environments serve individuals who may require assistance with daily living, chronic illness management, or cognitive impairments such as dementia. Therefore, LTC becomes inextricable from the lives of those receiving the care (Kane et al., 1998) and can benefit greatly from the application of a person-centered approach (Miller, 1997).

This holistic approach to care provision in LTC settings comes with many benefits for the person receiving care, their families, and healthcare workers. The involvement of patients, families, and caregivers in the co-creation of care plans and shared decision-making leads to improved health outcomes and higher satisfaction with the care received (The Health Foundation, 2012; Yee et al., 2021). In the context of person-centered dementia care in LTC settings, there were notable reductions in behavioral symptoms and psychotropic medication use among residents with dementia (Li & Porock, 2014). Healthcare workers in person-centered LTC environments reported greater job satisfaction and reduced intention to leave their positions (Choi et al., 2021). Person-centered care has also been tied to better distribution of resources, lowered costs, and expanded profit margins across stages of care delivery (NEJM Catalyst, 2017).

Culture Change Movement in LTC

What Is the Culture Change Movement?

To shift from the traditional institutional model of care to the application of person-centered care requires a robust **culture change**, a movement that gained popularity in the 1980s (Iyamu et al., 2022). Culture change requires a fundamental transformation in both the philosophy and practice of LTC, emphasizing health improvements and quality of life that are driven by and centered around the person receiving care (White-Chu et al., 2009). Various models of culture change have come to the forefront, such as Wellspring, Greenhouse, Eden Alternative, and the Live Oak Institute (Hemphill et al., 2023; White-Chu et al., 2009). Fundamental to culture change in LTC are the following elements: a home-like environment, strong and adaptive leadership, workforce reorganization, resident choice, and relationship-centered care (Corazzini et al., 2015; Dupuis et al., 2016; Evans, 2017; Iyamu et al., 2022; White-Chu et al., 2009).

Transforming the physical environment to feel more like a home—one that is nurturing, safe, and less clinical—is crucial, particularly for those residing in LTC facilities (Evans, 2017). Prioritizing private spaces and access to outdoor areas can create a more comfortable and supportive living experience (Iyamu et al., 2022). Creating a home-like environment is further enhanced by offering residents greater autonomy and choice. The move to LTC often triggers feelings of loss, particularly a sense of losing control and leaving behind the familiarity of home, largely due to the structured and hierarchical nature of care settings. However, by giving residents more autonomy, such as allowing them to choose their meals with buffet style dining—a more home-like environment can be re-created, making the transition smoother and providing a sense of normalcy (White-Chu et al., 2009). Resident autonomy is at the core of person-centered care, recognizing that each person leads a unique life and that a one-size-fits-all approach is inadequate (White-Chu et al., 2009). The focus is on delivering care that aligns with the specific needs, preferences, and values of each resident, ensuring they maintain control over their care and daily experiences.

The culture change movement also demands a rethinking of institutional operations, particularly in workforce management and care delivery. An important component is workforce re-design, which involves moving away from rigid top-down hierarchies that place unnecessary strain on staff (White-Chu et al., 2009). Instead, self-directed work teams offer a solution by giving staff greater autonomy over care practices and management (White-Chu et al., 2009). This empowerment reduces staff stress, which has been shown to enhance the staff's ability to provide person-centered care in LTC facilities (Chang et al., 2020). Additionally, a less stressed and more independent staff strengthens relationships among residents, families, and caregivers, contributing to a more collaborative and supportive care environment (Dupuis et al., 2016; Kokorelias et al., 2019; Ryan et al., 2008). Further, to effectively drive the culture change movement, managers and administrators must embrace adaptive leadership to navigate and address the complex challenges that arise (Corazzini et al., 2015). This approach is crucial in fostering the flexibility and innovation needed to transform traditional hierarchies, empower staff, and create a more resident-centered care environment.

Barriers and Facilitators of Culture Change

While LTC homes were progressing toward person-centered care, the COVID-19 pandemic halted this shift, pushing many facilities back toward a more medicalized, paternalistic model. Infection control measures, though important, were seen as conflicting with the goals of the culture change movement, undermining efforts to improve residents' quality of life (Iyamu et al., 2022). Strict protocols, such as cancelled visitations and social activities along with clinicians taking control of care to minimize COVID-19 risks, highlighted the shortcomings of LTC systems and their inability to fully balance resident-centered care with infection control during the crisis (Estabrooks et al., 2020; Iyamu et al., 2022). The pandemic highlighted the urgency for LTC facilities to find a sustainable balance between safeguarding health and maintaining the core principles of person-centered care.

Facilitators of culture change in LTC include interest holder engagement and strong collaborations between external partners and municipal governments (Hemphill et al., 2023). Hemphill et al. (2023) developed a unique LTC model for Toronto, called CareTO, through a co-creation process with interest holders. This process involved collaboratively defining the CareTO model and establishing priorities for implementation. Their findings demonstrate that engaging interest holders and fostering partnerships with external organizations and local governments are powerful strategies for driving implementation initiatives. These collaborations encourage deeper reflection, create a unified vision, and sharpen objectives, ultimately enhancing the success of culture change models.

Person-Centered Care for Persons with Dementia

People living with dementia comprise approximately 70% of the total LTC resident population in Canada (Iaboni et al., 2022). In addition to cognitive impairment, individuals with dementia often face comorbid conditions, such as physical health challenges (Livingston et al., 2020), making their healthcare needs complex to manage. Given the unique care needs of people living with dementia, person-centered care has become increasingly relevant. Equally important is the growing emphasis on family-centered care, as many residents, including people living with dementia, rely on family members (e.g., spouses, adult children, extended family, and friends) for support and involvement in their care (Gaugler, 2005).

Person- and family-centered care for dementia is vital for resident well-being, a positive patient and family experience, and driving better health outcomes. A systematic review and meta-analysis by Kim and Park (2017) demonstrated that person-centered care improved the quality of life for people living with dementia. A large majority of the studies included in this review were conducted in LTC settings, unveiling the applicability of this approach in such environments. In LTC, person-centered care can empower residents with or without dementia to take a more active role in their care, which enhances autonomy and independence. For instance, allowing residents to choose when and how they wish for certain care activities to be undertaken, such as bathing or meals, supports their dignity and personal preference.

Person-centered care also emphasizes continuity of care, where residents with and without dementia are cared for by consistent staff and family members who understand their unique preferences and needs (Cohen & Lindman, 2024). For example, consistent staffing for an individual or on a specific unit, such as memory care, allows staff to develop a deeper understanding of residents' preferred activities and routines. Fostering continuity of care requires comprehensive staff training, strong organizational leadership, and family involvement in care and decision-making. However, this can be hindered by insufficient resources, staff turnover, and limited funding (Ljungholm et al., 2022).

People living with dementia often face negative attitudes and low expectations, which pose significant obstacles to the application of person-centered care (Marulappa et al., 2022). Research suggests a relationship between care staff attitudes and the well-being of LTC residents, with negative staff attitudes correlating to worse resident outcomes (Gerritsen et al., 2019). To improve well-being of people with dementia living in LTC, staff must shift from disempowering practices to approaches that support residents' autonomy and capabilities (Willemse et al., 2015). To address this, there is an urgent need for staff training and education on the principles of person-centered care, the importance of family involvement, and the needs, preferences, and abilities of people living with dementia (Kim et al., 2024).

Special Considerations for Person-Centered Dementia Care

As person-centered care is personalized, care plans must be adapted to meet each individual's unique needs and preferences. This is especially important for people with dementia living in LTC, as well as for the families who provide them with support and care. Key principles that exemplify person-centered care include universal and inclusive design. While universal and inclusive design terms are often used interchangeably, they have distinct definitions, meanings, and implications.

Universal design is defined as *"the design of products and environments to be usable by all people, to the greatest extent possible, without the need for adaptation or specialized design"* (Burgstahler, 2009, p. 2). Universal design aims to develop a one-size-fits-all solution to suit the broadest range of consumers possible. An example of universal design in LTC is handrails and grab bars placed along hallways or within a resident's room. However, universal design has been critiqued for failing to adequately address the full spectrum of consumer diversity. Recent statistics indicate that universal design only encompasses approximately 80% of consumers, leaving the remaining 20% of "complex users" without a solution (Treviranus, 2021).

In contrast, **inclusive design** is described as *"a methodology that enables and draws on the full range of human diversity"* (Treviranus, 2021, p. 769). This approach emphasizes the importance of including and learning from people with diverse perspectives. For instance, implementing gender-neutral washrooms in LTC facilities serves as an example of inclusive design. Unlike universal design, which aims to accommodate as many users as possible, inclusive design aims to address the full range of human diversity, encompassing abilities, language, culture, gender, age, and other factors. The focus of inclusive design revolves around fostering empathy for users and adapting products, programs, environments, and services to accommodate a wide range of requirements, rather than adopting a one-size-fits-all approach. Regardless of fundamental differences, universal and inclusive design principles are closely related to person-centered care and have been effectively applied to people with dementia (Kenning, 2018).

As the recognition of inclusivity for diverse groups grows, so does the demand for person-centered solutions for people with dementia. Several innovative approaches to person-centered care for LTC residents living with dementia have emerged. These include interventions such as sensory stimulation (Backman et al., 2021), music therapy (Ray & Götell, 2018), reminiscence therapy (Saragih et al., 2022), and technology-based solutions (Alm et al., 2004; Hung et al., 2021). For instance, communication challenges and behavioral symptoms associated with dementia can be addressed through the creative application of technology. A recent scoping review highlighted that touchscreen tablets (e.g., iPads) could be used to foster social connections and reduce behavioral symptoms in dementia care settings and adult day programs (Hung et al., 2021). Similarly, a larger touchscreen computer called the Computer Interactive Reminiscing and Conversation Aid (CIRCA) can be used by people with dementia and their caregivers or staff to stimulate and maintain a conversation by promoting reminiscing (Alm et al., 2004). These approaches not only enhance the quality of care, but also promote meaningful engagement, ultimately improving the well-being of residents with dementia.

Health Equity and Health Disparities in LTC Settings

Traditionally, LTC environments have faced challenges in offering truly equitable care due to systemic disparities that affect access, quality, and outcomes for economically and socially marginalized populations (Scott et al., 2024). Health equity and health disparities are interconnected (Braveman, 2014; Braveman et al., 2018), yet distinct concepts central to addressing quality in LTC. **Health equity** is defined as a state in which *"everyone has a fair and just opportunity to be as healthy as possible,"* necessitating the removal of barriers such as poverty, discrimination, and inadequate access to resources, including quality healthcare, safe living conditions, and fair employment (Braveman et al., 2018, p. 2). In contrast, **health disparities** are measurable indicators that reflect our progress toward health equity, highlighting gaps in health outcomes that persist across demographic and socioeconomic groups (Braveman, 2014, p. 7). Thus, to advance health equity, LTC settings must address fairness and justice to reduce health disparities among economically and socially disadvantaged populations (Braveman, 2014; Braveman et al., 2018). These efforts are crucial for creating a supportive LTC environment that nurtures equitable health outcomes for all residents.

The culture change movement in LTC emphasizes a shift away from institutional, one-size-fits-all care models toward person-centered approaches that prioritize individual preferences, autonomy, and dignity. However, without addressing health disparities, even person-centered care risks reinforcing existing inequities. For example, racialized residents are more likely to reside in facilities with fewer resources, higher staff turnover, and lower standards of care, which can hinder person-centered practices. Additionally, social determinants of health—such as residents' socioeconomic status, cultural background, and access to supportive social networks—significantly influence the type and quality of care received, often disadvantaging those from marginalized backgrounds.

Promoting health equity within LTC requires integrating culturally competent care, actively reducing systemic barriers, and implementing policies that address these disparities at both provider and system levels. Providers trained in cultural competence and equipped to recognize and mitigate bias can better address the unique needs of diverse residents, ensuring that person-centered care genuinely reflects everyone's values, experiences, and health conditions. As the LTC sector continues to evolve, aligning person-centered care with health equity principles will be essential to transforming LTC into a more inclusive and just system.

Integrating health equity within LTC requires a collective responsibility among providers, policymakers, and communities, as emphasized by Martinez (2024). Martinez highlighted that *"Often, when contemplating the impact of racial disparities and racial health inequities, older adults are not considered. This in and of itself is an inequity"* (Martinez, 2024; p. 7). This work highlights the "potent" intersection of racism and ageism, which amplifies injustices, health disparities, and inequities for racialized older communities (Martinez, 2024; p. 7). To address these compounding challenges, Martinez advocates for a social justice approach, calling for political will, education, financial investment, and interdisciplinary collaboration—strategies that can be used to create a more equitable LTC system.

Within the person-centered care and culture change movement, the responsibility extends beyond providing individualized care to actively dismantle systemic barriers that perpetuate disparities. Integrating a social justice lens within LTC practice could empower providers and organizations to focus on both cultural competence and systemic reform, ensuring that each resident receives care that reflects their unique background and life experiences. By aligning person-centered care with equity and justice, LTC facilities can foster environments that address individual needs while tackling the broader social determinants of health, advancing a more inclusive and fairer standard of care for all.

Overcoming Barriers to Implementing Person-Centered Care

Barriers to person-centered care in LTC settings are multifaceted and stem from structural, systemic, and interpersonal challenges that hinder the delivery of high-quality, individualized care (Hower et al., 2019; Lloyd et al., 2018; Vennedey et al., 2020). Key obstacles include wage disparities, insufficient caregiver support, and chronic staffing issues, all of which demand focused and strategic interventions to ensure the successful implementation of person-centered care.

Understaffing in LTC facilities is a pervasive and widespread issue (Arjama et al., 2024), which overwhelms staff with excessive tasks, leaving little time for meaningful interactions with residents (Weinstein, n.d.). This often leads to a task-oriented rather than a person-centered approach to care (Berkovic et al., 2024; Dayeong et al., 2024). High staff turnover and shortages further exacerbate the problem by disrupting the continuity of care and weakening relationships between caregivers and residents (Mayo Clinic Proceedings, 2003). Addressing these staffing challenges requires targeted recruitment initiatives, increased staffing levels, and ongoing incentives to attract new workers (Fujisawa & Colombo, 2009). Implementing policies to ensure adequate staff-to-resident ratios can also contribute to a more stable and effective care environment (Perruchoud et al., 2021). In addition to improving care for residents, addressing staffing shortages enhances working conditions for staff themselves (Llena-Nozal et al., 2022). When staff have manageable workloads, they can engage more fully in their work, reduce burnout, and experience greater job satisfaction (Scales, 2021). This not only benefits the well-being of staff, but also enhances their ability to deliver the empathetic, person-centered care that is essential in LTC settings.

Wage disparity is another critical issue impacting the quality of care in LTC facilities (Kokorelias & Sinha, 2023). The disparity between wages for LTC workers and those in other healthcare sectors contributes to high turnover rates, workforce instability, and reduced staff morale (Kokorelias & Sinha, 2023; Lis & Boulhol, 2023). When LTC workers feel undervalued due to lower wages, their engagement in empathetic and person-centered care diminishes. Furthermore, the lack of competitive wages deters potential candidates from entering or remaining in the LTC workforce, exacerbating staffing shortages and compounding the challenges faced by these facilities (Kokorelias & Sinha, 2023). Addressing wage disparities requires dramatic shifts in policy and increased funding for LTC facilities to elevate wages to levels comparable with other healthcare sectors (Kokorelias & Sinha, 2023). By doing so, facilities can improve staff retention, reduce turnover, and foster a more stable and motivated workforce (Kokorelias & Sinha, 2023).

Insufficient support for caregivers, both paid and unpaid, also represents a significant barrier to person-centered care. Caregivers often face immense emotional and physical demands, and without adequate support systems, they are at risk of burnout (Broxson & Feliciano, 2020). Burnout among caregivers can severely impact the quality of care provided, as it may lead to neglect of residents' individual needs and preferences (Broxson & Feliciano, 2020; Gérain & Zech, 2022). To alleviate this issue, it is crucial to implement robust support systems, including access to mental health services, respite care, and educational resources that equip caregivers with the skills needed to deliver individualized care across the caregiving trajectory (Kokorelias et al., 2022). Enhanced support not only safeguards caregivers' well-being but also empowers them to be actively involved in the care process (Merrilees et al., 2020), promoting a collaborative approach to care between unpaid caregivers and paid LTC staff (Hoek et al., 2021).

Collaborative Approaches in Implementing Person-Centered Care

Multi-Disciplinary Team Approach

In order to implement person-centered care in LTC settings, there is a need for **interprofessional collaboration** to promote holistic health and well-being. Interprofessional collaboration involves a coordinated effort among care providers from diverse disciplines, working toward common goals such as enhancing resident care, improving access to healthcare interventions, or solving a specific problem (e.g., polypharmacy, recurrent falls). The interprofessional collaboration includes professionals from various disciplines, such as physicians, nurses, nursing aides, pharmacists, occupational therapists, physical therapists, recreation therapists, dietitians, and social workers. For example, consider a LTC resident with dementia who experiences recurring falls (*Mr. Y, man, aged 86*). An occupational therapist on the interprofessional team would conduct a comprehensive assessment and convey the results back to the team. This would help inform treatment plans from the physical therapist by prescribing rehabilitation exercises to Mr. Y for falls prevention. Additionally, the occupational therapist's assessment would inform the social worker's treatment plan by connecting Mr. Y and his family with relevant fall prevention education resources. The physical therapist's and social worker's treatment plans and findings would then feed back into the occupational therapist's future assessment and treatment plans, creating a holistic loop.

To ensure that multiple professionals truly collaborate in the coordination and delivery of resident care, assigning *case managers* for each resident and their families is crucial. The case manager plays a central role in facilitating cohesion within the interprofessional team by ensuring that roles are well-defined, and responsibilities are maximized (Hudon et al., 2019). A case manager is responsible for coordinating, evaluating, planning, and implementing services based on resident needs in close collaboration with other care providers (Hudon et al., 2019). For example, in the example of Mr. Y, a case manager would coordinate the efforts of the occupational therapist, physical therapist, and social worker. The case manager would assign complementary roles for each professional, ensure ongoing communication and feedback, monitor Mr. Y's progress and outcomes collaboratively, and facilitate debriefing once his care plan is established. This approach fosters integrated care and ensures that all professionals work together jointly for the benefit of the resident.

The benefits of interprofessional collaboration in health care have been well-documented. For example, interprofessional collaboration in care can improve resident outcomes by enhancing their quality of care, engagement, and safety (Morley & Cashell, 2017). Additionally, interprofessional collaboration has been shown to support person-centered care (McDonald & McCallin, 2010). Finally, interprofessional collaboration in care benefits healthcare staff working in LTC by boosting their satisfaction, productivity, impact, and retention (Morley & Cashell, 2017). When both residents and staff experience positive outcomes, the environment becomes more conducive to person-centered care. For instance, if Mr. Y is assigned a case manager who assembles an interprofessional team to address his recurrent falls, the team can collaboratively address all contributing factors, such as balance issues, medication management, and the need for environmental modifications. Each team member applies their specialized knowledge, ensuring that Mr. Y receives comprehensive, well-coordinated care aimed at preventing future falls, ultimately improving his well-being and safety.

Engagement of Residents and Families

The importance of resident and family engagement and inclusion in implementing and evaluating the effectiveness of person-centered care is crucial yet often overlooked. True interprofessional collaboration must include the involvement of residents and their families in decision-making and execution of care practices and approaches (McDonald & McCallin, 2010). The real-world impact of including residents and families in person-centered care has been documented in the literature (Siminoff, 2013). However, these impacts do not come without respective barriers. That is, cited barriers to implementing person- and family-centered care include organizational culture, the physical environment, as well as staff, time, and other constraints (Philibert et al., 2011). In the case of Mr. Y, he may have family members who juggle multiple responsibilities, such as young children and demanding jobs, making it challenging to involve them in consultations about care for Mr. Y's recurrent falls. Due to this, the family may be inadvertently left out of Mr. Y's care decisions, such as changes to his medication. Additionally, Mr. Y may face his own barriers to participating in his care. This could include a lack of capacity to consent for himself regarding treatment decisions due to dementia or speech difficulties, making it harder to express his symptoms or advocate for his needs and preferences.

Despite the proposed challenges in engaging residents and their families in person- and family-centered care, there remains an urgent need to optimize care outcomes and resident and family satisfaction. Barriers to the inclusion of residents and their families in person-centered care could be addressed by using alternate means of communication or strategies to ensure resident and family perspectives are included. A key mechanism to promote effective interprofessional care is clear communication with residents and families. This could include having information communicated to residents and families in alternate, more inclusive formats such as large-print documents, infographics, simplified verbal descriptions, or photos and videos. Effective communication not only ensures clarity, but also builds trust and fosters a collaborative partnership between the interprofessional care team, the resident, the family, and other key care partners.

In addition to tailoring person- and family-centered care plans, there is also importance in developing collaboration strategies to best suit the needs and preferences of each resident and their family. This may comprise meeting at different times of the day (e.g., early mornings, evenings, weekends), meetings in alternate formats (e.g., in-person, over the phone, videoconference), and meeting either together (the resident *and* family) or separately. It may also involve incorporating culturally specific practices, recognizing that family involvement in a resident's care decisions can vary based on cultural and familial preferences and norms. Flexibility and personalization are key in coordinating, communicating, delivering, and evaluating care. For example, in Mr. Y's family, it may be customary for his spouse to be more involved in care decision-making than his children. However, if his spouse has a busy schedule, this may be harder to achieve. As a result, there is a need to set clear expectations between all parties—clinicians, family, and Mr. Y himself—regarding how his care will be managed and how decisions will be communicated to ensure everyone remains informed and involved in the process.

Conclusion

In conclusion, person-centered care is a critical approach in LTC settings, particularly for individuals with dementia, who often have complex and evolving care needs. The shift toward this model emphasizes holistic care, autonomy, and the inclusion of families as partners in care, contributing to improved health outcomes, quality of life, and satisfaction for both residents and their families. Culture change movements within LTC facilities further support this transformation by creating environments that feel more like home, empowering residents, and fostering collaborative care. However, implementing person-centered care requires strong leadership, adequate resources, consistent staffing, and continuous family involvement.

As the population ages, the need for LTC will continue to grow, emphasizing the importance of evolving care practices to meet the diverse and dynamic needs of older adults. By advancing a model rooted in person-centered and culturally competent care, LTC settings can lead in establishing a compassionate standard that honors the diverse backgrounds, values, and experiences of all residents. This commitment not only shapes the future of care but also reaffirms our collective dedication to health equity, ensuring dignity and quality of life for all older adults.

References

Alm, N., Astell, A., Ellis, M., Dye, R., Gowans, G., & Campbell, J. (2004). A cognitive prosthesis and communication support for people with dementia. *Neuropsychological Rehabilitation, 14*(1-2), 117–134.

Arjama, A.-L., Suhonen, R., & Kangasniemi, M. (2024). Ethical issues in long-term care settings: Care workers' lived experiences. *Nursing Ethics, 31*(2–3), 213–226. https://doi.org/10.1177/09697330231191277

Backman, C., Demery-Varin, M., Cho-Young, D., Crick, M., & Squires, J. (2021). Impact of sensory interventions on the quality of life of long-term care residents: A scoping review. *BMJ Open, 11*(3), e042466. https://doi.org/10.1136/bmjopen-2020-042466

Berkovic, D., Macrae, A., Gulline, H., Horsman, P., Soh, S.-E., Skouteris, H., & Ayton, D. (2024). The delivery of person-centered care for people living with Dementia in residential aged care: A systematic review and meta-analysis. *The Gerontologist, 64*(5). https://doi.org/10.1093/geront/gnad052

Braveman, P. (2014). What are health disparities and health equity? We need to be clear. *Public Health Reports, 129*(1_suppl2), 5–8. https://doi.org/10.1177/00333549141291S203

Braveman, P., Arkin, E., Orleans, T., Proctor, D., Acker, J., & Plough, A. (2018). What is health equity? *Behavioral Science & Policy, 4*(1), 1–14. https://doi.org/10.1177/237946151800400102

Broxson, J., & Feliciano, L. (2020). Understanding the impacts of caregiver stress. *Professional Case Management, 25*(4), 213–219. https://doi.org/10.1097/NCM.0000000000000414

Burgstahler, S. (2009). Universal design: Process, principles, and applications. *DO-IT*.

Caregiver and clinician shortages in an aging nation. Mayo Clinic Proceedings; 2003. Elsevier.

Chang, H., Gil, C., Kim, H., & Bea, H. (2020). Person-centered care, job stress, and quality of life among long-term care nursing staff. *Journal of Nursing Research, 28*(5), e114. https://doi.org/10.1097/JNR.0000000000000398

Choi, J., Kim, D. E., & Yoon, J. Y. (2021). Person-centered care environment associated with care staff outcomes in LTC facilities. *Journal of Nursing Research, 29*(1), e133. https://doi.org/10.1097/JNR.0000000000000412

Cohen, E., & Lindman, I. (2024). Importance of continuity of care from a patient perspective - a cross-sectional study in Swedish health care. *Scandinavian Journal of Primary Health Care, 42*(1), 195–200. https://doi.org/10.1080/02813432.2023.2299119

Corazzini, K., Twersky, J., White, H. K., Buhr, G. T., McConnell, E. S., Weiner, M., & Colón-Emeric, C. S. (2015). Implementing culture change in nursing homes: An adaptive leadership framework. *The Gerontologist, 55*(4), 616–627. https://doi.org/10.1093/geront/gnt170

Dayeong, K., Young-Rim, C., Ye-Na, L., et al. (2024). Nurses' Shared Subjectivity on Person-Centered Care for Behavioral and Psychological Symptoms of Dementia in Nursing Homes. *Journal of Nursing Research*. 10. 1097

Dupuis, S., McAiney, C. A., Fortune, D., Ploeg, J., & de Witt, L. (2016). Theoretical foundations guiding culture change: The work of the partnerships in dementia care alliance. *Dementia, 15*(1), 85–105. https://doi.org/10.1177/1471301213518935

Estabrooks, C. A., Straus, S. E., Flood, C. M., Keefe, J., Armstrong, P., Donner, G. J., Boscart, V., Ducharme, F., Silvius, J. L., & Wolfson, M. C. (2020). Restoring trust: COVID-19 and the future of long-term care in Canada. *FACETS, 5*(1), 651–691. https://doi.org/10.1139/facets-2020-0056

Evans, B. J. (2017). Person-centered care and culture change. *Caring for the Ages, 18*(8), 6. https://doi.org/10.1016/j.carage.2017.07.007

Fujisawa, R., & Colombo, F. (2009). *The long-term care workforce: Overview and strategies to adapt supply to a growing demand*. In *The long-term care workforce: Overview and strategies to adapt supply to a growing demand*. OECD Publishing.

Gaugler, J. E. (2005). Family involvement in residential long-term care: A synthesis and critical review. *Aging and Mental Health, 9*(2), 105–118. https://doi.org/10.1080/13607860412331310245

Gérain, P., & Zech, E. (2022). A harmful care: The association of informal caregiver burnout with depression, subjective health, and violence. *Journal of Interpersonal Violence, 37*(11–12), NP9738–NP9762. https://doi.org/10.1177/0886260520983259

Gerritsen, D. L., van Beek, A. P. A., & Woods, R. T. (2019). Relationship of care staff attitudes with social well-being and challenging behavior of nursing home residents with dementia: A cross sectional study. *Aging & Mental Health, 23*(11), 1517–1523. https://doi.org/10.1080/13607863.2018.1506737

Håkansson Eklund, J., Holmström, I. K., Kumlin, T., Kaminsky, E., Skoglund, K., Höglander, J., Sundler, A. J., Condén, E., & Summer Meranius, M. (2019). "Same same or different?" A review of reviews of person-centered and patient-centered care. *Patient Education and Counseling, 102*(1), 3–11. https://doi.org/10.1016/j.pec.2018.08.029

Hemphill, J., MacGregor, L., Austen, A., Calay, R., Kikuta, S. C., Dockery, J., Sheppard, C. L., & Hitzig, S. L. (2023). The process of implementing culture change across a city-operated long-term care home and the importance of stakeholder engagement. *Healthcare Management Forum, 36*(6), 414–419. https://doi.org/10.1177/08404704231188961

Hoek, L. J., van Haastregt, J. C., de Vries, E., Backhaus, R., Hamers, J. P., & Verbeek, H. (2021). Partnerships in nursing homes: How do family caregivers of residents with dementia perceive collaboration with staff? *Dementia (London, England), 20*(5), 1631–1648. https://doi.org/10.1177/1471301220962235

Hower, K. I., Vennedey, V., Hillen, H. A., Kuntz, L., Stock, S., Pfaff, H., & Ansmann, L. (2019). Implementation of patient-centred care: Which organisational determinants matter from decision maker's perspective? Results from a qualitative interview study across various health and social care organisations. *BMJ Open, 9*(4), e027591–e027591. https://doi.org/10.1136/bmjopen-2018-027591

Hudon, C., Chouinard, M. C., Pluye, P., El Sherif, R., Bush, P. L., Rihoux, B., et al. (2019). Characteristics of case management in primary care associated with positive outcomes for frequent users of health care: A systematic review. *Annals of Family Medicine, 17*(5), 448–458. https://doi.org/10.1370/afm.2419

Hung, L. L., Chow, B., Shadarevian, J., O'Neill, R., Berndt, A., Wallsworth, C., et al. (2021). Using touchscreen tablets to support social connections and reduce responsive behaviours among people with dementia in care settings: A scoping review. *Dementia-International Journal of Social Research & Practice, 20*(3), 1124–1143. https://doi.org/10.1177/1471301220922745

Iaboni, A., Quirt, H., Engell, K., Kirkham, J., Stewart, S., Grigorovich, A., et al. (2022). Barriers and facilitators to person-centred infection prevention and control: Results of a survey about the Dementia Isolation Toolkit. *BMC Geriatrics, 22*(1), 74. https://doi.org/10.1186/s12877-022-02759-4

Iyamu, I., Plottel, L., Snow, M. E., Zhang, W., Havaei, F., Puyat, J., Sawatzky, R., & Salmon, A. (2022). Culture change in long-term care-post COVID-19: Adapting to a new reality using established ideas and systems. *Canadian Journal on Aging / La Revue Canadienne Du Vieillissement, 42*(2), 351–358. https://doi.org/10.1017/S0714980822000344

Kane, R. A., Kane, R. L., & Ladd, R. C. (1998). *The heart of long term care*. Oxford University Press.

Kenning, G. (2018). Reciprocal design: Inclusive design approaches for people with late stage dementia. *Design for Health, 2*(1), 142–162. https://doi.org/10.1080/24735132.2018.1453638

Kim, D., Choi, Y.-R., Lee, Y.-N., & Chang, S. O. (2024). Nurses' shared subjectivity on person-centered care for behavioral and psychological symptoms of dementia in nursing homes. *The Journal of Nursing Research, 32*(3), 1–10. https://doi.org/10.1097/jnr.0000000000000611

Kim, S. K., & Park, M. (2017). Effectiveness of person-centered care on people with dementia: A systematic review and meta-analysis. *Clinical Interventions in Aging, 12*, 381–397. https://doi.org/10.2147/cia.s117637

Kogan, A. C., Wilber, K., & Mosqueda, L. (2015). Person-centered care for older adults with chronic conditions and functional impairment: A systematic literature review. *Journal of the American Geriatrics Society, 64*(1), e1–e7. https://doi.org/10.1111/jgs.13873

Kokorelias, K. M., Gignac, M. A., Naglie, G., Rittenberg, N., MacKenzie, J., D'Souza, S., & Cameron, J. I. (2022). A grounded theory study to identify caregiving phases and support needs across the Alzheimer's disease trajectory. *Disability and Rehabilitation, 44*(7), 1050–1059. https://doi.org/10.1080/09638288.2020.1788655

Kokorelias, K. M., Gignac, M. A. M., Naglie, G., & Cameron, J. I. (2019). Towards a universal model of family centered care: A scoping review. *BMC Health Services Research, 19*(1), 564. https://doi.org/10.1186/s12913-019-4394-5

Kokorelias, K. M., & Sinha, S. K. (2023). Commentary: Minding the gap--why wage parity is crucial for the care of older canadians. *Healthcare Policy, 19*(1). https://doi.org/10.12927/hcpol.2023.27160

Latimer, T., Roscamp, J., & Papanikitas, A. (2017). Patient-centredness and consumerism in healthcare: An ideological mess. *Journal of the Royal Society of Medicine, 110*(11), 425–427. https://doi.org/10.1177/0141076817731905

Li, J., & Porock, D. (2014). Resident outcomes of person-centered care in long-term care: A narrative review of interventional research. *International Journal of Nursing Studies, 51*(10), 1395–1415. https://doi.org/10.1016/j.ijnurstu.2014.04.003

Lis, M., & Boulhol, H. (2023). Work and wages in long-term care today. In *Beyond applause? Improving working conditions in long-term care*. Organization for Economic Cooperation & Development.

Livingston, G., Huntley, J., Sommerlad, A., Ames, D., Ballard, C., Banerjee, S., et al. (2020). Dementia prevention, intervention, and care: 2020 report of the Lancet Commission. *Lancet, 396*(10248), 413–446. https://doi.org/10.1016/s0140-6736(20)30367-6

Ljungholm, L., Edin-Liljegren, A., Ekstedt, M., & Klinga, C. (2022). What is needed for continuity of care and how can we achieve it? - Perceptions among multiprofessionals on the chronic care trajectory. *BMC Health Services Research, 22*(1), 686. https://doi.org/10.1186/s12913-022-08023-0

Llena-Nozal, A., Rocard, E., & Sillitti, P. (2022). Providing long-term care: Options for a better workforce. *International Social Security Review (English Edition), 75*(3–4), 121–144. https://doi.org/10.1111/issr.12310

Lloyd, B., Elkins, M., & Innes, L. (2018). Barriers and enablers of patient and family centred care in an Australian acute care hospital: Perspectives of health managers. *Patient Experience Journal, 5*(3), 55–64. https://doi.org/10.35680/2372-0247.1270

Martinez, O. N., Jr. (2024). Who is responsible for addressing racial disparities and health equity in older adults? *Public Policy & Aging Report, 34*(1), 6–8. https://doi.org/10.1093/ppar/prad030

Marulappa, N., Anderson, N. N., Bethell, J., Bourbonnais, A., Kelly, F., McMurray, J., et al. (2022). How to implement person-centred care and support for dementia in outpatient and home/community settings: Scoping review. *BMC Health Services Research, 22*(1), 541. https://doi.org/10.1186/s12913-022-07875-w

McDonald, C., & McCallin, A. (2010). Interprofessional collaboration in palliative nursing: What is the patient-family role? *International Journal of Palliative Nursing, 16*(6), 286–289. https://doi.org/10.12968/ijpn.2010.16.6.48832

Merrilees, J. J., Bernstein, A., Dulaney, S., Heunis, J., Walker, R., Rah, E., Choi, J., Gawlas, K., Carroll, S., Ong, P., Feuer, J., Braley, T., Clark, A. M., Lee, K., Chiong, W., Bonasera, S. J., Miller, B. L., & Possin, K. L. (2020). The care ecosystem: Promoting self-efficacy among dementia family caregivers. *Dementia (London, England), 19*(6), 1955–1973. https://doi.org/10.1177/1471301218814121

Miller, N. A. (1997). Patient centered long-term care. *Health Care Financing Review, 19*(2), 1–10.

Morley, L., & Cashell, A. (2017). Collaboration in health care. *Journal of Medical Imaging and Radiation Sciences, 48*(2), 207–216. https://doi.org/10.1016/j.jmir.2017.02.071

NEJM Catalyst. (2017). What is patient-centered care? *Catalyst Carryover, 3*(1). https://doi.org/10.1056/CAT.17.0559

Pan American Health Organization. (2019). Number *of older adults with LTC needs will triple by 2050, PAHO warns*. https://www.paho.org/en/news/1-1-2019-number-older-adults-long-term-care-needs-will-triple-2050-paho-warns

Perruchoud, E., Weissbrodt, R., Verloo, H., Fournier, C.-A., Genolet, A., Rosselet Amoussou, J., & Hannart, S. (2021). The impact of nursing staffs' working conditions on the quality of care received by older adults in long-term residential care facilities: A systematic review of interventional and observational studies. *Geriatrics (Basel), 7*(1), 6. https://doi.org/10.3390/geriatrics7010006

Philibert, I., Patow, C., & Cichon, J. (2011). Incorporating patient- and family-centered care into resident education: Approaches, benefits, and challenges. *Journal of Graduate Medical Education, 3*(2), 272–278. https://doi.org/10.4300/jgme-03-02-34

Ray, K. D., & Götell, E. (2018). The use of music and music therapy in ameliorating depression symptoms and improving well-being in nursing home residents with dementia. *Frontiers in Medicine (Lausanne), 5*, 287. https://doi.org/10.3389/fmed.2018.00287

Ryan, T., Nolan, M., Reid, D., & Enderby, P. (2008). Using the senses framework to achieve relationship-centred dementia care services: A case example. *Dementia, 7*(1), 71–93. https://doi.org/10.1177/1471301207085368

Saragih, I. D., Tonapa, S. I., Yao, C. T., Saragih, I. S., & Lee, B. O. (2022). Effects of reminiscence therapy in people with dementia: A systematic review and meta-analysis. *Journal of Psychiatric and Mental Health Nursing, 29*(6), 883–903. https://doi.org/10.1111/jpm.12830

Scales, K. (2021). It is time to resolve the direct care workforce crisis in long-term care. *The Gerontologist, 61*(4), 497–504. https://doi.org/10.1093/geront/gnaa116

Scott, M. M., Ménard, A., Sun, A. H., Murmann, M., Ramzy, A., Rasaputra, P., Fleming, M., Orosz, Z., Huynh, C., Welch, V., Cooper-Reed, A., & Hsu, A. T. (2024). Building evidence to advance health equity: A systematic review on care-related outcomes for older, minoritised populations in long-term care homes. *Age and Ageing, 53*(4), afae059. https://doi.org/10.1093/ageing/afae059

Siminoff, L. A. (2013). Incorporating patient and family preferences into evidence-based medicine. *BMC Med Inform Decis Mak, 13*(3), S6. https://doi.org/10.1186/1472-6947-13-s3-s6

The Health Foundation. (2012). *Evidence: Helping people share decision-making*. https://www.health.org.uk/publications/helping-people-share-decision-making

The Health Foundation. (2016). *Person-centered care made simple: What everyone should know about person-centered care*. https://www.health.org.uk/sites/default/files/PersonCentredCareMadeSimple.pdf

Treviranus, J. (2021). Inclusive design - valuing difference, recognizing complexity: Introduction. In M. H. Rioux, A. Buettgen, E. Zubrow, & J. Viera (Eds.), *Handbook of disability: Critical thought and social change in a globalizing world* (pp. 1–24). Springer Nature Singapore. https://doi.org/10.1007/978-981-16-1278-7_98-2

Vennedey, V., Hower, K. I., Hillen, H., Ansmann, L., Kuntz, L., & Stock, S. (2020). Patients' perspectives of facilitators and barriers to patient-centred care: insights from qualitative patient interviews. *BMJ Open, 10*(5), e033449–e033449. https://doi.org/10.1136/bmjopen-2019-033449

Weinstein, D. (n.d.). Nursing homes during COVID-19: How better working conditions for CNAs can improve the well-being of residents. *Undergraduate Academic Journal, 12*.

White-Chu, E. F., Graves, W. J., Godfrey, S. M., Bonner, A., & Sloane, P. (2009). Beyond the medical model: The culture change revolution in long-term care. *Journal of the American Medical Directors Association, 10*(6), 370–378. https://doi.org/10.1016/j.jamda.2009.04.004

Willemse, B. M., Downs, M., Arnold, L., Smit, D., de Lange, J., & Pot, A. M. (2015). Staff–resident interactions in long-term care for people with dementia: The role of meeting psychological needs in achieving residents' well-being. *Aging & Mental Health, 19*(5), 444–452. https://doi.org/10.1080/13607863.2014.944088

Yee, J., Ribeiro Souza, M. C. M., Horta, N. D. C., & Kartoz, C. (2021). Person-centered care for older adults living in long-term care facilities: A systematic literature review. *Journal of Public Health Issues and Practices, 5*(2). https://doi.org/10.33790/jphip1100184

Chapter 14
Extending the Age-Friendly Movement to Long-Term Care

Patricia Oh, Mary Lou Ciolfi, and Kimberly Snow

The global age-friendly community (AFC) movement champions policies, services, and infrastructure that foster active, healthy, and engaged aging across all aspects of civic life. The initiative aims to create environments where people of all ages and abilities are respected as valued members of the community who contribute to and benefit from their community. AFCs focus on multiple key aspects of community life. The growth of AFCs and their success over the past decade has corresponded with similar person-centered paradigm shifts in healthcare delivery. Age-friendly healthcare systems (AFHS) is an innovative approach that highlights the importance of a person-centered, person-directed focus in the healthcare sector, including hospitals, acute care settings, and long-term care (LTC) organizations. The AFC movement has overlapped with and amplified the thirty-plus year, incremental, steady progress in patient and person-centered healthcare delivery.

Despite a challenging history, LTC organizations—nursing homes and assisted living communities—play a vital role in supporting AFCs in offering residential living options so that community members managing chronic illness or disability can live with dignity and purpose. The integration of care organizations with

P. Oh (✉) · M. L. Ciolfi
Center on Aging Policy Research and Analysis, University of Maine Center on Aging, Bangor, ME, USA

Consortium for Aging Policy Research and Analysis, University of Maine Center on Aging, Bangor, ME, USA
e-mail: patricia.oh@maine.edu; marylou.ciolfi@maine.edu

K. Snow
Center on Aging Policy Research and Analysis, University of Maine Center on Aging, Bangor, ME, USA

Catherine Cutler Institute, Muskie School of Public Service, University of Southern Maine, Portland, ME, USA
e-mail: kimberly.i.snow@maine.edu

K. K. Bhattacharyya (ed.), *Health Promotion in Long-Term Care Facilities*,
https://doi.org/10.1007/978-3-031-91038-8_14

community services and initiatives—a key goal of age-friendly long-term care—presents opportunities for AFHS and AFCs to collaborate in enhancing the care experiences of LTC residents, family care partners, and professional caregivers. This chapter considers the evolution of AFCs, person-centered LTC, and the advantages of implementing age-friendly long-term care (AFLTC). The chapter describes how AFCs in the United States have partnered with long-term care and explores how emerging technologies may expand opportunities for older residents to age in their preferred communities. It concludes with recommendations for promoting integration between AFC and AFLTC.

Collaboration between age-friendly communities (AFCs) and age-friendly long-term care organizations could better address the evolving needs of an aging population. However, empirical evidence on AFC engagement with LTC systems and the promotion of technology to help people remain safely and comfortably at home is limited. This chapter aims to expand this knowledge by examining a sample of AFCs from the AARP Network of Age-Friendly States and Communities. We explore current efforts to embed meaningful age-friendly, person-centered care in LTC and the challenges facing those efforts. We also explore ways in which AFCs promote smart technology and equip community members to use it, highlighting the nature and prevalence of reported engagement between AFCs and AFLTC.

Background

Global Age-Friendly Community Movement

The global Age-Friendly Community (AFC) movement aims to create more equitable, inclusive communities across multiple sectors to improve the natural (e.g., outdoor spaces), built (e.g., transportation), social (e.g., civic engagement), and service environments (e.g., healthcare) for aging (Mondal et al., 2021; WHO, 2018). To structure the approach, AFCs commit to a five-year cycle of continuous improvement: (1) engage and understand, (2) plan, (3) act, and (4) measure (WHO, 2019). Based on the success of the age-friendly movement, other sectors (e.g., healthcare, higher education) developed comprehensive approaches to support and equip older adults to live active, healthy, meaningful lives (Sixsmith et al., 2023). Despite sharing a focus on age-friendly, efforts in each sector have often been siloed, with few collaborations between the different approaches to making.

Defining Age-Friendly Communities

AFCs are geographically defined areas that actively value, engage, and equip older people in community development to ensure that residents of all ages and abilities can achieve optimal health and well-being through policy, services, and infrastructure that effectively accommodate diverse and evolving needs (Greenfield et al., 2015; WHO, 2007). AFCs foster collaboration among community members, informal groups, local and regional organizations, and municipal government across multiple sectors to facilitate the planning and implementation of improvements in the built, social, service, natural, and policy environments to promote healthy aging across the lifespan. AFCs uniquely position older residents as change agents, actively including them in planning and implementation. This approach challenges ageism, a significant barrier to healthy aging, by leveraging the skills, contributions, goals, and preferences of older residents to build on community strengths and needs to create an environment where people with diverse aging experiences can thrive (Greenfield et al., 2022).

Development of the Age-Friendly Community Movement

The WHO launched the age-friendly movement in 2010 as part of its efforts to promote active, healthy, and engaged aging (WHO, 2018). Since then, over 1600 communities across 53 countries have joined the WHO Global Network of Age-Friendly States and Communities (WHO-GNAFCC), with more than half (900 as of September 2024) concentrated in the United States (U.S.) (W. Armbruster, personal communication, September 10, 2024). In 2012, AARP became an organizational affiliate of the WHO-GNAFCC to manage and promote AFCs in the U.S. and continues to provide technical assistance to members of the AARP Network of Age-Friendly States and Communities (AARP NAFSC) and link AFCs with other sectors in the age-friendly ecosystem, including age-friendly health systems, public health, and home and community-based services.

To develop a comprehensive "all-of-community" approach for AFCs, the WHO conducted an extensive study that included focus groups with more than 2000 older adults, care partners, and service providers across 33 cities in 22 countries (WHO, 2007). Based on their findings, researchers identified eight domains of livability that older community members deemed crucial for healthy, engaged aging. These domains span the built/natural (housing, transportation, outdoor spaces, and public buildings), social (civic engagement and employment, social participation, respect, and social inclusion), and service environments (community and health services, communication, and information). The policy environment is also key to AFC development since it crosses all the domains. The AARP Network of Age-Friendly States and Communities (NAFSC) adopts a flexible approach to membership, encouraging each AFC to tailor its initiatives to their community context. This adaptability allows communities to focus on select domains, consolidate multiple domains into a single category, or introduce additional focus areas, such as elder abuse prevention or disaster preparedness, to address locally relevant concerns (Black & Oh, 2022).

Age-Friendly Focus: Community Supports and Health Services

The movement envisions strengthening community health and provides a catalyst for partnerships between AFCs and healthcare sectors. Collaboration offers the healthcare sector a tool to promote health and well-being across ages, abilities, and life experiences. While all domains of livability intersect with healthcare, the community supports and health services domain has the most overlap encompassing a broad mix of formal and informal services (Lowen et al., 2015), including food security, emergency preparedness, elder abuse prevention, services for people living with dementia and care partners, wellness promotion, and telehealth. Age-friendly communities use different strategies to approach the community supports and health services domain, including partnering with healthcare services (e.g., offering scholarships for CNA licensing), advocacy (e.g., working with a dental school to bring a clinic to a remote area), raising awareness of or expanding existing programs (e.g., facilitating telehealth access), and developing new services (e.g., providing/installing smart home devices) (AARP, n.d.). While the WHO-GNAFCC acknowledges needs that can accompany advanced old age and multiple chronic conditions (WHO, 2018), programmatic emphasis in the U.S. and elsewhere is often on promoting active, healthy, and engaged aging (e.g., AARP, 2018), rather than on meeting the needs of people with multiple chronic illnesses or disability requiring services and supports to live safely at home. Despite programmatic guidelines, a growing number of AFCs have developed programs to link older residents with technology to allow people to age in their homes, have developed initiatives to support the long-term care workforce, and/or are partnering with long-term care organizations to integrate residents with the community.

Age-Friendly Health Systems

Like AFC work in the community supports and health services domain, Age-Friendly Health Systems (AFHS) aims to enhance the lives of older people by providing better care and services and by removing barriers to participation. In 2017, the John A. Hartford Foundation and the Institute for Healthcare Improvement launched the AFHS movement, organizing healthcare delivery into four primary domains referred to as the 4Ms: what matters, medication, mentation, and mobility. The goal of the 4Ms approach is to align delivered care with the wishes and goals of the older adult and to improve the quality of care by integrating services among the four domains.

Within a few years of the launch of age-friendly health systems, there was a call to apply the framework to the LTC sector (Edelman et al., 2021). In 2024, the Institute for Healthcare Improvement (IHI) published an updated AFHS guide for AF nursing homes (IHI, 2024). Since the COVID-19 pandemic and the subsequent National Academies of Science, Engineering, and Medicine (NASEM, 2022) report, *The National Imperative to Improve Nursing Home Quality: Honoring Our*

Commitment to Residents, Families, and Staff (2022), there is a renewed focus on delivering age-friendly, person-centered long-term care.

Person-Centered Care

The early models of a person-centered approach in LTC include the Eden Alternative (1994) and the Wellspring Model (1997), which accompanied the culture change movement in LTC to shift away from the traditional institutional look and feel of nursing home care. After 2020, the outsized impact of the COVID-19 pandemic on older adults living in nursing homes led to alarm among residents and families, long-term care sector experts, and policymakers. In 2021, the National Academies of Science, Engineering, and Medicine (NASEM) convened national experts to study the issue. NASEM's 2022 report, *The National Imperative to Improve Nursing Home Quality: Honoring Our Commitment to Residents, Families, and Staff*, lays our seven improvement goals anchored in a central premise: quality care must balance resident autonomy with safety while prioritizing individual choice in daily life (NASEM, 2022).

In addition to the work of the MFC, LTC communities are increasingly adopting the AFHC framework, which emphasizes a comprehensive and integrated approach to care and services in recognition that nursing homes and assisted living communities are each resident's home and resident preferences for all aspects of daily life can and should be consistently collected and honored (Institute for Healthcare Improvement, 2024). AFLTC acknowledges the difficulty of coordinating care across multiple departments—nursing, dietary, activities, housekeeping, and facilities management—and offers implementation tools that incorporate the evidence-based *Plan-Do-Study-Act* quality improvement model. Many LTC organizations already use several person-centered approaches, such as gathering life story information at admission and allowing full choice in the timing of waking, retiring, meals, ablutions, and activities and outings. The AF framework encourages homes to build on existing structures, processes, and practices, deepen their knowledge of each resident, and question underlying ageist and other intersectional assumptions that often result in fundamental inequities of ability, age, gender, race, LGBTQ+ status, class, and other social groups. For LTC residents, the geographic and social fabric of the cities and towns where LTC communities are situated can provide residents with a vital bridge to their personal histories, lived experiences, and interests, helping maintain continuity of identity and social engagement. Collaboration between community-based groups and LTC communities requires overcoming barriers to popular awareness that LTC residents are a vital part of the community, including the need for education about aging (Bhattacharyya et al., 2022).

The Challenges of High-Quality Age-Friendly Care

While there is broad consensus across sectors—but particularly among the consuming public and resident advocacy groups—that the care in our nation's nursing homes and assisted living communities should be higher quality and more person-centered, there are long-standing systemic factors that stand in the way of meaningful reform, including Medicaid reimbursement rates, the aging of the population, and workforce factors. Ageist beliefs and attitudes about older people, particularly those with physical and cognitive changes requiring residential care placement, lie at the heart of our collective failure to address systemic barriers and bring age-friendly, age-positive reform to LTC settings. While new tools are emerging to address ageism among LTC workers (Gendron et al., 2021) and the public (Burnes et al., 2019), widespread change is needed. Our society has long marginalized older people, particularly people with physical or cognitive limitations (Kang & Kim, 2022) and, consequently, we have denied them meaningful choice autonomy, including the freedom to make choices that hold benefit for the individual even though there may be a potential risk of harm.

Studies have long established that the loss of choice among nursing home residents leads to decreased quality of life (Kane et al., 1997). Autonomy and personal choice are associated with human dignity and recognition by others as having inherent value and worth (Dong et al., 2021), a basic human right (Ibrahim & Davis, 2013). Loss of feelings of dignity is associated with a lack of attention to and honoring of resident choice and preference and generates psychosocial harm, feelings of anger, and frustration (Behrens et al., 2022) and has deep and lasting impact. Technology can help connect people living in a community with friends and neighbors so that they are able to participate in community life. Similarly, AFCs can be a conduit connecting LTC communities to the broader community. Dignity is enhanced when residents of LTC communities have the option to connect to their community in a way that is comfortable and in the way that they desire.

Emergence and Use of Home Technology to Support Aging-in-Place

Research consistently shows that older adults prefer to age in their own homes and communities (Binette & Farago, 2021). Technology adoption may help delay or prevent admission to an LTC setting (Choi et al., 2021; Jachan et al., 2021). Age-friendly communities have promoted the use of smart home technologies as part of their work in both the housing and community support and health services domain (Zhou et al., 2024). While the research is mixed on the effectiveness of smart home technology (e.g., virtual personal assistants, smart switches) in delaying transitions to supportive housing or residential care settings for individuals living with illness or disability that qualify them for state-subsidized in-home care (Facchinetti et al.,

2023; Liu et al., 2019), new evidence suggests that this technology improves the quality of life for this population. Tech adopters report a greater sense of achievement and safety (Aggar et al., 2023). Even a short delay in transitioning to more supportive environments benefits older adults and their communities. However, a move to a more supportive setting may eventually become necessary when technology and community services can no longer meet an individual's requirements.

Smart home technology has evolved from an initial focus on basic appliances (e.g., television remote control) to encompass many devices that leverage the Internet of Things (IoT) and artificial intelligence, creating interconnected living environments. Research has shown that smart home technology may assist older adults in aging comfortably and safely and remaining socially connected to their families and communities (Facchinetti et al., 2023; Moreno et al., 2023; Hill et al., 2015). Voice-activated devices like Amazon Echo and Google Home offer hands-free control of smart home functions to help older adults perform tasks such as adjusting lighting, making phone calls, and accessing entertainment such as music playlists (O'Brien, 2020). Smart home technologies, including thermostats, stoves, lighting, and security systems, assist older adults in controlling their home environment (Fritz et al., 2016). These devices can be programmed to adapt to individual routines, enhancing comfort and safety. Sensors can detect motion, contact, light, temperature, and movement within the home to help track ADLs, falls, and entry or exit from the home Facchinetti et al., 2023). Wearable technologies and home health monitoring devices enable continuous tracking of health metrics, such as gait speed, heart rate, and medication adherence. This data can be shared with healthcare providers and family members, facilitating proactive health management (Zhong & Rau, 2020).

Older Adult Adoption of Smart Technologies

Although evidence supports smart home technology's positive impact on quality of life and ability to age in place (Aggar et al., 2023; Popejoy et al., 2022) and older adults are interested in health monitoring technologies (Wang et al., 2019), uptake of these devices is still low. A recent AARP survey found older adults (50+) own most types of smart devices (e.g., smartphones, tablets, home assistants, wearables) at about the same rate as younger adults (18–49), but across both age groups, only about one-quarter of adults use smart home technology (Kakulla, 2024). The most common types of smart home technology used by older adults are home security devices such as front door cameras (32%), window or door alarms (17%), and automatic timers or shut-off for appliances, lights, and thermostats.

Another survey found that less than one-third of adults ages 50–80 currently use a mobile health app to monitor their exercise, nutrition, weight, sleep, or blood pressure (Malani et al., 2022). Although 17% of survey respondents reported having type 2 diabetes, only 11% of these reported using a mobile health app together with a CGM patch on their skin to track their blood sugar. These results indicate that although health apps are often promoted to assist in managing and monitoring chronic health conditions, older adults have not widely adopted this technology.

Barriers to the Uptake of Technology

Barriers and challenges to older adults' adoption of smart technology include perceptions of benefit and need for the technology, cost, lack of interest, lack of knowledge of how to use it, and concerns about personal control, security and privacy and may vary by type of technology (Harris et al., 2022; Hawley-Hague et al. 2014; Lee & Coughlin, 2015; Tural et al., 2021). For example, a scoping review of the literature showed attitudes toward surveillance-type of technologies for falls prevention are much different from wearable technologies with the former being less acceptable, in general, than the latter. However, the perceived need for technology can overcome concerns about privacy and control (Arthanat et al., 2019; Hawley-Hague et al., 2014).

Steele et al. (2009) found cost a top factor in older adults' attitudes toward adopting wireless sensor technology in the home. Older adults were not only concerned with the upfront cost but also the cost of maintaining the system. Technology programs that have an upfront cost and a cost for ongoing use may be unattractive to some who do not see the economic value, even when the technology has the potential to avert expensive emergency room and hospital services. High upfront and ongoing costs can put technology out of reach of many older adults on limited incomes, creating inequities among those who benefit from these innovations (Fang, 2022).

Healthcare providers may contribute to lower rates of adoption of smart technologies, especially telehealth and smartphone apps, through their own ageist attitudes about older adults' capacity to use the technology (Mace et al., 2022). Similarly, ageism in technology development that has focused on younger end users leaves older adults with different motor skills, vision, and hearing unable to access technology that could be useful to them.

Facilitators to Uptake of Technology

The motivation to adopt and continue to use smart technology is related to older adults' attitudes around control over their own lives and environments, affordability, independence, and perceived need for technology. Positive messaging around the benefits of smart technology and ensuring it is simple to use, reliable, safe, and customizable to individual needs may support greater adoption of smart home technologies by older adults (AARP, n.d.; Hawley-Hague et al., 2014; Lee & Coughlin, 2015; Marston et al., 2019; Zhou et al., 2024).

Zhou, Qian, and Kaner describe the goal of a smart home is "to provide a safer, convenient, and comfortable living space." Yet, they note that many smart home technologies are not designed with older adults in mind or consider their physical needs, creating less practical and convenient functionality. The easier the technology is to use, the greater the adoption by older people. Including older adults as end users in the design of smart home and digital health technologies may help ensure they can easily access these devices (Mace et al., 2022; Sumner et al., 2021; Zhou et al., 2024).

Adequate instruction on how to use the technology and ongoing technology support is critical to help older adults master and continue to use smart home technology (Gell et al., 2021; Gleason & Suen, 2022; Koon et al., 2020;). Instruction needs to account for different learning styles and needs among older adults, such as their level of digital literacy preferences for reading manuals to learn about new technologies and devices (Steele et al., 2009; Tsai et al., 2012). Programs and policies addressing economic and geographic disparities in broadband access and disparities in digital literacy will ensure equal access to the benefits of these technologies as they age in their communities.

Age-Friendly Communities: Equipping Older People to Age in Their Communities Through Technology and Partnerships with LTC

The availability of convenient and accessible CSHS is critical for shaping the perception of municipal age-friendliness (e.g., Choi, 2021) and improving the health and well-being of people aging with a disability or chronic illness (Miskimmin et al., 2019; Zamora et al., 2020). Studies have shown that AFCs collaborate with AFHC (Bhattacharyya et al., 2022; Liebzeit et al., 2023) working collaboratively to advance healthcare goals (Black & Oh, 2022; Oh & White, 2022), which includes the availability of long-term care options. Although studies have looked at the role of CSHS to bolster the age-friendliness of communities and collaboration with AFHC, few have looked at the extent and nature of AFC collaboration with AFLTC

Methods

We explored evidence of AFC initiatives in the CSHS domain to learn the extent, range, and type of activities reported by NAFSC members to extend the ability of community members to AIP and to explore how AFCs collaborate with LTC organizations. We then synthesized results for an enhanced understanding of age-friendly community engagement in CSHS, with a focus on activities to enhance AIP and to partner with local LTC organizations.

Research Design and Analysis

This study, using methods developed and explicated in Oh & White (2022), employed directed content analysis to examine 102 progress reports submitted by members of the AARP Network of Age-Friendly States and Communities (NAFSC). These reports, required as part of network membership, are publicly available on the AARP NAFSC website (https://www.aarp.org/livable-communities/network-age-friendly-communities/). Our analysis examined initiatives that enhanced access to technology, enabling older residents with chronic illness, disability, or dementia to live safely and comfortably in the community—either at home or, when that is no longer possible, in a long-term care (LTC) organization.

Sample and Data Collection

To maintain membership in AARP NAFSC, members submit a progress report documenting the work they have accomplished in the three years following their age-friendly assessment and development of the action plan. Of the 900 active members of NAFSC on October 01, 2024, 102 submitted progress reports that were publicly available on the AARP member website. These reports covered 127 communities, with 10 reports detailing regional initiatives comprised of two to nine municipalities collaborating on age-friendly goals.

Progress reports were submitted by AFCs located across 28 states, with 19 in the West region, 26 in the South, 17 in the Midwest, and 40 in the Northeast. Communities that met the inclusion criteria ranged from small rural communities of less than 1000 residents to large urban areas with more than nine million. We excluded AFCs that had not submitted a progress report to AARP, ensuring a focus on communities actively engaged in the reporting process.

Results

Of 102 progress reports submitted to AARP, nearly all (93%, $n = 95$) planned activities, programs, services, or advocacy as part of their approach to increasing the availability of and access to CSHS, and 32 (31%) indicated reported some engagement with LTC or promotion of technology or other supports to help people extend their ability to age in place (AIP) safely and comfortably in their homes.

Community Support and Health Services

AFCs play a crucial role in enhancing the quality of life for older community members through access to CSHS. A comprehensive analysis of the progress reports indicated that AFCs built on community strengths, most often by partnering with other groups and organizations, to promote health, wellness, and independence by residents with diverse life experiences, abilities, resources, and needs. This overview details the most common approaches adopted by AFCs in their efforts to connect residents to CSHS. Most commonly (see Table 14.1), AFCs promoted access to local and regional services and programs (e.g., partnered to develop a community navigator program), increased awareness of healthy lifestyles (e.g., hosted a Healthy Brain training), provided access to technology (e.g., launched a Tech Handy Helper program that installs virtual assistants or trains people to participate in Tele-Health visits), and created, advocated, or promoted caregiver supports. A few communities also developed initiatives to promote AIP by community members with multiple chronic illnesses or a disability (24%) or to improve LTC environments (12%) (see Table 14.1).

Partnerships in CSHS and LTC The effectiveness of AFCs to support AIP and improve LTC environments often hinged on their organizational structure, strategic partnerships, and alignment with regional health plans. AFCs with initiatives to extend AIP or coordinate with LTC organizations were likelier to describe a dedicated planning team leading the work in CSHS. Specifically, 67% of the 27 communities with a domain planning team described such initiatives, compared with 9% of the 75 communities without a CSHS planning team. Nearly all (93%) of the CSHS domain teams included at least one representative from healthcare (e.g., nurse, hospital administrator) or an LTC organization (e.g., healthcare center, retirement community, assisted living). A smaller proportion (30%) included higher education, typically someone in healthcare or related fields. Partnerships with public health and other healthcare services increased opportunities for AFCs to align their work with other community health plans. For example, among AFCs with AIP or LTC initiatives that partnered with healthcare, 48% had goals overlapping with their Community Health Improvement Plan, compared to only 2% without this focus.

Progress reports typically detail one or two activities to extend AIP or coordinate AFC with LTC organizations. However, a few AFCs, generally with healthcare and LTC representation on the core leadership team, described up to six distinct activities encompassing multiple approaches to improve LTC environments and extend AIP. For example, one such AFC described continuing education for LTC staff, development of an assisted living housing option, training on telehealth devices, evidence-based wellness programs, a community health worker initiative, and telepsychiatry access for area nursing homes.

Cross-sector leadership of AFC work in CSHS provides the resources and skills that AFCs need to implement comprehensive initiatives and align their goals with broader community health plans. These teams, particularly when they include diverse representation from healthcare, long-term care organizations, and higher education, drive more comprehensive and innovative approaches in CSHS. The alignment of AFC CSHS initiatives with broader community health improvement plans further amplifies their impact and positions the AFC to leverage emerging opportunities to develop additional programs, services, and activities to equip older community members to age in their homes and to improve LTC environments.

Table 14.1 Summary of activities in the Community Supports and Health Services Domain

Community Supports and Health Services Activity	% Progress reports address issue area ($n = 102$)
Policy change	16.7
Address economic security	38.9
Promote health knowledge and skills	77.8
Increase access to community services	83.3
Wellness initiative	66.7
Dementia-related activity, service, education	50.0
Activity, program or service for people with dementia	38.9
Education about dementia-friendly practices	33.3
Formally joins Dementia-Friendly America©	5.6
Activities, programs, or services for informal caregivers	50.0
Promote and advocate for caregiver-friendly policies	22.2
Programs or services for informal caregivers	44.4
Funding for services	16.7
Address food security	50.0
Elder mistreatment initiative	33.3
Public Service initiative	83.3
Crime prevention and awareness	44.4
Fire prevention and home safety	50.0
Emergency preparedness	61.1
Advanced Care and End of Life Planning	33.3
Access to services, programs, or activities to promote safe aging at home, collaborate with long-term care organizations, or improve long-term care environments	$n = 32$
Promote aging at home/equip residents for aging in place	75.0
Increase access to or promote telehealth/telemedicine	21.9
Equip or educate about SMART home devices	34.4
Community health care worker/paramedicine	9.4
Program or service to reduce readmission	22.2
Increase access to primary or specialty care	28.1
Program, service, or activity to improve Long-Term Care Organization	56.3
Development of long-term care housing	21.9
Advocate or promote age-friendly health care	16.7
Recruit health care workers	27.8
Continuing education for health care workers	15.6
Program, service, or activity to facilitate connections between LTC residents and community members	21.9
Partnership with Long-Term Care organizations	34.4
Long-Term Care organization—steering committee.	10.7
Long-Term Care organization—resource partner with age-friendly	15.6

Programs and Services to Equip Residents to Adapt Their Environment to Age in Place Equipping older adults to age in their homes as long as possible is crucial for maintaining quality of life, independence, and a sense of belonging. AFCs often built on initiatives in other domains (e.g., housing, communication, and information) to create programs that meet the needs of people aging in the community with cognitive impairment, chronic illness, or other disability that required adaptation of the home environment for the individual to age safely and comfortably in their own home for as long as possible. Home chore and repair programs, volunteer transportation initiatives, and COVID-19 inspired social engagement initiatives most often led to the creation of a program or service to equip people to age in place when environmental adaptations were needed. Less often, an initiative in the CSHS domain led to the implementation of a new program. For example, in one AFC, a community paramedicine initiative led to the development of a home visitor program that linked people to essential and social resources.

Technology Access to technology and confidence using available technology is critical for older people to age in their homes as long as possible. About 2:3 of AFCs described initiatives to increase access to technology. More AFCs described work to increase confidence using technology (e.g., educational events about digital devices, telehealth training) than did increasing access (e.g., hot-spot rental programs, providing notebooks or smart home devices). Often, training initiatives were intergenerational, with high school or college students providing one-on-one guidance to use devices, and were made possible through partnerships with libraries, higher education, and service organizations (e.g., Key Club, Circle K International). Initiatives that provided technology to older adults also included education. For example, one AFC had a "Tech Handy Helper Program" that purchased SMART technology needed by community members, and a volunteer provided personalized setups and instructions on how to use the devices confidently.

Initiatives to Equip Community Members to Age in Their Own Homes Overall, more communities reported successful initiatives to extend AIP than to improve LTC environments (see Table 14.1). AFCs with initiatives to extend AIP reported success by (1) educating community members about SMART home devices or by providing and installing the devices (e.g., virtual assistant; smart smoke detectors); (2) increasing access to primary or specialty care (e.g., transportation, mobile health clinic); (3) programs or services to reduce readmission (e.g., community referrals for social engagement and transportation). AFCs also reported telehealth initiatives and implementing community nursing or paramedicine programs (see Table 14.1). Less frequently, AFCs described programs to increase access to Home and Community-Based Services, implement a housing navigator program, and partner to start a helpline, most often for mental health support. One AFC matched residents with robotic pets. AFC initiatives to extend the time community members could age in their own homes were often complex and multi-faceted, requiring collaboration between two or more partners. For example, an emergency paramedicine program required intersectoral cooperation between multiple municipal departments (e.g., public health; emergency services) as well as engagement by multiple sectors (e.g., healthcare services; higher education).

Initiatives to Improve LTC Environments The involvement of community members in LTC housing plays a vital role in enhancing the quality of life for residents. Collaborations between AFCs and LTC organizations described in the progress reports involved up to seven different LTC organizations and led to innovative approaches that addressed workforce shortages, created new housing options, and encouraged community members of all ages to engage with LTC residents.

AFCs that developed initiatives to improve LTC environments reported active engagement with the aging and health services sectors, with up to 7 partners with connections to LTC organizations. Among the 18 communities that described such approaches, 39% focused on improving long-term care through workforce initiatives, 44% described initiatives to develop supportive housing options, and 50% shared successful outreach to LTC organizations to include residents in community life. While it was less common for AFCs to report collaboration with LTC organizations to improve care, 16% described advocacy for AFHC.

Frequently reported activities to support the workforce were continuing education opportunities (e.g., behavioral health/dementia training, LGBTQ+ trauma-informed care) and recruiting health care workers (e.g., ESL and scholarships for CNAs, support for nursing students). AFCs that advocated to increase the supply of assisted living generally worked with the municipality to convert an existing structure for use as a small assisted living facility (under 20 beds) or to expand assisted living options to people aging with intellectual disabilities or people living with mental illness. Outreach to facilitate community connections between residents of long-term care organizations and community members most commonly took the form of: (1) promoting intergenerational exchanges (e.g., intergenerational game afternoons, recruiting young people as volunteers); (2) creating cultural opportunities (e.g., an art exhibit located in a facility, a concert by a traditional band that is open to the public); and, (3) providing opportunities outside a facility (e.g., rickshaw bicycle rides; transportation to social opportunities). Occasionally, AFCs collaborated with long-term care organizations on disaster preparedness initiatives.

These collaborative approaches demonstrate how community involvement can transform LTC environments. By fostering these connections, AFCs not only improve the immediate living conditions for residents but also create a more integrated and supportive ecosystem for older adults, ultimately contributing to a more age-inclusive community.

Future Directions

Age-Friendly Communities

The AFC movement is gaining momentum and has forged diverse partnerships across community sectors. Local initiatives increasingly focus on building community resilience, addressing social isolation, and developing programs and services for people living with disabilities and with cognitive changes. The shift builds on work AFCs have completed to make the built environment more accessible for all ages and abilities and to develop programs that address home safety (e.g., volunteer home repair programs, tech handy helpers). By moving from making the built environment more age-friendly to focusing on improvements to the service environment to create or expand programs and services for people living with chronic illness, disability, and cognitive changes, AFCs are creating new opportunities for collaborations among health care systems, long-term care communities, age-friendly volunteers, and other groups and organizations dedicated to age-inclusive community development. Examples can be seen in Massachusetts, where most AFCs include a dementia-friendly focus and are involved in ageism awareness campaigns, and in Maine, where half of the AFCs include dementia inclusion and age-inclusive messaging in their action plans. The focus on dementia inclusion and on ageism raises awareness in the population of broad issues of aging, including aging with a condition that requires care in a long-term care community.

Age-Friendly Long-Term Care

The future of continued efforts to improve and strengthen age-friendly, person-centered LTC initiatives depends in large part on federal and state policymakers. Meaningful AFLTC requires training, resources, improved staffing, and in many cases, physical plant upgrades given the age and institutional look and feel of many nursing homes. The cost of these investments will be considerable, and currently, there are no obvious federal champions for widespread reform nor any public appetite for the associated costs. That said, grassroots efforts fueled the post-COVID regulatory changes, allowing family members to be considered "essential workers" so they could not be denied access to loved ones during a public health emergency (Montesanti et al., 2023). Given the philanthropic support for nursing home reform, the visible efforts of the Moving Forward Coalition (Moving Forward Nursing Home Quality Coalition, 2024), and the availability of resources to support age-friendly care in nursing homes, the movement is likely to sustain, and hopefully gain, momentum in upcoming years. The Biden-Harris Administration has made it a policy priority to improve nursing home quality with several initiatives (The White House, 2022), and this support may precipitate future policy activity, including policy support for age-friendly, person-centered LTC. In addition, the growth of the

Reframing Aging Initiative to build the public's skills in recognizing and addressing ageism in societal structures, interpersonal exchanges, and in attitudes toward our own aging will undoubtedly result in public demands for system improvements and coordination between AFC and LTC that reflect anti-ageism values.

Technology Support for Age-Friendly Living

Older adults are as likely to use smartphones, tablets, and other communication technology as their younger counterparts (Kakulla, 2024). Yet, there are barriers to widespread adoption of these technologies to enhance health and well-being, such as cost, perceived lack of usefulness or need, and difficulty using the technology to its full potential. Health monitoring apps that have complicated interfaces need to be simplified for older adults and caregivers alike to maximize their utility. As AFCs become more ubiquitous and public perceptions of older adults' abilities and willingness to use technology change to reflect reality, tech developers should realize they have an interest in ensuring their products meet the needs of a growing market that differs from younger customers.

Promising technology developments that may help us interact with our communities, maintain our homes, and improve our health and well-being include driverless cars, robotic lawnmowers, over-the-counter hearing aids, computer gaming equipment supporting safe movement, watchbands integrated with a smartwatch allowing the wearer to turn appliances on and off with a move of their hand, and lighting systems that adjust when they sense movement in the room (Berlyn, 2023; Berlyn, 2024). While these advancements have the potential to help preserve our independence, they are not without concerns for the safety of the user and those around them, affordability, and ease of use for people with different cognitive abilities and digital literacy.

Policy Implications: Call to Action

To Promote Collaboration and Effectiveness in Community Supports and Health Services

The complexity and multi-faceted nature of successful AFC initiatives underscore the importance of creating policy frameworks and incentives that encourage cross-sector collaboration. The AFC progress reports suggested that planning teams with representation by older residents, local government, healthcare, higher education, and LTC promote partnerships on AIP and LTC initiatives. Collaborations benefit AFCs, which can tap into the skills and resources of partnering organizations. Strategic alignment with AFC also allows partners to advance their own goals in the community. However, it takes time and requires organizations to invest resources into AFC before they can realize organizational and collaborative benefits. This may involve developing guidelines and funding mechanisms that reward cross-sector partnerships in CSHS.

AFCs, especially in rural areas, depend on older volunteers to plan, implement, and provide ongoing coordination for programs, services, and activities to equip older residents for AIP. Although many studies point to the intrinsic and extrinsic benefits of volunteering, emerging evidence suggests that strategic investment in volunteer infrastructure substantially amplifies the scope and effectiveness of community programs. Enhanced local, state, and federal funding for AFCs and their volunteer networks has the potential to expand the reach and impact of initiatives that both support older adults in aging in place and enhance long-term care (LTC) environments.

To Promote Age-Friendly, Person-Centered Long-Term Care

For fundamental reform, policymakers must address several complex structural and cost issues. Currently, 70% of the nation's nursing homes are for-profit (Statista, 2023), which has resulted in largely invisible, hard-to-entangle ownership structures that pose obstacles for regulatory oversight and accountability. At the same time, smaller homes and nonprofit homes are burdened by regulations that are sometimes misaligned with quality-of-care incentives. Further, while it recognized the undisputed need for more staffing in LTC to meet resident needs, the new CMS staffing rule (89 Fed. Reg. 40876, 2024) was controversial because there are insufficient workers to meet labor demands in many areas of the country. The failure to hire workers is often a demographic issue or a cost issue, the latter being a product of inadequate reimbursement given the high percentage of Medicaid residents in nursing homes.

Finally, policymakers can support greater awareness of and training for anti-ageism skill development. Despite efforts made over the past decade, many policymakers and members of the public remain unaware of the definition and manifestation of ageism in society. Yet, historic ageism and the long-standing marginalization of older adults are the root cause of many systemic inequities in the modern day. Until this root cause is addressed, we may be unable to achieve the just and equitable society we seek.

To Promote the Use and Development of Smart Technology

Smart technology can assist older people to live safely and comfortably in their communities and potentially delay or avert the need to move to a formal care setting. However, access to affordable technology devices and broadband services is not universal nor is digital literacy required to use them effectively. AFCs are well-positioned to provide ongoing technical instruction to older adults and advocate for increased access to broadband for all community members. They can educate older adults about the benefits of smart technology in their everyday lives. Encouraging the inclusion of end users in the technology design process and developing measurable outcomes that demonstrate its benefits will help older adults have a voice in the process and increase adoption of and build the evidence for smart tech as a key tool for AIP.

Conclusion

The global age-friendly community (AFC) movement aims to create environments where people of all ages and abilities can thrive through improved policies, services, and infrastructure. Based on an analysis of 102 progress reports from the AARP Network of Age-Friendly States and Communities, most US AFCs (93%) planned activities to increase access to CSHS, with about one-third specifically focused on helping people age in place through technology adoption or improving LTC environments. The most successful approaches involved dedicated planning teams with representatives from healthcare, LTC organizations, and higher education, allowing AFCs to align their work with broader community health plans.

While technology like smart home devices and health monitoring systems can help older adults age safely at home, adoption remains relatively low due to barriers including cost, perceived lack of need, privacy concerns, and difficulty of use. AFCs have worked to address these challenges through programs providing both technology access and education, often through intergenerational partnerships. Additionally, some AFCs have developed innovative collaborations with LTC facilities to improve workforce training, create new housing options, and better integrate facility residents with the broader community. Future progress will require policy support for cross-sector collaboration, structural reforms in long-term care, and initiatives to make technology more accessible and user-friendly for older adults.

References

AARP. (2018). *AARP Roadmap to Livability Collection*. Retrieved October 25, 2024 from https://www.aarp.org/livable-communities/tool-kits-resources/info-2017/roadmap-to-livability-collection.html

AARP. (n.d.). *AARP Livable Communities Map*. AARP. Retrieved October 25 from https://livablemap.aarp.org/#/view=list/f7=1,2,3

Aggar, C., Sorwar, G., Seton, C., Penman, O., & Ward, A. (2023). Smart home technology to support older people's quality of life: A longitudinal pilot study. *International Journal of Older People Nursing, 18*(1), e12489. https://doi.org/10.1111/opn.12489

Arthanat, S., Wilcox, J., & Macuch, M. (2019). Profiles and predictors of smart home technology adoption by older adults. *OTJR (Thorofare N J), 39*(4), 247–256. https://doi.org/10.1177/1539449218813906

Behrens, L. L., Boltz, M., Sciegaj, M., Kolanowski, A., Jones, J. R., Paudel, A., & Van Haitsma, K. (2022). Nursing staff perceptions of outcomes related to honoring residents'"risky" preferences. *Research in Gerontological Nursing, 15*(6), 271–281. https://pmc.ncbi.nlm.nih.gov/articles/PMC10189806/pdf/nihms-1884299.pdf

Berlyn, D. (2023). *Tech innovations that are improving the way we age*. National Council on Aging. Retrieved October 25, 2024 from https://www.ncoa.org/article/tech-innovations-that-are-improving-the-way-we-age/

Berlyn, D. (2024). *How AI and new technology could support healthy aging*. National Council on Aging. Retrieved October 25, 2024 from https://www.ncoa.org/article/how-ai-and-new-technology-could-support-healthy-aging/

Bhattacharyya, K. K., Molinari, V., Black, K., & Whitbourne, S. K. (2022). Creating age-friendly nursing homes: The time is now. *Gerontology & Geriatrics Education, 44*(4), 613–630. https://doi.org/10.1080/02701960.2022.2106981

Binette, J., & Farago, F. (2021). *Where we live, where we age: Trends in home and community preferences*. In *2021 Home and community preferences survey: A national survey of adults age 18-plus*. AARP Research. Retrieved from https://www.aarp.org/pri/topics/livable-communities/housing/2021-home-community-preferences/

Black, K., & Oh, P. (2022). Assessing age-friendly community progress: What have we learned? *Gerontologist, 62*(1), 6–17. https://doi.org/10.1093/geront/gnab051

Burnes, D., Sheppard, C., Henderson, C. R., Jr., Wassel, M., Cope, R., Barber, C., & Pillemer, K. (2019). Interventions to reduce ageism against older adults: A systematic review and meta-analysis. *American Journal of Public Health, 109*(8), e1–e9.

Choi, Y. J. (2021). Understanding aging in place: Home and community features, perceived age-friendliness of community, and intention toward aging in place. *The Gerontologist, 62*(1), 46–55. https://doi.org/10.1093/geront/gnab070

Choi, Y. K., Thompson, H. J., & Demiris, G. (2021). Internet-of-things smart home technology to support aging-in-place: Older adults' perceptions and attitudes. *Journal of Gerontological Nursing, 47*(4), 15–21. https://doi.org/10.3928/00989134-20210310-03

Dong, D., Cai, Q., Zhang, Q. Z., Zhou, Z. N., Dai, J. N., Mu, T. Y., ... & Shen, C. Z. (2021). Dignity and its related factors among older adults in long-term care facilities: A cross-sectional study. *International Journal of Nursing Sciences, 8*(4), 394–400. https://www.sciencedirect.com/science/article/pii/S2352013221000843

Edelman, L. S., Drost, J., Moone, R. P., Owens, K., Towsley, G. L., Tucker-Roghi, G., & Morley, J. E. (2021). Editorial: Applying the age-friendly health system framework to long term care settings. *The Journal of Nutrition, Health & Aging, 25*(2), 141–145. https://doi.org/10.1007/s12603-020-1558-2

Facchinetti, G., Petrucci, G., Albanesi, B., De Marinis, M. G., & Piredda, M. (2023, Jan 10). Can smart home technologies help older adults manage their chronic condition? A systematic literature review. *International Journal of Environmental Research and Public Health, 20*(2). https://doi.org/10.3390/ijerph20021205

Fang, M. L. (2022). *Future of agetech: Transdisciplinary considerations for equity, intersectionality, sustainability, and social justice*. In Proceedings of the 15th International Conference on Pervasive Technologies Related to Assistive Environments, Corfu, Greece. https://doi.org/10.1145/3529190.3534757

Fritz, R. L., Corbett, C. L., Vandermause, R., & Cook, D. (2016). The influence of culture on older adults' adoption of smart home monitoring. *Gerontechnology, 14*(3), 146–156. https://doi.org/10.4017/gt.2016.14.3.010.00

Gell, N., Hoffman, E., & Patel, K. (2021, Dec 9). Technology support challenges and recommendations for adapting an evidence-based exercise program for remote delivery to older adults: Exploratory mixed methods study. *JMIR Aging, 4*(4), e27645. https://doi.org/10.2196/27645

Gendron, T., Cimarolli, V. R., Inker, J., Rhodes, A., Hennessa, A., & Stone, R. (2021, Jul-Sep). The efficacy of a video-based intervention to reduce ageism among long-term services and supports staff. *Gerontology and Geriatrics Education, 42*(3), 316–330. https://doi.org/10.1080/02701960.2021.1880904

Gleason, K., & Suen, J. J. (2022). Going beyond affordability for digital equity: Closing the "Digital Divide" through outreach and training programs for older adults. *Journal of the American Geriatrics Society, 70*(1), 75–77. https://doi.org/10.1111/jgs.17511

Greenfield, E. A., Black, K., Oh, P., & Pestine-Stevens, A. (2022, Jan 14). Theories of community collaboration to advance age-friendly community change. *Gerontologist, 62*(1), 36–45. https://doi.org/10.1093/geront/gnab136

Greenfield, E. A., Oberlink, M., Scharlach, A. E., Neal, M. B., & Stafford, P. B. (2015). Age-friendly community initiatives: Conceptual issues and key questions. *Gerontologist, 55*(2), 191–198. https://doi.org/10.1093/geront/gnv005

Harris, M. T., Blocker, K. A., & Rogers, W. A. (2022, May). Older adults and smart technology: Facilitators and barriers to use. *Frontiers in Computer Science, 4*. https://doi.org/10.3389/fcomp.2022.835927

Hawley-Hague, H., Boulton, E., Hall, A., Pfeiffer, K., & Todd, C. (2014, Jun). Older adults' perceptions of technologies aimed at falls prevention, detection or monitoring: A systematic review. *International Journal of Medical Informatics, 83*(6), 416–426. https://doi.org/10.1016/j.ijmedinf.2014.03.002

Hill, R., Betts, L. R., & Gardner, S. E. (2015., 2015/07/01). Older adults' experiences and perceptions of digital technology: (Dis)Empowerment, wellbeing, and inclusion. *Computers in Human Behavior, 48*, 415–423. https://doi.org/10.1016/j.chb.2015.01.062

Ibrahim, J. E., & Davis, M. C. (2013). Impediments to applying the 'dignity of risk'principle in residential aged care services. *Australasian Journal on Ageing, 32*(3), 188–193. https://doi.org/10.1111/ajag.12014

Institute for Healthcare Improvement. (2024). *Age-friendly health systems: Guide to care of older adults in nursing homes*. IHI. Retrieved from https://241684.fs1.hubspotusercontent-na1.net/hubfs/241684/IHI-Age-Friendly-Guide-Nursing-Homes_March28-2022.pdf

Jachan, D. E., Müller-Werdan, U., Lahmann, N. A., & Strube-Lahmann, S. (2021, Mar 24). Smart@home - supporting safety and mobility of elderly and care dependent people in their own homes through the use of technical assistance systems and conventional mobility supporting tools: A cross-sectional survey. *BMC Geriatrics, 21*(1), 205. https://doi.org/10.1186/s12877-021-02118-9

Kakulla, B. (2024). *2024 Tech trends and adults 50+*. AARP Research. Retrieved from https://www.aarp.org/content/dam/aarp/research/topics/technology/internet-media-devices/2024-tech-trends-adults-50-plus.doi.10.26419-2Fres.00772.001.pdf

Kane, R. A., Caplan, A. L., Urv-Wong, E. K., Freeman, I. C., Aroskar, M. A., & Finch, M. (1997). Everyday matters in the lives of nursing home residents: Wish for and perception of choice and control. *Journal of the American Geriatrics Society, 45*(9), 1086–1093.

Kang, H., & Kim, H. (2022). Ageism and psychological well-being among older adults: A systematic review. *Gerontology and Geriatric Medicine, 8*, 23337214221087023. https://doi.org/10.1177/23337214221087023

Koon, L. M., McGlynn, S. A., Blocker, K. A., & Rogers, W. A. (2020). Perceptions of digital assistants from early adopters aged 55+. *Ergonomics in Design, 28*(1), 16–23. https://doi.org/10.1177/1064804619842501

Lee, C., & Coughlin, J. F. (2015). Perspective: Older adults' adoption of technology: An integrated approach to identifying determinants and barriers. *Journal of Product Innovation Management, 32*(5), 747–759. https://doi.org/10.1111/jpim.12176

Liebzeit, D., Krupp, A., Bunch, J., Tonelli, S., Griffin, E., McVeigh, S., et al. (2023). Rural age-friendly ecosystems for older adults: An international scoping review with recommendations to support age-friendly communities. *Health Science Reports, 6*(5), e1241. https://doi.org/10.1002/hsr2.1241

Liu, P., Li, G., Jiang, S., Liu, Y., Leng, M., Zhao, J., et al. (2019, Sep-Oct). The effect of smart homes on older adults with chronic conditions: A systematic review and meta-analysis. *Geriatric Nursing (New York, N.Y.), 40*(5), 522–530. https://doi.org/10.1016/j.gerinurse.2019.03.016

Lowen, T., Davern, M. T., Mavoa, S., & Brasher, K. (2015, 2015/10/02). Age-friendly cities and communities: Access to services for older people. *Australian Planner, 52*(4), 255–265. https://doi.org/10.1080/07293682.2015.1047874

Mace, R. A., Mattos, M. K., & Vranceanu, A. M. (2022, Dec 30). Older adults can use technology: Why healthcare professionals must overcome ageism in digital health. *Translational Behavioral Medicine, 12*(12), 1102–1105. https://doi.org/10.1093/tbm/ibac070

Malani, P., Kullgren, J., Solway, E., Lee, P., Aikens, J., Richardson, C., et al. (2022). *National poll on healthy aging: Mobile health app use among older adults*. University of Michigan, Institute for Healthcare Policy & Innovation. Retrieved October 25, 2024 from. https://doi.org/10.7302/4019

Marston, H. R., Genoe, R., Freeman, S., Kulczycki, C., & Musselwhite, C. (2019, Jul 4). Older adults' perceptions of ICT: Main findings from the technology in later life (till) study. *Healthcare (Basel), 7*(3). https://doi.org/10.3390/healthcare7030086

Miskimmin, C., Shooshtari, S., Menec, V., Duncan, K. A., Martin, T., & Stoesz, B. M. (2019). Age-friendly communities for older persons with intellectual disabilities. *Quality in Ageing and Older Adults, 20*(4), 206–218. https://doi.org/10.1108/QAOA-11-2018-0058

Mondal, S., Van Belle, S., & Maioni, A. (2021, May 17). Learning from intersectoral action beyond health: A meta-narrative review. *Health Policy and Planning, 36*(4), 552–571. https://doi.org/10.1093/heapol/czaa163

Montesanti, S., MacKean, G., Fitzpatrick, K. M., & Fancott, C. (2023, Mar 31). Family caregivers as essential partners in care: Examining the impacts of restrictive acute care visiting policies during the COVID-19 pandemic in Canada. *BMC Health Services Research, 23*(1), 320. https://doi.org/10.1186/s12913-023-09248-3

Moreno, A., Scola, M. C., Sun, H., Durce, H., Couve, C., Acevedo, K., & Gutman, G. M. (2023). A systematic review of gerontechnologies to support aging in place among community-dwelling older adults and their family caregivers. *Frontiers in Psychology, 14*, 1237694. https://doi.org/10.3389/fpsyg.2023.1237694

Moving Forward Nursing Home Quality Coalition. (2024). *A guide to addressing resident goals, preferences, and priorities (GPP)*. The Coalition. Retrieved from https://nursinghomeactionguides.org/addressing-residence-goals/

National Academies of Science, Engineering, and Medicine. (2022). *The national imperative to improve nursing home quality: Honoring our commitment to residents, families, and staff*. National Academies Press. Retrieved from https://doi.org/10.17226/26526

O'Brien, K., Liggett, A., Ramirez-Zohfeld, V., Sunkara, P., & Lindquist, L. A. (2020). Voice-controlled intelligent personal assistants to support aging in place. *Journal of the American Geriatrics Society, 68*(1), 176–179. https://agsjournals.onlinelibrary.wiley.com/doi/pdfdirect/10.1111/jgs.16217

Oh, P., & White, L. J. (2022, Winter). Approaches to community supports and health services in U.S. Age-friendly communities: Focus on advance care and end-of-life planning. *Journal of Aging Life Care, 32*(2), 11–17.

Popejoy, L., Zaniletti, I., Lane, K., Anderson, L., Miller, S., & Rantz, M. (2022, May-June). Longitudinal analysis of aging in place at tiger place: Resident function and well-being. *Geriatric Nursing (New York, N.Y.), 45*, 47–54. https://doi.org/10.1016/j.gerinurse.2022.02.030

Sixsmith, J., Makita, M., Menezes, D., Cranwell, M., Chau, I., Smith, M., et al. (2023, May 11). Enhancing community participation through age-friendly ecosystems: A rapid realist review. *Geriatrics (Basel), 8*(3). https://doi.org/10.3390/geriatrics8030052

Steele, R., Lo, A., Secombe, C., & Wong, Y. K. (2009, Dec). Elderly persons' perception and acceptance of using wireless sensor networks to assist healthcare. *International Journal of Medical Informatics, 78*(12), 788–801. https://doi.org/10.1016/j.ijmedinf.2009.08.001

Sumner, J., Chong, L. S., Bundele, A., & Wei Lim, Y. (2021, Sep 13). Co-designing technology for aging in place: A systematic review. *Gerontologist, 61*(7), e395–e409. https://doi.org/10.1093/geront/gnaa064

The White House. (2022, February 28). *Fact sheet: Protecting seniors by improving safety and quality of care in the nation's nursing homes*. The White House. Retrieved October 2024 from https://www.whitehouse.gov/briefing-room/statements-releases/2022/02/28/fact-sheet-protecting-seniors-and-people-with-disabilities-by-improving-safety-and-quality-of-care-in-the-nations-nursing-homes/

Tsai, W.-C., Rogers, W. A., & Lee, C.-F. (2012, 08). Older adults' motivations, patterns, and improvised strategies of using product manuals. *International Journal of Design, 6*(2), 55-65.

Tural, E., Lu, D., & Austin Cole, D. (2021, Jan-Dec). Safely and actively aging in place: Older adults' attitudes and intentions toward smart home technologies. *Gerontol Geriatr Med, 7*, 23337214211017340. https://doi.org/10.1177/23337214211017340

Wang, J., Du, Y., Coleman, D., Peck, M., Myneni, S., Kang, H., & Gong, Y. (2019, May 15). Mobile and connected health technology needs for older adults aging in place: Cross-sectional survey study. *JMIR Aging, 2*(1), e13864. https://doi.org/10.2196/13864

WHO Global Network for Age-friendly Cities and Communities. (2019). *Membership in the Global Network of Age-Friendly Cities and Communities*. World Health Organization. Retrieved from https://www.who.int/publications/m/item/membership-in-the-global-network-of-age-friendly-cities-and-communities-(gnafcc)

World Health Organization. (2007). *Global age-friendly cities: A guide*. WHO. Retrieved from https://www.who.int/publications/i/item/9789241547307

World Health Organization. (2018). *The global network for age-friendly cities and communities: Looking back over the last decade, looking forward to the next* (WHO/FWC/ALC/18.4). WHO. Retrieved from https://iris.who.int/bitstream/handle/10665/278979/WHO-FWC-ALC-18.4-eng.pdf

Yang, J. (2023). *Distribution of nursing homes in the U.S. 2003-2023, by ownership type*. Statista. Retrieved October 25, 2024 from https://www.statista.com/statistics/716813/distribution-of-nursing-homes-in-us-by-ownership-type/

Zamora, F. M. V., Kloseck, M., Fitzsimmons, D. A., Zecevic, A., & Fleming, P. (2020., 2020/01/02). Use of community support and health services in an age-friendly city: The lived experiences of the oldest-old. *Cities & Health, 4*(1), 107–116. https://doi.org/10.1080/23748834.2019.1606873

Zhong, R., & Rau, P. P. (2020, Mar-Apr). Are cost-effective technologies feasible to measure gait in older adults? A systematic review of evidence-based literature. *Archives of Gerontology and Geriatrics, 87*, 103970. https://doi.org/10.1016/j.archger.2019.103970

Zhou, C., Qian, Y., & Kaner, J. (2024). A study on smart home use intention of elderly consumers based on technology acceptance models. *PloS One, 19*(3), e0300574. https://doi.org/10.1371/journal.pone.0300574

Chapter 15
Potentials of Health Promotional Practices in Long-Term Care

Sean N. Halpin and Joshua Saul

The schedule shifts at 11 am every weekday in a large (90+ bed) assisted living facility in Atlanta. Echoes of preaching from the church service fade away and are replaced by the Motown and Soul music of Marvin Gaye and James Brown. About half of the residents in attendance ease their bodies from the chairs and slowly exit, some under their own power, others assisted by walkers and wheelchairs. A few might even do a little jig as they return to their rooms. The remaining residents store their Bibles and begin an instructor-led chair exercise program. The instructor, a spirited younger woman, often encourages residents with ebullient banter and personalized callouts, making everyone feel included and motivated. Exercisers lift and stretch their arms and legs in unison, gestures designed to be performed by all residents regardless of their ability level. Some residents share smiles and laughter with each other and the instructor, while others sing along with familiar tunes. As such, the forum provides more than physical exercise; it also provides a cognitive workout by engaging memory, attention, and problem-solving skills, a mood boost, and it fosters a sense of belonging, all crucial factors for maintaining overall well-being.

Long-term care settings worldwide repeat the above scene, sometimes substituting chair exercises for other physical exercises, mind–body practices, or even traditional Chinese medicines. In one case, a memory care home offers meditation to its residents, intending to reduce stress and improve memory. Elsewhere, acupuncturists apply their trade to residents of extra care housing to reduce anxiety, manage pain, and increase overall well-being. In other settings, practitioners apply the same holistic approach through yoga, tai chi, and qigong, enhancing flexibility and

S. N. Halpin (✉)
GenOmics and Translational Research Center, RTI International,
Research Triangle Park, NC, USA
e-mail: snhalpin@rti.org

J. Saul
Sun Wellness Holistic Healthcare, Sandy Springs, GA, USA

K. K. Bhattacharyya (ed.), *Health Promotion in Long-Term Care Facilities*,
https://doi.org/10.1007/978-3-031-91038-8_15

balance and promoting mental focus. Likewise, music therapy evokes memories and improves mood, involves residents in singing, playing instruments, and listening to music to reminisce, stimulate their minds, and provide emotional release. These diverse practices underscore the commitment of long-term care facilities to adopting innovative methods to promote health in their older adult residents.

It is well-documented that many forms of cognitive and physical performance decline with age in adulthood (Handing et al., 2020). Beyond lack of demonstrated efficacy, there are many drawbacks to managing late-life cognitive decline using a Western medical model, such as the risk of institutionalization and isolation, adverse effects of prescription medication, and the high cost of the associated therapy (Nagata et al., 2022; Halpin et al., 2020; Halpin, 2018; Halpin et al., 2017). However, alternatives exist in exercise and mind–body practices. Indeed, in recent years, alternatives such as exercise and mind–body practices have gained significant traction. The number of adults in the United States practicing mind–body activities has doubled in the last decade, highlighting a shift toward holistic health approaches (Bhattacharyya et al., 2020; Wang et al., 2019). As a researcher and a clinician, we have seen firsthand how long-term care settings support the physical, cognitive, and emotional needs and health of their residents by integrating holistic healthcare practices. Regular physical activity, mind–body activity, and traditional Chinese medicines help preserve mobility, cognition, and improve quality of life (QoL).

In this chapter, we delve into sampling each method used to promote health and well-being in long-term care. First, we will explore the benefits of exercise with a focus on functional fitness, including strength training, flexibility and balance, and aerobic exercises. Second, we will review mind–body practices, music therapy, and traditional Chinese medicine techniques, including meditation, movement-based therapies, and acupuncture. We will also review the synergistic effect of engaging with multiple approaches in a long-term care setting. Next, we will consider how the practices mentioned above directly impact QoL. Last, we will summarize key points and provide suggestions for further reading.

Exercise and Physical Activity

After 30 min, Otis Redding croons through the speakers, "Sittin' on the dock of the bay; Wastin' time," announcing that today's chair exercises are over. The instructor unplugs her phone, which doubles as a music player, from the speakers and replaces the podium at the front of the room while residents file away. A centenarian with short white hair ambles out, smiling toward her friends. She has just finished stretching her muscles, and now, she tells a nearby direct-care worker that she is looking forward to afternoon meditation. Three residents aged 70 to 99 years old remain in the room, waiting in wheelchairs for staff to help them ambulate. Most, with eyes downcast and not speaking, will return to their rooms for naps. Like many long-term care facilities, residents' abilities range widely here. Some remain physically independent and cognitively sharp, while others have greater needs. Staff encourage all residents, regardless of their current ability, to engage in exercise. Regular exercise helps maintain muscle mass, joint health, and cardiovascular function, especially in older age (Bao et al., 2020). Moreover, these benefits ensure that residents can participate in their community, maintain social ties, and challenge their cognition (Bender et al., 2021). In the following paragraphs, we will touch on multiple exercise and physical activity components, including cardiovascular fitness, strength, flexibility, and balance.

Cardiovascular Fitness

Cardiovascular fitness refers to the ability of the heart, lungs, and circulatory system to supply oxygen and nutrition to the body during sustained movement, such as getting dressed or walking to the bingo room (Colcombe et al., 2004). It encompasses aerobic and anaerobic components, each playing a role in overall health and well-being. The aerobic system refers to activities that require oxygen and is important not only for physical tasks like active movement between different areas in the facility but also for cognitive health, as improved cardiovascular fitness increases blood flow and oxygen to the brain. For long-term care residents, maintaining cardiovascular fitness is crucial to sustaining the ability to perform daily tasks independently. Improved cardiovascular health not only supports physical movement but also enhances cognitive function, which allows residents to better engage in social activities and maintain a connection with their community, reducing feelings of isolation. Adequate aerobic capacity ensures residents can engage in activities without excessive fatigue, promoting an active and engaged lifestyle with improved memory and mental clarity. The anaerobic system instead pertains to short bursts of activity where energy is produced without relying on oxygen—and is activated for activities requiring strength and quick reactions such as transferring from the bed to a chair, climbing a few stairs, or avoiding falls. Anaerobic activities are important for maintaining muscle strength but are less efficient and do not work well over longer periods of time.

The maximum amount of oxygen a person's body can process, termed VO_2 max, provides a key predictor of the person's functional cardiovascular limit, including the capacity to participate in everything from daily activities to more vigorous demands (Mandsager et al., 2018). Further, lower levels of VO_2 max are predictive of increased mortality, with those in the bottom quarter having a four times higher chance of mortality compared to those in the top quarter (Mandsager et al., 2018). The actual VO_2 max number can be calculated by a clinician or a scientist, often using tests that require physical exertion from the participant through intensive exercise on a treadmill or a stationary bicycle. Yet, a person's calculated VO_2 max number is less important than the concept that an increased ability to process oxygen increases capacity for daily activities. For example, a resident sitting in the weekday morning church service often has their body relaxed and stationary. Their breathing will slow as they focus on the preacher, requiring lower levels of oxygen consumption. In this case, even someone with a lower maximum oxygen consumption level can often participate in the morning church service. Alternately, the resident who stands and begins to walk swiftly down the hall will experience a quickening of their heartbeat and respiration, activities that require greater amounts of oxygen to perform. A resident with a higher VO_2 max will walk quickly down the hall with ease and may even have a conversation without pausing for breath. This resident with a higher VO_2 max will rely on their efficient aerobic system—as swift walking does not tax their cardiovascular capacity. A resident with a lower VO_2 max will reach their ceiling of cardiovascular capacity quicker, resulting in their switching over to the less efficient anaerobic system. They may be unable to walk briskly, need frequent pauses, and have challenges speaking as their voice competes with the need for increased oxygen.

Strength

Muscular strength refers to the ability of the muscles to exert force during physical activity, an important concept for maintaining independence into older adulthood (Jochem et al., 2019). Muscular strength is important for holding the body upright, standing up from a chair, and bathing oneself. It includes isotonic and isometric components, working in concert to perform daily activities. The isotonic system involves contracting muscles during movement, such as when walking up or down stairs and transferring from a bed to a chair. The isometric system instead involves muscle contraction without movement and is important during tasks requiring stability, such as maintaining one's posture while holding a heavy object, like a book, for an extended period of time. Both isotonic and isometric components are important for maintaining muscle tone and preventing falls.

As with cardiovascular capacity, those with lower levels of strength experience more than double the risk of mortality compared to those with higher strength (Jochem et al., 2019). As such, having an extra reserve of strength is protective, allowing for greater daily functional abilities. For example, a person who has the strength to lift heavy objects from the floor without assistance will have no problem retrieving a newspaper that fell on the floor. Now imagine a person whose leg muscles have atrophied to the degree of uncomfortable squatting down to pick something up. When lifting things up from the ground, the adage to "lift with your legs" is often repeated, and with good reason. The leg muscles are much larger and often stronger than those in the upper body. If a person were to lift something heavy from the floor by curving their back and pulling up with their arms, thus using their smaller upper body muscles to lift the heavy object, they are more likely to be injured. When needing to pick up the newspaper from the floor, that same person will have a lower muscular strength reserve not just in their legs but likely throughout their body and be more prone to injury. Alternately, someone with higher levels of muscular reserve, even if not lifting with their stronger leg muscles, will still have a measure of muscle to protect their body from injury when retrieving the newspaper from the floor. Maintaining muscular strength also promotes independence in daily self-care routines. In long-term care, where many residents experience physical decline, maintaining strength can mean the difference between requiring assistance for basic activities and remaining self-sufficient. This independence is not only physically beneficial but also contributes significantly to residents' emotional well-being and sense of dignity, as they are able to participate more actively in communal life. Tasks such as dressing, bathing, and grooming require a certain level of strength and dexterity. Further, sufficient muscular strength allows residents to participate fully in recreational and social activities, such as exercise classes, gardening, and games. Residents who can perform these activities independently not only preserve their dignity but also experience a greater sense of autonomy and confidence.

Flexibility and Balance

Flexibility describes the ability of the joints to move through a full range of motion. Maintaining flexibility and balance not only helps perform everyday tasks like reaching for items or tying shoes but also contributes to cognitive health by requiring coordination and focus, which strengthen executive function and mental agility. As with cardiovascular fitness and strength described above, flexibility can be broken down into multiple components, including static and dynamic flexibilities. Static flexibility involves holding a stretch for an extended time and is important for sitting comfortably throughout a meal and maintaining an upright posture. Adequate static flexibility helps residents perform activities without discomfort or strain. Alternately, dynamic flexibility involves movement-based stretches during activities like walking or participating in exercise classes. Dynamic flexibility is also important for maintaining joint health, preventing stiffness, and avoiding injuries (Holland et al., 2002). For residents in long-term care, improving flexibility and balance reduces the likelihood of falls, a leading cause of injury among older adults. This results in greater confidence in mobility, allowing residents to easily navigate their environment and enhancing their QoL by reducing fear of injury.

Balance is closely related to flexibility but is often overlooked in traditional physical fitness. Nevertheless, balance is essential for all ages, especially older adults in long-term care settings. Balance is the ability to maintain one's center of mass over its base of support, whether standing still or moving. Good balance is vital for everyday tasks, such as walking, standing up from a seated position, and reaching for objects without falling. Balance encompasses both static and dynamic components, each playing a role in overall health and well-being. Static balance involves the ability to hold oneself in one position with no or minimal movement—for example, standing in the shower while washing oneself. Dynamic balance instead involves movement such as carrying a glass of water while walking. Both flexibility and balance are important for moving freely and confidently, participating in social and recreational activities, and performing daily self-care tasks easily and safely.

The Power of Exercise and Physical Activity

In addition to structured exercise classes, residents in long-term care facilities can participate in various practical physical activities that not only support cardiovascular health, muscular strength, and flexibility but also help preserve cognitive functions like memory, attention, and problem-solving. Engaging in these activities helps maintain their independence and fosters a sense of community and well-being.

Gardening One such activity is gardening. Gardening provides a multifaceted workout that can be tailored to the abilities of each resident. For those with more mobility, tasks such as digging, planting, and weeding involve cardiovascular exertion, muscle use, and joint flexibility. For residents with limited mobility, container gardening or assisting with lighter tasks like watering plants can still offer physical and mental health benefits. The repetitive motions involved in gardening also help with both static and dynamic balance, as residents need to reach, bend, and move around the garden area, enhancing their stability and coordination. Gardening also allows residents to spend time outside the facility in nature.

Walking Walking is another excellent activity that residents can easily incorporate into their daily routine. Whether a leisurely stroll around the facility's grounds or a more structured walking club, this low-impact exercise promotes cardiovascular fitness and leg strength. Walking on different surfaces, such as pavement, grass, or indoor hallways, can further challenge and improve dynamic balance. Residents can also benefit from social interactions during group walks, which provide an opportunity for meaningful engagement and support.

Chair Exercises Seated exercises can be highly effective for residents with varying levels of mobility. These exercises often include a combination of cardiovascular, strength, and flexibility components. Simple movements like seated leg lifts, arm circles, and ankle rotations help maintain muscle tone and joint flexibility. Additionally, seated exercises can include resistance bands or light weights to enhance muscular strength. This type of activity is inclusive and can be done in a group setting, fostering a sense of camaraderie among residents.

Dancing Another valuable activity is dancing, which can range from simple movements to more structured classes like line dancing or ballroom dancing. Dancing not only provides a fun and engaging way to exercise but also offers substantial cardiovascular benefits. It requires coordination, rhythm, and balance, making it an excellent way to improve dynamic balance and flexibility. Dancing can also be adapted to suit different ability levels, from standing dances to seated movements that still engage the core and limbs.

Tai Chi, Qigong, and Yoga Tai chi, qigong, and yoga (along with other practices discussed in Section 2) are particularly beneficial for improving flexibility, balance, and strength. Tai chi, a martial art that originated as one of the pillars of Traditional Chinese Medicine, with its slow and deliberate movements, helps enhance dynamic balance and coordination while promoting mental relaxation and focus. Yoga, on the other hand, commonly combines static stretches with strength-building poses, which are excellent for joint flexibility and muscular endurance. Both practices emphasize mindful movement and can be modified to suit the needs of each resident, whether they are performed standing, sitting, or using a support or prop for stability. Yoga can be performed in a chair, as is done in many healthcare settings, for less mobile residents.

Everyday Tasks Lastly, everyday tasks such as folding laundry, setting the table, or light housekeeping can also be turned into physical activity. These chores require various movements, from bending and reaching to lifting and carrying, which can help maintain flexibility and muscle strength. Encouraging residents to participate in these tasks not only keeps them active but also promotes a sense of purpose and involvement in their daily environment.

Mind–Body Practices and Traditional Chinese Medicine

Shortly after lunch, the assisted living home takes on a tranquil atmosphere. The soft sound of chimes and gentle flute music fills the air. An 85-year-old stores her walker within reach and finds her spot near a window in the common room. She sits in a comfortable chair, feet flat on the floor, hands resting on her lap. The afternoon sun casts a warm glow, enhancing the peaceful ambiance. The resident closes her eyes and takes a deep breath as she begins her daily meditation practice. Guided by the Activities Director, she inhales and exhales, focusing on the rhythm of her breath. The guided meditation lets her visualize a serene garden with blooming flowers and a rippling stream. A soft smile forms on her lips. After about twenty minutes, a gentle bell sound concludes the session. She opens her eyes, stretches her arms and legs, and joins her friends nearby. The practice not only relaxes her body but also invigorates her mind, leaving her feeling refreshed. Along with exercise, staff encourage residents to engage in meditation and other mind–body techniques. Mind–body techniques involve a range of practices where "the mind is directed to have an impact on physical functioning and promote health" (Esch et al., 2024, p2), and thus are used to improve overall well-being and address various health conditions. Below, we explore key methods within mind–body practices, including relaxation techniques, movement-based therapies, music therapy, and traditional Chinese medicine. Each of these methods offers unique benefits and contributes to a holistic approach to health and wellness.

Meditation

Meditation is often identified as the most common form of mind–body practice, likely due to its many iterations and low barrier of entry (Halpin et al., 2020; Halpin et al., 2018). Meditation comprises interrelated practices, including mindfulness meditation, progressive muscle relaxation, and guided imagery, all meant to increase mental awareness. The practices promote relaxation, enhanced emotional well-being, and improved QoL through a focus on breathing, bodily sensations, thoughts, and feelings. Broadly, meditation can be subdivided into two approaches: (1) concentrative/introspective practices and (2) mindfulness practices (Krebs, 2015). Concentrative/introspective practices focus on a sound, image, or bodily sensation and are often incorporated into other mind–body practices, such as yoga. Focusing on a single element is meant to help practitioners cultivate deep concentration and mental clarity. Alternately, mindfulness practices, also referred to as transcendental, involve open monitoring of the practitioners' thoughts, feelings, bodily sensations, and surroundings without judgment. In long-term care settings, meditation has proven beneficial for managing stress, reducing symptoms of anxiety and depression, and enhancing overall emotional well-being (Myint et al., 2024). For residents in long-term care, meditation offers more than just mental clarity—it is a powerful tool for managing stress and improving emotional resilience. Regular practice helps reduce anxiety, improve mood, and offers a non-pharmacological method to cope with feelings of loneliness or depression.

Mindfulness Meditation

Mindfulness meditation involves focusing attention on the present moment and cultivating awareness of thoughts, feelings, and bodily sensations without judgment. Often, mindfulness meditation begins in a comfortable seated position. The individual closes their eyes or softens their gaze and brings their attention to their breath—noticing sensations such as their breathing pattern and anchoring themselves in the present moment. As the mind wanders, participants are asked to bring their focus back to their breath gently. Over time, the practice helps participants develop greater awareness of their thoughts and demotions, helping them respond to life's challenges with greater clarity. For older adults, it can help reduce anxiety, improve mood, and enhance overall mental health (Li & Bressington, 2019). Further, regular mindfulness practice can lower stress levels, improve sleep, and boost cognition, making it an invaluable addition to care (Li & Bressington., 2019).

Progressive Muscle Relaxation

Progressive muscle relaxation involves systematically tensing and relaxing individual muscle groups. In a typical session, an individual is guided through a series of exercises focusing on one body part at a time. For example, they may lay or sit in a relaxing position and begin by focusing on the muscles in their forehead, first tensing and then gradually releasing the tension while paying close attention to the contrast between tension and relaxation. The process is repeated throughout the body, starting from the head and working down to the feet. The goal is to help practitioners become aware of physical tension and how to release it, contributing to a sense of calm. In long-term care facilities, where sleep disturbances are common among residents, progressive muscle relaxation has been shown to improve sleep quality. By regularly practicing this technique, residents can experience more restful nights, which in turn positively impacts their mood, energy levels, and overall QoL. Progressive muscle relaxation can improve mental health, reduce tension, and improve the sleep quality of older adults (Hayati et al., 2020).

Guided Imagery

Guided imagery is a technique that uses mental visualization to help practitioners relax, reduce stress and pain, and enhance overall well-being (Cole, 2021). During a guided imagery session, participants often listen to a trained facilitator either in person or through a pre-recorded audio guide. The facilitator leads them through a series of vivid, descriptive scenarios, such as walking through a familiar and comforting environment (e.g., a serene garden). The imagery engages the senses and encourages practitioners to imagine the sights, sounds, smells, and feelings associated with the imagined scene. For older residents in long-term care settings, guided imagery may offer the added benefit of providing an outlet for reminiscence or personal reflection (Bryant et al., 2005). Further, it can be especially useful in settings where residents may face physical limitations or cognitive decline, as it provides a non-invasive way to cultivate a positive mental state (Elsegood & Wongpakaran, 2012).

Movement-based Therapies

One of the oldest forms of movement-based therapies was the creation of yoga. Yoga was originally developed in ancient India as a practice system involving breathing techniques and meditation to calm the mind with body exercises designed to support the physical demands of spiritual devotion. Thanks to the appearance of yoga studios in Western society, which focus more exclusively on Hatha yoga, yoga has become synonymous with postures and physical exercises focusing on strength and flexibility rather than relaxation or specific medical ailments. Many forms of physical yoga (Vinyasa, Ashtanga, Yin, Iyengar, etc.) fall under the Hatha yoga category, most commonly called "yoga." When examining all forms of yoga practice and their associated health benefits, many postures and exercises can be adapted from standing or floor positions to seated positions for residents in long-term care medical settings “Chair yoga” is a gentle form of meditation that can be performed along with other yoga styles that do not require significant strength but instead focus on the slow, easy movement of the body and major joints.

Other forms of gentle body movement that have gained popularity in the West are tai chi (Tie-chee) and qigong (Chee-gong). Both were originally developed in ancient China, but Tai Chi originated as a martial art that focused on slow, meditative movements to develop strength while practicing motion that taught self-defense. Tai Chi is practiced in countries around the globe, but in China, elderly practitioners wake early most mornings to meet in social groups and practice in parks across the country. Qigong is also based on slow movements of the body, but the focus is more on strengthening the function of specific organs or organ systems. Both involve aspects of mindfulness in practice, often called “moving meditation.” They are ideal practices for residents in a long-term care setting who need slower, low-impact, controlled movements or have limited mobility.

Expressive Therapies

Expressive therapies include activities that help practitioners use creative expression to explore emotions and develop self-awareness. In long-term care, older adults often use these therapies to connect with their emotions, memories, and sense of identity and to form new social bonds. Therapy techniques focus on music, art, dance/movement, and drama, all providing outlets for self-expression. Below, we highlight two forms of expressive therapy: music therapy and art therapy.

Music Therapy

Practitioners across the health spectrum use music therapy in various ways to affect a person's physical, mental, and emotional well-being during the treatment of illness or injury (Biley, 1992). While music as a therapy is relatively new in healthcare and more rigorous studies are needed, relaxing music therapy demonstrated measurably lower blood pressure, heart rate, respiratory rate, and arterial pressure (Mofredj et al., 2016). The opposite is also true. Several studies have shown that engaging with more exciting music motivates residents’ movement and activity; this is seen anecdotally in long-term care facilities when residents are encouraged to get up and dance. The right song has residents clapping their hands, moving their hips, and enjoying the experience of sharing some rhythm with others. Music therapy offers another tool that is low cost, low risk, non-pharmacologic, and easy to implement with residents regardless of their health status.

Art Therapy

Art therapy has also emerged as a valuable therapeutic tool, harnessing the creative process to support psychological and physical well-being (Stephenson, 2021). The techniques allow participants to explore their personal creativity through various mediums such as painting, drawing, and sculpture, offering a safe space for self-expression and reflection. While art therapy is still a developing field, research has shown that creating art can reduce anxiety, alleviate symptoms of depression, and improve overall QoL (Bosman et al., 2021).

Traditional Chinese Medicine Techniques

Traditional Eastern medicines refer to the various traditional medical systems originating in India, China, Korea, and other East Asian countries. Traditional Chinese Medicine (TCM) is often the most recognized and widely studied. Acupuncture refers to one technique in the TCM medical system, including acupuncture, Chinese herbology, meditation, tai chi and qigong or other martial arts, and Tui Na, which refers to Asian bodywork and massage. Acupuncture involves the shallow insertion of very thin, solid (filiform) needles into specific body areas. Insertion along pathways of major nerves or nerve branches and manual or electrical manipulation of these small needles excite nerves that correspond with specific brain regions and stimulate a wide range of targeted body responses. Needles are usually retained at the point of insertion for anywhere from 15–30 min, depending on the condition. Physical response can include the release of endogenous endorphins for pain relief and regulating the Vagus nerve in counterbalancing the "fight-or-flight" mechanism as a reaction to stress.

The use of acupuncture in geriatric care or for any residents involved in long-term care has several benefits. For example, it is easily administered, safe compared to Western treatments (Allen et al., 2022), and often embraced by older adults, especially those who have had trouble finding medications to ease their other symptoms (Halpin et al., 2014; Halpin et al., 2014; Halpin & Len, 2020). The current Western model of medicine emphasizes surgical intervention or drug therapy as a means of managing residents' symptomology. For older adults, this often leads to a complex treatment program and polypharmacy, both of which have inherent risks. As of 2010, it is estimated that almost 40% of seniors aged 65 or older take five or more prescription medications, with the expectation this number will continue to rise as the population ages and residents experience multiple comorbidities (Charlesworth et al., 2015). Modalities that do not add additional prescriptions to resident care while providing measurable and/or perceived improvement to resident well-being are invaluable tools.

Acupuncture is also useful as a tool in long-term care because it has a low barrier to participation. Residents can be treated anywhere, in various positions, including sitting in a wheelchair or reclining in a bed. Various methods can be utilized based on what body region is accessible to the practitioner. For example, the resident's arms and legs can be used in distal or balance method acupuncture, the ear in auricular acupuncture, and the hands in Korean hand therapy.

Acupuncture is a gentle therapeutic modality, as discomfort from needle insertion and needle retention is typically non-existent or minimal for most residents. It is also very safe when practiced by an appropriately licensed acupuncturist (National Certification Commission for Acupuncture and Oriental Medicine, 2024). It is a minimally invasive therapy and poses little risk of injury or infection. Common adverse reactions are usually limited to mild soreness after treatment and minor bruising (Bäumler et al., 2021). Very rarely, severe adverse reactions can occur and could include nerve damage or organ injury, including pneumothorax. While serious adverse events are rare, when they do occur, they can be fatal, which highlights the need for an adequately trained and licensed acupuncturist.

Acupuncture has been proven to be an effective therapeutic modality in treating many conditions that pertain to geriatric and long-term care. It is an incredibly effective modality for managing acute and chronic pain, post-surgical pain, orthopedic injuries, and arthritis. Many studies have shown that participants receiving acupuncture release endogenous opioids, endorphins, and corticosteroids that serve as natural pain modulators to maintain or improve the healing process (Patil et al., 2016). Acupuncture continues to prove itself effective at helping manage psycho-emotional conditions such as stress, anxiety, and depression as a non-drug therapy and adjuvant to conventional therapy. This is particularly important as antidepressant use is a major cause of the notable increase in polypharmacy in geriatrics (Charlesworth et al., 2015). While it can be difficult to create objective measurements for evaluating efficacy related to psychologically oriented conditions, results from many studies point to favorable outcomes (Pilkington et al., 2007; Huang et al., 2018).

Enhancing Quality of Life for Residents and Staff

As the day progresses, a resident in his late sixties sits comfortably in a small community room, his hands resting calmly in his lap as he looks out over the garden. Nearby, other residents relax after a day filled with activities tailored to support body, mind, and spirit. Some are still chatting quietly after a group yoga session, while others exchange a few words with staff as they wrap up a day of shared meals, walks, and music. This scene reflects more than a routine; it's a holistic approach to well-being designed to enhance QoL for both residents and the long-term care staff.

QoL represents a multidimensional construct essential to the residents' and staff's well-being. Maintaining QoL requires addressing physical, cognitive, and emotional challenges for residents facing aging-associated issues. Integrating mind–body practices, physical exercise, and TCM offers a holistic approach that can enhance QoL for both residents and caregivers by addressing these interconnected needs. For residents, practices such as yoga, tai chi, meditation, and guided imagery provide benefits extending beyond symptom relief, supporting autonomy, dignity, and emotional resilience—all of which can increase their ability to participate in meaningful activities that promote interpersonal connectedness (Bhattacharyya et al., 2022). For staff, incorporating these interventions within routine care not only improves residents' well-being but also contributes to a more sustainable caregiving experience, reducing burnout and fostering satisfaction as staff observe the positive impact on residents' daily lives (Ball et al., 2009).

A focus on health-promoting practices supports a shift away from traditional, often medication-dependent models of care, instead promoting a framework that centers on the root causes of many age-related issues. Engaging residents through physical, cognitive, and emotional support can foster a caring environment that addresses the holistic needs of older adults, enhancing QoL and supporting well-being across multiple domains.

Physical Well-Being and Functional Independence

For older adults, maintaining functional independence means performing physical tasks and retaining self-reliance. Activities that improve strength and flexibility, such as chair exercises, offer residents a path to greater independence. A resident who can lift themselves from a chair, walk across a room without assistance, or participate in group activities will experience enhanced physical well-being that directly contributes to their QoL. Incorporating physical activity into daily routines benefits residents at all levels of ability, allowing everyone to participate in a way that supports physical health and nurtures a sense of community. This approach to physical well-being in long-term care offers more than just physical maintenance; it provides a gateway to independence, social engagement, and a more fulfilling day-to-day experience.

Cognitive Health and Emotional Resilience

Mind–body practices like meditation, mindfulness, and guided imagery provide meaningful support for cognitive and emotional resilience in older adults. These practices engage the mind, helping residents manage stress, reduce symptoms of anxiety and depression, and sharpen cognitive skills such as focus and memory. For example, guided meditation encourages them to stay present, allowing them to develop a gentle awareness of thoughts and feelings. This awareness can become a vital tool for managing emotional challenges that arise in long-term care, offering an outlet for inner calm and acceptance.

Engaging in these cognitive practices offers more than momentary relaxation. Studies show that regular mindfulness and meditation can improve residents' ability to process and retain information, fostering mental clarity and enhancing overall cognitive function (Han et al., 2023). Such practices not only reduce the cognitive strain associated with aging but also contribute to emotional well-being, helping residents cultivate a resilient mindset that supports a positive outlook.

For many residents, these practices build a greater sense of control over their thoughts and emotions, empowering them to navigate daily challenges with poise and adaptability. The emotional benefits extend to social relationships as well, as residents who participate in group sessions or engage in expressive therapies—such as music or art—find opportunities to share memories, explore their emotions, and connect with others in a meaningful way. Together, these practices form a foundation for cognitive health and emotional resilience, enhancing QoL and enriching the daily experience for residents.

Social Engagement and Community Integration

Social engagement plays an important role in enhancing the QoL for residents in long-term care, as meaningful relationships contribute to emotional well-being and a sense of purpose (Park et al., 2012). Group activities such as gardening, chair yoga, or music therapy create natural opportunities for residents to interact, fostering bonds that reduce feelings of loneliness and isolation. Shared experiences, whether through hands-on projects or collaborative games, help build a sense of camaraderie and community, offering residents a sense of place and connection that is essential to emotional resilience.

These social interactions extend beyond companionship; they foster emotional support and encourage active participation in the community. For residents, having a circle of friends or activity companions enhances their day-to-day experiences, adding depth and variety to their routines. Furthermore, activities that integrate both residents and caregivers—such as group yoga sessions or storytelling circles—build trust and mutual respect, enriching the overall atmosphere of the facility.

Encouraging social engagement not only benefits individual residents but also strengthens the community as a whole, creating a vibrant and supportive environment where everyone feels valued. This focus on community integration, facilitated through structured group activities, offers residents a platform for meaningful social connections, enriching their lives with friendship, laughter, and a sense of belonging.

Autonomy and Purposeful Living

Autonomy and purposeful living are essential elements of QoL, especially in a long-term care setting where residents often face limitations in their independence. Providing opportunities for residents to engage in familiar, purposeful tasks—such as folding laundry, setting tables, or assisting with gardening—helps them retain a sense of agency. No matter how small, each task allows residents to exercise choice and feel valued.

Supporting autonomy is about fostering a care environment that respects residents' preferences and encourages active engagement. By engaging in daily routines, residents can maintain a connection to their own identity and self-worth. For some, this might mean organizing an activity; for others, it could be taking part in an art project or helping prepare a meal. These moments of purposeful engagement not only provide emotional fulfillment but also reduce the dependency which can erode self-esteem over time. Encouraging autonomy and purposeful living transforms the care experience from one of passive care to active involvement, empowering residents to shape their daily lives. This approach supports a deeper sense of meaning, confidence, and satisfaction, enriching their experience and fostering a holistic QoL in the long-term care setting.

Conclusion

As the day ends, the assisted living home residents settle down for the night. Many will have engaged in one or more of the exercises, mind–body practices, or Traditional Chinese Medicine techniques described above. There exist a myriad of benefits to integrating exercise and mind–body practice into long-term care routines. Regular exercise, tailored to the resident's ability, helps maintain mobility, reduces fall risk, and improves cardiovascular health. Mind–body practices like meditation, guided imagery, and progressive muscle relaxation not only reduce stress but also improve mental health, leading to overall well-being. For residents in long-term care, the integration of exercise and mind–body practices provides more than just physical benefits. These practices contribute to a holistic approach to well-being that addresses emotional and social health as well. By incorporating these techniques, long-term care facilities can foster a sense of community, encourage independence, and improve residents' overall QoL. Traditional Chinese Medicine, such as acupuncture, offers strategies that can address chronic pain and support emotional balance (Patil et al., 2016; Huang et al., 2018). In concert, these practices contribute to an integrated approach to health, addressing both the body and the mind, offering older adults a higher QoL.

As these fields evolve, so too do ways to enhance care. Emerging trends such as integrating monitoring technology, guiding exercise routines, and personalized mind–body techniques are ripe for exploration. Future research should focus on the long-term impacts of these practices, including their effectiveness in diverse groups and how to tailor them to different needs and preferences. Exploring synergies between modern medicine and the above strategies could also lead to innovative approaches for supporting physical, emotional, and cognitive health. Many long-term care facilities already support one or more of these practices. By incorporating exercise and mind–body practices into their care models, facilities provide residents with tools to manage stress, maintain physical and cognitive health, and improve overall well-being.

In conclusion, integrating exercise, mind–body practices, and Traditional Chinese Medicine, such as acupuncture, into long-term care is beneficial and necessary. As our population ages, the demand for holistic, person-centered care has continued to grow. By embracing these practices, we ensure long-term care residents receive the comprehensive care they service, promoting longevity and independence.

References

Allen, J., Mak, S. S., Begashaw, M., Larkin, J., Miake-Lye, I., Beroes-Severin, J., et al. (2022). Use of acupuncture for adult health conditions 2013 to 2021: A systematic review. *JAMA Network Open, 5*(11), e2243665–e2243665. https://doi.org/10.1001/jamanetworkopen.2022.43665

Ball, M. M., Lepore, M. L., Perkins, M. M., Hollingsworth, C., & Sweatman, M. (2009). "They are the reason I come to work": The meaning of resident–staff relationships in assisted living. *Journal of Aging Studies, 23*(1), 37–47. https://doi.org/10.1016/j.jaging.2007.09.006

Bao, W., Sun, Y., Zhang, T., Zou, L., Wu, X., Wang, D., & Chen, Z. (2020). Exercise programs for muscle mass, muscle strength, and physical performance in older adults with sarcopenia: A systematic review and meta-analysis. *Aging and Disease, 11*(4), 863–873. https://doi.org/10.14336/AD.2020.0526

Bäumler, P., Zhang, W., Stübinger, T., & Irnich, D. (2021). Acupuncture-related adverse events: Systematic review and meta-analyses of prospective clinical studies. *BMJ Open, 11*(9), e045961. https://doi.org/10.1136/bmjopen-2020-045961

Bender, A. A., Halpin, S. N., Kemp, C. L., & Perkins, M. M. (2021). Barriers and facilitators to exercise participation among frail older African American assisted living residents. *Journal of Applied Gerontology, 40*(3), 268–277. https://doi.org/10.1177/0733464819866071

Bhattacharyya, K. K., Hueluer, G., Meng, H., & Hyer, K. (2020). Mind-body practices in U.S. adults: Prevalence and correlates. *Complementary therapies in medicine, 52*, 102501. https://doi.org/10.1016/j.ctim.2020.102501

Bhattacharyya, K. K., Molinari, V., & Hyer, K. (2022). Self-reported satisfaction of older adult residents in nursing homes: Development of a conceptual framework. *The Gerontologist, 62*(8), e442–e456.

Biley, F. (1992). Use of music in therapeutic care. *British Journal of Nursing, 1*(4), 178–180.

Bosman, J. T., Bood, Z. M., Scherer-Rath, M., Dörr, H., Christophe, N., Sprangers, M. A., & van Laarhoven, H. W. (2021). The effects of art therapy on anxiety, depression, and quality of life in adults with cancer: A systematic literature review. *Supportive Care in Cancer, 29*, 2289–2298.

Bryant, F. B., Smart, C. M., & King, S. P. (2005). Using the past to enhance the present: Boosting happiness through positive reminiscence. *Journal of Happiness Studies, 6*(3), 227–260. https://doi.org/10.1007/s10902-005-3889-4

Charlesworth, C. J., Smit, E., Lee, D. S., Alramadhan, F., & Odden, M. C. (2015). Polypharmacy among adults aged 65 years and older in the United States: 1988–2010. *Journals of Gerontology Series A: Biomedical Sciences and Medical Sciences, 70*(8), 989–995. https://doi.org/10.1093/gerona/glv013

Colcombe, S. J., Kramer, A. F., Erickson, K. I., Scalf, P., McAuley, E., Cohen, N. J., et al. (2004). Cardiovascular fitness, cortical plasticity, and aging. *Proceedings of the National Academy of Sciences, 101*(9), 3316–3321. https://doi.org/10.1073/pnas.0400266101

Cole, L. (2021). The impact of guided imagery on pain and anxiety in hospitalized adults. *Pain Management Nursing, 22*(4), 465–469. https://doi.org/10.1016/j.pmn.2021.03.003

Elsegood, K. J., & Wongpakaran, N. (2012). The effects of guided imagery on affect, cognition, and pain in older adults in residential care: A randomized controlled study from Thailand. *Research in Gerontological Nursing, Gerontological Nursing, 5*(2), 114–122. https://doi.org/10.3928/19404921-20120110-03

Esch, T., Stefano, G. B., & Michaelsen, M. M. (2024). The foundations of mind-body medicine: Love, good relationships, and happiness modulate stress and promote health. *Stress and Health*. Advance online publication. https://doi.org/10.1002/smi.3387

Halpin, S. N. (2018). Declining with purpose: Resilience despite cognitive decline. *Life Span and Disability, 21*(1), 89–108. https://doi.org/10.1093/geroni/igy023.1795

Halpin, S. N., Carruth, E. C., Rai, R. P., Edelman, J. E., Fiellin, D. A., Gibert, C., et al. (2018). Complementary and alternative medicine among persons living with HIV in the era of combined antiretroviral treatment. *AIDS and Behavior, 22*, 848–852. https://doi.org/10.1007/s10461-017-1961-x

Halpin, S. N., Dillard, R. L., & Puentes, W. J. (2017). Socio-emotional adaptation theory: Charting the emotional process of Alzheimer's disease. *The Gerontologist, 57*(4), 696–706. https://doi.org/10.1093/geront/gnw176

Halpin, S. N., Ge, L., Mehta, C. C., Gustafson, D., Robertson, K. R., Rubin, L. H., Sharma, A., Vance, D., Valcour, V., Waldrop-Valverde, D., & Ofotokun, I. (2020). Psychosocial resources and emotions in women living with HIV who have cognitive impairment: Applying the socio-emotional adaptation theory. *Research and Theory for Nursing Practice, 34*(1), 49–66. https://doi.org/10.1891/RTNP-D-20-00016

Halpin, S. N., Huang, W., & Perkins, M. M. (2014). Physicians' influence on veterans' decision to use acupuncture. *Patient Education and Counseling, 97*(2), 211–215. https://doi.org/10.1016/j.pec.2014.08.006

Halpin, S. N., & Len, K. (2020). Complementary and alternative medicine in an online support group for people with Alzheimer's disease. *Gerontechnology, 19*(4), 1–9. https://doi.org/10.4017/gt.2020.19.04.403.00

Halpin, S. N., Perkins, M. M., & Huang, W. (2014). Determining attitudes toward acupuncture: A focus on older U.S. veterans. *The. Journal of Alternative and Complementary Medicine, 20*(2), 118–122. https://doi.org/10.1089/acm.2013.0177

Halpin, S. N., Potapragada, N. R., Bergquist, S. H., & Jarrett, T. (2020). Use and factors associated with non-disclosure of complementary and alternative medicine among older adults. *Educational Gerontology, 46*(1), 18–25. https://doi.org/10.1080/03601277.2020.1696202

Han, Y. M., Chan, M. M., Choi, C. X., Law, M. C., Ahorsu, D. K., & Tsang, H. W. (2023). The neurobiological effects of mind–body exercise: a systematic review and meta-analysis of neuroimaging studies. *Scientific Reports, 13*(1), 10948.

Handing, E. P., Leng, X. I., Kritchevsky, S. B., & Craft, S. (2020). Association between physical performance and cognitive function in older adults across multiple studies: A pooled analysis study. *Innovation in Aging Aging, 4*(6), igaa050. https://doi.org/10.1093/geroni/igaa050

Hayati, A., Saberi, L. F., Yaghoubi, T., Pourasghar, M., Mousavinasab, N., & Taraghi, Z. (2020). The effect of progressive muscle relaxation on depressive symptoms in elderly people. *Journal of Nursing and Midwifery Sciences, 7*(4), 248–254.

Holland, G. J., Tanaka, K., Shigematsu, R., & Nakagaichi, M. (2002). Flexibility and physical functions of older adults: A review. *Journal of Aging and Physical Activity, 10*(2), 169–206. https://doi.org/10.1123/japa.10.2.169

Huang, W., Johnson, T. M., Kutner, N. G., Halpin, S. N., Weiss, P., Griffiths, P. C., & Bliwise, D. L. (2018). Acupuncture for treatment of persistent disturbed sleep: A randomized clinical trial in veterans with mild traumatic brain injury and posttraumatic stress disorder. *The Journal of Clinical Psychiatry, 80*(1), 353. https://doi.org/10.4088/JCP.18m12300

Jochem, C., Leitzmann, M., Volaklis, K., Aune, D., & Strasser, B. (2019). Association between muscular strength and mortality in clinical populations: A systematic review and meta-analysis. *Journal of the American Medical Directors Association, 20*(10), 1213–1223. https://doi.org/10.1016/j.jamda.2019.05.015

Krebs, L. U. (2015). Mind-body interventions. *Oncology Nursing Society*. https://www.ons.org/sites/default/files/publication_pdfs/Mind-Body_Interventions.pdf

Li, S. Y. H., & Bressington, D. (2019). The effects of mindfulness-based stress reduction on depression, anxiety, and stress in older adults: A systematic review and meta-analysis. *International Journal of Mental Health Nursing, 28*(3), 635–656. https://doi.org/10.1111/inm.12571

Mandsager, K., Harb, S., Cremer, P., Phelan, D., Nissen, S. E., & Jaber, W. (2018). Association of cardiorespiratory fitness with long-term mortality among adults undergoing exercise treadmill testing. *JAMA Network Open, 1*(6), e183605. https://doi.org/10.1001/jamanetworkopen.2018.3605

Mofredj, A., Alaya, S., Tassaioust, K., Bahloul, H., & Mrabet, A. (2016). Music therapy: A review of the potential therapeutic benefits for the critically ill. *Journal of Critical Care*. https://doi.org/10.1016/j.jcrc.2016.05.02

Myint, K. M., DeMaranville, J., Wongpakaran, T., Peisah, C., Arunrasameesopa, S., & Wongpakaran, N. (2024). Meditation moderates the relationship between insecure attachment and loneliness: A study of long-term care residents in Thailand. *Medicina, 60*(4), 622. https://doi.org/10.3390/medicina60040622

Nagata, T., Shinagawa, S., Inamura, K., & Shigeta, M. (2022). Pathogenesis and personalized interventions for pharmacological treatment-resistant neuropsychiatric symptoms in Alzheimer's disease. *Journal of Personalized Medicine, 12*(9), 1365. https://doi.org/10.3390/jpm12091365

National Certification Commission for Acupuncture and Oriental Medicine. (2024, August 24). Educational requirements for NCCAOM certification. *NCCAOM*. https://www.nccaom.org/certification/nccaom-certification-eligibility/educational-eligibility/

Park, N. S., Zimmerman, S., Kinslow, K., Shin, H. J., & Roff, L. L. (2012). Social engagement in assisted living and implications for practice. *Journal of Applied Gerontology, 31*(2), 215–238.

Patil, S., Sen, S., Bral, M., Reddy, S., Bradley, K. K., Cornett, E. M., et al. (2016). The role of acupuncture in pain management. *Current Pain and Headache Reports, 20*(1), 1–8. https://doi.org/10.1007/s11916-016-0566-5

Pilkington, K., Kirkwood, G., Rampes, H., Cummings, M., & Richardson, J. (2007). Acupuncture for anxiety and anxiety disorders: A systematic literature review. *Acupuncture in Medicine, 25*(1-2), 1–10. https://doi.org/10.1136/aim.25.1-2.1

Stephenson, R. C. (2021). *Art therapy and creative aging: Reclaiming elderhood, health, and wellbeing*. Routledge.

Wang, C. C., Li, K., Choudhury, A., & Gaylord, S. (2019). Trends in yoga, tai chi, and qigong use among US adults, 2002-2017. *Am J Public Health, 109*(5), 755–761. https://doi.org/10.2105/AJPH.2019.304998

Index

A
Acupuncture, 204, 213, 214, 217, 218
Adrenalin, 5
Advance care planning (ACP), 100–101, 103
Age-friendly communities (AFCs), 181–184, 189–198
Age-friendly health system (AFHS), 2, 181, 182, 184
Ageism, 122, 141, 172, 183
Aging in Place, 1, 6, 49, 57, 142, 155–161, 186–189, 192, 197
Allegations, 15, 17, 19
Antipsychotic medications, 32, 34, 36, 78, 80
APOE, 27
Assisted living facilities, 1, 6, 9, 10, 61, 103, 123, 140, 143, 144, 148, 151, 194, 203

B
Behavioral and psychological symptoms of dementia (BPSD), 31, 32, 35
Benzodiazepines, 30, 31
Black, Indigenous, and People of Color (BIPOC), 50

C
Caregiver disparities, 115
CareTO model, 169
Centers for Medicare & Medicaid Services (CMS), 11, 14, 16–18, 32–34, 36, 51, 67, 89, 104, 105, 197
Certification and Survey Provider Enhanced Reports (CASPER), 13
Cognitive impairment, 9, 18, 25–27, 29, 30, 42, 45, 46, 111, 112, 115, 116, 127, 139, 157, 167, 169, 193
Compassionate Communities model, 99
Complement, 4, 17, 97, 102
Complementary and alternative, 18
Consumer complaints, 11, 14–19
COVID-19, 6, 49, 51–54, 62–67, 70, 114, 124, 130, 165, 168, 184, 185, 193
Cultural competence, 123–125, 131, 151, 172
Cultural humility, 123–124, 131
Culture change, 2, 3, 6, 165–176, 185

D
Danish healthcare, 55
DASH diets, 26
Deficiency citations, 11–13, 15–17
Dementia, 6, 9, 27, 41, 51, 71, 78, 111, 127, 139, 158, 166, 184
Dementia citizenship, 33, 41–46
Dementia village (DV), 127
Deprescribing, 34–36
Diagnostic and Statistical Manual of Mental Disorders, Fifth Edition (DSM-5), 25, 111
Direct care workers (DCWs), 3, 49–57, 77, 86, 87
Donabedian's SPO model, 12
Disasters, 6, 61–72, 183, 194

E
Eden Alternative, 167, 185
Electronic health records (EHRs), 54, 55

K. K. Bhattacharyya (ed.), *Health Promotion in Long-Term Care Facilities*,
https://doi.org/10.1007/978-3-031-91038-8

F
Facilities, 15
Fight-or-flight, 213
Five Aspects Meal Model (FAMM), 127
Five-star rating, 16, 18
Flexibilities, 98, 130, 142, 168, 176, 203–205, 207–209, 211, 215

G
Gamma-aminobutyric acid (GABA), 30
Gardening, 18, 151, 207, 208, 216
Graduate from hospice, 98
Guided imagery, 210, 211, 214–215, 217

H
Health, 2, 9, 25, 41, 49, 61, 77, 98, 111, 123, 137, 156, 167, 182, 204
Health disparities, 111–116, 143, 171, 172
Health equities, 6, 112, 113, 115–116, 143, 171, 172, 176
Health inequities, 138, 172
Health Information Technology (HIT), 44
Health-promoting palliative care (HPPC), 99
Health promotion, 1–6, 49–57, 61–71, 78–80, 85, 88, 98–99, 131, 137–152, 161
Home, 1, 44, 50, 61, 78, 102, 113, 123, 137, 155, 167, 182, 203
Home care, 50–52, 56, 102, 130, 138, 142, 144, 145, 147–149, 151, 158
Hospice care, 98, 101–106, 108
Hurricane Sandy, 63

I
Immediate jeopardy, 15
Inclusive design, 170
Individual trauma, 66
Interprofessional collaboration, 174, 175
Intersectionality, 138–143
Isotonic system, 206

J
Jeopardy, 1

L
Long-term care (LTC), 1–6, 9–19, 25–36, 41–47, 49–57, 61–71, 77–85, 88–90, 97–108, 111–116, 121–131, 137–152, 155–161, 165, 181–198, 203–218

M
Meals-on-Wheels, 149
Medicaid, 10–13, 16, 53, 82, 85, 86, 104, 105, 139, 145, 186, 197
Medical ageism, 122
Medicare, 10, 11, 16, 34, 104, 105, 108
Medication Appropriateness Index (MAI), 44
Meditation, 203, 204, 209–215, 217
Mediterranean diet, 26
Memory care, 129, 138, 141, 144–146, 148, 169, 203
Mild cognitive impairment (MCI), 27
Minimum Data Set (MDS), 18, 34, 127
Moral distress, 83
4Ms model, 2
8Ms framework, 3
Music therapy, 18, 171, 204, 209, 212, 216

N
National Academies of Sciences, Engineering, and Medicine (NASEM), 79, 86, 139, 140, 144–146, 148, 150–152, 184, 185
Neurocognitive disorders, 25, 111–113
Nursing home compare, 9, 140, 160
Nursing homes, 1, 3, 6, 9–19, 26, 27, 29, 31, 33–35, 41–45, 50–56, 61, 62, 65, 68, 77–90, 103, 104, 137–140, 143–152, 160, 181, 184–186, 191, 195, 197

O
Omnibus Budget Reconciliation Act (OBRA), 10

P
Palliative care, 6, 97–108
Personal protective equipment (PPE), 67, 77, 81
Person-centered care, 2, 3, 6, 19, 46, 49, 53, 54, 57, 68, 124, 143, 150, 151, 165–176, 182, 185–186, 218
Place, 1, 49, 64, 86, 102, 121, 150, 155, 165, 187, 216
Polypharmacy, 6, 14, 25–36, 41–47, 174, 213, 214
Prescribing cascade, 29
Psychological first aid, 68–69, 72

Q
Qigong, 203, 209, 212, 213
Quality, 2, 10, 33, 49, 78, 99, 112, 122, 138, 159, 171, 185, 211
Quality of care, 2–6, 9–19, 41, 43, 47, 51, 54, 55, 67, 79, 108, 111, 113, 114, 131, 138, 139, 141, 143, 144, 149, 150, 171–174, 184, 197
Quality of life (QoL), 2–6, 9–19, 42–43, 51, 53–55, 57, 61, 64, 65, 97, 99–101, 103, 104, 112–114, 121–131, 137, 140, 141, 143, 144, 147–150, 152, 155–158, 160, 167–169, 176, 186, 187, 190, 193, 194, 204, 214–217

R
Recertification surveys, 11, 14
Reframing Aging Initiative, 196
Religious holidays, 129
Residential comfort, 159, 161
Residential normalcy, 159
Re-traumatization, 67, 68
Roleless role, 121

S
Selective optimization with compensation (SOC) model, 6
SiMbA study, 44
SMART technologies, 182, 187–188, 193, 197–198
Social determinants of health (SDOH), 2, 6, 113, 114, 126, 137–152, 171, 172
Successful aging, 121, 122, 157

T
Tai chi, 203, 209, 212–214
Tech Handy Helper Program, 191, 193
Technologies, 53, 64, 107, 121, 142, 155, 171, 182, 217
Telehealth, 66, 70–72, 102, 184, 188, 191–193
Transformational leadership, 87
Trauma-informed care (TIC), 66–68, 71, 194
Tuskegee Experiment, 126

U
United States Office of Inspector General, 15
Understaffing, 42, 77, 90, 172
Universal design, 170
U.S. Bureau of Labor Statistics (BLS), 50, 51, 86
US GAO, 11, 15–17

V
Vagus nerve, 213
Voice-activated devices, 187
VO_2 max, 205, 206

W
Wages, 51, 172, 173
Walking, 151, 205–208, 211
Welfare technologies, 56
What matters, 2, 3, 18, 184
World Health Organization (WHO), 2, 5, 6, 12, 49, 61, 97–99, 106, 112, 122, 124, 130, 137, 138, 182–184

Y
Yoga, 18, 203, 209–212, 214, 216
Young old, 122

The manufacturer's authorised representative in the EU is Springer Nature Customer Service Centre GmbH, Europaplatz 3, 69115 Heidelberg, Germany. If you have any concerns regarding our products, please contact ProductSafety@springernature.com

Printed and bound by CPI Group (UK) Ltd, Croydon, CR0 4YY
01/10/2026
02225864-0006